Building Motivational Interviewing Skills

Applications of Motivational Interviewing
Stephen Rollnick and William R. Miller, Series Editors

Since the publication of Miller and Rollnick's classic *Motivational Interviewing*, MI has become hugely popular as a tool for facilitating many different kinds of positive behavior change. This highly practical series demonstrates MI approaches for a range of applied contexts and with a variety of populations. Each accessible volume reviews the empirical evidence base and presents easy-to-implement strategies, illuminating concrete examples, and clear-cut guidance on integrating MI with other interventions.

Motivational Interviewing in the Treatment of Psychological Problems
*Hal Arkowitz, Henny A. Westra, William R. Miller,
and Stephen Rollnick, Editors*

Motivational Interviewing in Health Care:
Helping Patients Change Behavior
Stephen Rollnick, William R. Miller, and Christopher C. Butler

Building Motivational Interviewing Skills: A Practitioner Workbook
David B. Rosengren

Building Motivational Interviewing Skills

A Practitioner Workbook

David B. Rosengren

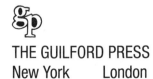

THE GUILFORD PRESS
New York   London

© 2009 The Guilford Press
A Division of Guilford Publications, Inc.
72 Spring Street, New York, NY 10012
www.guilford.com

Printed in the United States of America

This book is printed on acid-free paper.

Last digit is print number: 9   8   7   6   5   4   3

Library of Congress Cataloging-in-Publication Data

Rosengren, David B.
    Building motivational interviewing skills : a practitioner workbook / David B.
Rosengren.
        p.   cm. — (Applications of motivational interviewing)
    Includes bibliographical references and index.
    ISBN 978-1-60623-299-6 (pbk. : alk. paper)
    1. Motivational interviewing.   2. Counseling.   3. Interviewing in mental
health.   I. Title.
    BF637.I5R67 2009
    158′.39—dc22
                                                                            2009016131

For Nancy Ann

About the Author

David B. Rosengren, PhD, is a Research Scientist at the University of Washington's Alcohol and Drug Abuse Institute; a clinical research specialist for the Prevention Research Institute, Lexington, Kentucky; a motivational interviewing (MI) consultant and trainer; and a clinical psychologist in private practice. His primary research and clinical interests are motivation, the process of change, and training methods. Dr. Rosengren has provided MI training since 1993, including serving as a master trainer for the Motivational Interviewing Network of Trainers (MINT). He has authored numerous book chapters and journal articles on MI-related topics.

Series Editors' Note

During the past decade, the method of motivational interviewing (MI) has spread across the globe at a surprising rate. It is being applied with a wide array of populations in health care, corrections, addiction and mental health treatment, and social services. The demand to learn MI has outpaced the reach of the many hundreds of trainers now teaching it in at least 38 languages.

An unfortunate consequence of such rapid dissemination is that misunderstandings of the method easily arise, and the quality of service delivery can suffer. In some ways MI is simple, but mastering it is neither quick nor easy. We have likened the process to that of learning to play a musical instrument or a skillful sport. Reading and lectures can take you a certain distance, but ultimately it is practice that shapes and improves skill in MI. As in music or sport, it helps to receive good feedback and coaching along the way. We also recognize that currently, such expert supervision is not readily available in many areas.

How then to help people who want to learn the method of MI? That is the purpose for which this book was written. Over the years the Motivational Interviewing Network of Trainers (MINT) has developed quite an array of useful training methods to help people in learning MI (see *www.motivationalinterview.org*). David Rosengren has been one of MINT's most creative and generous contributors in this regard, and in this book he draws together his experience in training thousands of people in MI. He has done an excellent job of balancing content and practice: both clarifying important key concepts in MI and providing helpful aids for developing skill in this method.

This book is not meant to replace good feedback and coaching where it is available. To the contrary, it contains a wealth of material that is useful in training, coaching, and learning this method. For those without immediate access to an expert coach, it offers practical methods that can be used by individuals or groups attempting to improve their professional skill. For those fortunate enough to have good MI supervision and coaching available, the clear presentation and methods in this book will also prove useful in the learning process.

We are pleased, therefore, with the publication of this next volume in The Guilford Press series Applications of Motivational Interviewing. It is a unique contribution to the series, and we hope that it will help and encourage you as you gain skill in this broadly applicable method for calling forth people's own motivations for change.

WILLIAM R. MILLER, PhD
STEPHEN ROLLNICK, PhD

Preface

Motivational Interviewing (MI), an empirically supported clinical method (e.g., Project MATCH, 1997a, 1998a), has experienced an explosion of interest in treatment, intervention, and research settings. With that steep climb in interest comes a corresponding demand for opportunities to learn MI. There are a variety of methods to meet that demand. Training by expert MI trainers is an important initial tool, but too often does not include either follow-up coaching or ongoing feedback on trainee skills. Prior MI texts have rich contextual material, but do not provide opportunities to practice skills. Videos allow opportunities to observe models, but are primarily passive observational tools. Interactive web and DVD materials are starting to appear, but remain in their infancy. Missing in all of these materials is a text that allows the learner to review basic concepts and opportunities to practice skills, alone, with others, and with clients.

This workbook fills that void. It provides overviews of concepts and skill areas and is grounded in experiential learning. Through engaging activities and practice opportunities readers will test their knowledge, learn skills, and refine techniques for using MI. For someone new to MI, this book will provide an introduction to concepts. For a recent workshop attendee, this workbook will provide opportunities to refine skills, deepen understanding, and check progress. For an experienced MI provider, the material here will offer the chance to learn additional techniques and become more adroit in skills. It also provides guidelines for establishing an MI learning group.

A companion to Miller and Rollnick's (2002) second edition of *Motivational Interviewing*, this book is built on my 16 years of experience in training practitioners and MI trainers in the skills of MI, as well as my research studying the acquisition of MI skills. It offers a user-friendly option for that trainee question "Where can I learn more?"

Acknowledgments

It is easy to think of writing as a solitary process, but this conveniently ignores the many hands and heads that make an idea bloom into a manuscript and finally a book. I owe thanks to many. Terri Moyers brought me into this project when it was only a seed and graciously allowed me to cultivate it when her path went elsewhere. Editorial guidance was critical. At The Guilford Press, Kitty Moore started with me and Jim Nageotte finished this meandering; Kitty was a great inspiration and Jim a great guide. Thanks also to the many others at Guilford who brought this book to conclusion. Bill Miller and Steve Rollnick have given much in their work on MI generally and to me particularly. Steve gave me the very helpful advice to make my writing time sacred rather than another burden on an already (too) busy schedule. Bill provided the repeated readings and shepherding that this process needed. It was a bit like having my own graduate seminar with Bill Miller. How great is that? The result is evident: a much better volume where the wisdom is his and the mistakes are mine.

Then, of course, there are the many members of MINT who've contributed so much to the MI method, training, and research. Editing has reduced all of the names that appeared in early versions, but I am well aware of how this work stands on your shoulders. The richness of ideas, the generosity of spirit, and enthusiasm for your work make me glad to be a part of your ranks and certainly better for it. Your wisdom and friendships are something I hold dear.

Even with all of those other things, family and friends made this work possible. Friends are ballast in my life and I am richly blessed to have Ed, Rhonda, Catherine, David, Colleen, Stuart, Dudley, and Candace to keep me upright and headed in the right direction. In contrast to the common complaint, I am delighted to spend time with my in-laws. Andy and Ida provide support in things large and small, as well as being great company. My brother, Todd, and sister, Nancy, gave me the usual sibling grief, but also far more care and compassion than a brother can rightfully expect. I've spent far too much time away from their good and honest company—in Lake Woebegon. My parents first taught me about listening and the value of being truly heard. They've given so many gifts to me it is hard to be thankful enough. In reverse, my children have put up with a pale imitation of those role models. Kate, Michael, and Sophia permitted me to hole up in the office early in the morning and late at night, endured my grouchiness, and loved me all the same. You're my joy. And, finally, there is my wife, Stephanie, who asked me what I dreamt and when I couldn't answer, suggested that was a problem; then she held me to account to do something about it. Although all others played roles, your love, spirit, and support made it happen—all of it. Thank you!

Contents

Chapter 1

Introduction

Motivational interviewing (MI) is coming of age. A review of funding by the National Institutes of Health in October 2008 showed 180 research projects using either MI or motivational enhancement therapy (a manualized form of MI used originally in Project MATCH [Matching Alcohol Treatment to Client Heterogeneity; Miller, Zweben, DiClemente, & Rychtarik, 1992]). The empirical support for MI has begun to accumulate across problem behaviors (see Burke, Arkowitz, & Dunn, 2002; Hettema, Steele, & Miller, 2005) and beyond its origins in the treatment of addictive behavior. There is clear specification of the intervention elements (Miller & Rollnick, 1991, 2002), applications to settings beyond addictions (Arkowitz, Westra, Miller, & Rollnick, 2008; Rollnick, Miller, & Butler, 2008), manuals available for interventions (Project MATCH, Project COMBINE [Combining Medication and Behavioral Intervention]), and supervision manuals (MIA-Step [Motivational Interviewing Assessment: Supervisory Tools for Enhancing Proficiency]; Martino et al., 2006). There are some tantalizing hints about what may be some of the critical elements in effective MI sessions (Amrhein, Miller, Yahne, Palmer, & Fulcher, 2003; Moyers et al., 2007). Miller (2005) has been working toward specification of a theory of MI, and *Motivational Interviewing* was completely rewritten for the second edition to address this depth and breadth of research. Finally, there are researchers, including myself, beginning to study best practices in skill acquisition.

Several authors describe research (e.g., Baer et al., 2009; Miller, Yahne, Moyers, Martinez, & Pirritano, 2004; Miller et al., 2008) showing that a 2-day workshop on MI is a fine introduction to the concepts. Indeed, individuals can become much more "MI consistent" after such training. However, to remain proficient individuals need additional practice, coaching, and feedback on that practice.

There are many ways to gain this additional practice, such as participating in follow-up training and receiving feedback from supervisors and consultants. Miller et al. (2004) note that their model for teaching MI has shifted from a focus on specific techniques to one of "learning to learn" (p. 1059). That is, prior training emphasized the teaching of skills, as well as the importance of receiving feedback in the initial acquisition of skills. Recent findings suggest that learners do need ongoing feedback, and most clinicians do not have immediate access to this level of consultation. Miller and Moyers (2006) liken this situation to hitting golf balls in the dark: One may know how the swing feels, but there is no information about what happened and what adjustments need to be made. Fortunately, there is a feedback source readily accessible: our clients. So Miller et al. (2004) now emphasize learning how to observe clients. Client response to practitioner behavior (e.g., increased change talk or increased resistance) signals when we are practicing in an MI-consistent or MI-inconsistent way. In this way the client becomes an ongoing source of feedback (i.e., a teacher) receiving good or less-good MI practice.

Other methods for learning MI are available. For example, videotapes of MI demonstrations are available, and researchers are working on the development of video, DVD, computer-based, and web-based assessment and training. My colleagues and I recently described work for the Video Assessment of Simulated Encounters—Revised (VASE-R; Rosengren, Baer, Hartzler, Dunn, & Wells, 2005; Rosengren, Hartzler, Baer, Wells, & Dunn, 2008), a system that allows evaluation of learners' MI skills in five domains. Still missing from these resources is a manual to assist learners in the development and practice of MI skills without outside expertise and without prior experience in skill evaluation. Thus, the inspiration for this workbook was born.

Purpose

This manual is meant for practitioners across a variety of intervention and professional spectrums. Although I use the conventions of "practitioner" and "client" for convenience, this manual would be equally applicable for corrections workers, paraprofessionals, peer counselors, physicians, dental hygienists, diabetes educators, chemical dependency professionals, counselors, as well as a host of others working in helping situations. The common denominators would be *people struggling with the possibility of change* and *"helpers" engaged with these people in that struggle.*

The book serves as an adjunct to the second edition of Miller and Rollnick (2002) *Motivational Interviewing (MI-2)*, as well as the more recent books in this MI series: *Motivational Interviewing in the Treatment of Psychological Problems* (Arkowitz et al., 2008) and *Motivational Interviewing in Health Care: Helping Patients Change Behavior* (Rollnick et al., 2008). In these texts, the authors review the context, practice, and applications of MI to a variety of treatment populations and settings. They also discuss learning techniques and other conceptual issues. But they don't provide practice opportunities; that is the focus of this book.

The reader is not required to have read MI-2 to use this book. Each chapter provides an overview of concepts to which a trainee would be exposed if he or she took one of my standard 2- or 3-day workshops. For people already familiar with MI, this information will serve as a review; for those new to MI, it will introduce the concepts. However, in either case, reading MI-2 will deepen your understanding of MI, as well as the value of this book.

This book does not follow the organization of the MI-2 book. Instead, it reflects the order of concepts I use in standard workshops, building logically on prior concepts and providing an organizational structure for understanding MI for those readers new to the topic. However, chapters are freestanding, and for those already familiar with the concepts or who tend to work in a nonlinear fashion, the workbook is an a la carte menu.

Miller and Rollnick (2002) use Phase I and II to describe the MI process. Phase I goals are to raise the importance of a change, enhance confidence, and resolve ambivalence. During Phase II the practitioner seeks to solidify the client's commitment to change and to negotiate a change plan. Chapters 3–9 address skills used in Phase I, and Chapters 10 and 11 focus on Phase II.

Finally, although this book is obviously a verbal–linguistic effort, it is written in a manner that addresses multiple intelligences and learning styles (Silver, Strong, & Perini, 2000). There are a range of learning activities, some of which may work better for different types of learners. While I encourage you to try all, don't feel compelled to do so.

Specific Goals

This book has three aims. First, the reader has an opportunity to "see" MI concepts applied in the many clinical and training examples sprinkled through the text. These examples are based on my 20 years of work as a psychologist and 15 years as an MI trainer. Although the visual image and the richness of the verbal exchange from a case are not present in a written text, the reader does have the advantage of examining the interchanges at a leisurely rate and "hearing" the thoughts of the practitioner. Often, gleaning the subtleties of interchanges requires more than one hearing, and this format allows the luxury of that repetition.

Second, this workbook provides practice opportunities for you and others. The exercises allow you to try out and refine your skills. Some of these activities are things you can do alone, but others require interaction with others, including specific opportunities to work with a partner. The exercises could also be used as part of an MI study group. There are worksheets for all exercises, included at the end of each chapter. I encourage you to keep completed sheets, as some may be used again for later activities. You are free to copy and use these worksheets for your skill development.

Third, this workbook includes some activities that you can use with clients. Although they may be presented in one chapter, exercises can serve multiple purposes and can be used at different points. Still, these exercises are not MI. Although the design is congruent with MI principles, how the practitioner uses these materials determines whether they are MI consistent. Thus, before using these in a helping situation with another, the reader will have some experience with the forms and can alter them to the needs of the situation.

Chapter Organization

The first and last chapters have a somewhat different organization from the remaining ones. Whereas this chapter provides an introduction, the last chapter affords a brief overview of research and recommendations about learning MI. Chapters 2–11 share the format described below.

- *Opening.* A clinical example illustrates the challenges to be explored in the chapter. Through a combination of description and dialogue, the reader experiences a clinical or life situation that grounds the learning in real interchanges, and then is asked, "Where would you go next?"

- *A Deeper Look.* This portion introduces the concepts that underlie a given chapter. For example, Chapter 3 contains a discussion of what reflective listening is, how it works, and the subtleties in its application. For a reader new to the area this information lays a basic foundation for the experiential work that follows; for the more experienced MI practitioner, it is a review that illustrates nuances that I have learned through my years using, researching, and training others in MI.

- *Concept Quiz—Test Yourself!* This brief test is meant to be a fun check on your grasp of the material just reviewed. For the experienced practitioner, the quiz may serve as a measure for whether a review of *A Deeper Look* is in order. Answers and explanations follow the quiz.

- *In Practice.* This component integrates conceptual material back into clinical exchanges. You observe MI in practice with emphasis on how the skills can be applied.

- *Try This!* This section contains practice opportunities. The form and number vary by chapter, but these do not require an ongoing practice partner. However, some exercises will involve skill practice with others (e.g., friends and family, coworkers, the barista at the local coffee shop). Don't worry—you won't be asked to do therapy with your brother-in-law, though you might be asked to *try* to understand his weird thinking in an empathy exercise.

Although some of the exercises may seem simple, this does not necessarily make them easy. Often, with greater skill comes greater complexity. Reflective listening is an excellent example of how practice can improve depth, direction, and diversity in use. Similarly, working through an exercise one time does not make you proficient. You might want (or need) to practice the skill several times before you feel comfortable with it. Consider making copies of the forms before you try them out; this way you will be able to retry exercises with a fresh slate. In my training experience, really excellent MI practitioners rarely find a practice opportunity that is too basic for them. There's simply too much room to refine skills. Bill Miller notes an analogy in karate: There is always room for improvement in a *kata*, no matter what one's belt level.

- *Partner Work.* Although the exercises in this book can be done as a solo project, it may also be quite helpful to work through them with a friend or colleague, or as part of a study/practice group. Learning with others allows for discussion, practice, and direct feedback that might not otherwise be available. Each chapter provides exercises specifically designed for partner practice. These activities often mirror what can be done with clients and thus provide a dress rehearsal—with feedback—before the curtain goes up!

- *Other Thoughts. ...* These are all the odds and ends that trainers and practitioners collect over years of practice but that don't always fit neatly into the other packages. For example:

> "When doing a double-sided reflection, consider ending with the side that emphasizes change. This strategy allows you to segue naturally into the area you are working toward."

These are the things that I jot down as margin notes when I am learning from others—things that I want to remember but that don't necessarily fit into neat categories. This section also includes discussion of issues that are still being debated by MI trainers and experts, allowing you to observe some of the nuance that occurs in such interchanges.

Backmatter

The backmatter contains information that you'll find useful in working your way through this book and for pursuing more learning about MI.

- *Establishing an MI Learning Group.* In addition to using a partner, you might consider setting up an MI learning group. Appendix A contains specific suggestions for how you might do this. You do not need to be an expert in MI to lead such a group, only someone who is willing to make the group happen. This appendix contains recommendations for a potential leader of an MI group, including practical suggestions about arranging an organizational meeting and structuring the group. I encourage you to look it over.
- *Additional Resources.* This appendix provides information on books, videos, websites, and other materials you might find helpful in learning about MI. For example, in this area you'll find information about where can you get copies of video materials.
- *References and Index.* These areas include references cited in the text as well as an index for quick referencing of terms.

A Word about Wording

In a book like this, there is always a concern about how to refer to the person doing the changing and the person assisting with the change. Given that this book is designed to address a range of helping situations, there is no perfect phrasing for all circumstances. So, I have chose to use the terms *client* and *practitioner* throughout and hope that you can translate this language into your situation. Also, I have chosen to use plural forms of pronouns to avoid alternating gender throughout the text. In situations where this was unavoidable, I used both male and female references.

So Who Am I, Anyway?

I am a clinical psychologist who, in retrospect, has been pursuing the issue of client motivation since before I received my PhD in 1988. I learned that I could conceptualize client issues, develop well-considered plans, and implement empirically supported treatments, but none of this meant that clients would do it—whatever *it* was. This impasse set me on a search for answers and eventually to the doorstep of MI in 1990.

Since then, my research career has focused primarily on the use of brief interventions in the process of outreach, engagement, and intervention. Over this time I participated in research looking at alcohol and drug use, HIV risk behavior, driving practices and DUI risk, and prevention of alcohol-affected births. My work has taken place in street outreach, detox units, assessment centers, treatment programs, client homes, and over the phone. Recently my interest has shifted to models of effective MI training and methods for evaluating skill acquisition. My role in these projects, in addition to working as an investigator, has often been to serve as an MI trainer, supervisor, and consultant.

In 1993 I attended the inaugural training of new trainers (TNT) event that Miller and Rollnick held in Albuquerque, New Mexico. In that meeting I volunteered to start a newsletter. From that humble beginning and the efforts of many have emerged an international collection of MI trainers known as the Motivational International Network of Trainers (MINT). This organization has hundreds of members spread across six continents and hosts an international meeting each year.

In the past 15 years I have trained or presented MI material to a wide range of groups and professions. A consistent question following this work has been, "How do I learn more?" Now I have a concrete answer—try this workbook.

Chapter 2

Foundations of MI

Opening

"Well, I can see where this MI would be helpful with folks who are highly verbal and not too bad off, but not with the folks that we work with. These people are meth addicts, and there is something about that drug that is different. These people become antisocial. They lie and steal. They'll scam you, if you don't confront them. It just won't work with them." Rick was on a roll now.

Several heads nodded in agreement. If this had been a Baptist revival instead of an MI training session, there would have been a chorus of "Amens!" The counterargument began to flood my mind. The data about methamphetamine users and MI effectiveness said differently. I hear this concern arise—in one form or another—regularly in trainings. I also thought about people I know who struggle with alcohol and drugs, including meth. They weren't the person being described. The man raising this objection, chatty and opinionated, had been a thorn in my side throughout this training experience. Rick struggled to understand MI and apply the skills, raised objections continually, and cared deeply about his clients. But he was irritating, and I wanted to confront him—I mean, *really* confront him and show him he was wrong! I opened my mouth and said. . . .

We are at a crossroads here: a situation that often arises in treatment, consultations, and training, in which a person raises objections, and we would rather not deal with them. In fact, we may be annoyed, irritated, or frustrated, just as I was. So, we have a choice. Do we offer facts? Counter the arguments? Ignore the objections? Dismiss the concerns because of the messenger? Use the group to address Rick? Weigh in with our expertise? Or do we respond in a manner that focuses on his reasons for concern? Do we try to understand what is driving this behavior? The choice we make lies at the heart of the underlying philosophy and principles of MI. This chapter introduces the elements of MI, describes the spirit of MI, and provides opportunities to observe how this spirit interplays with the elements of MI.

A Deeper Look

Readiness to Change

Clients differ in their readiness to change. This statement is not a revelation to most of you. In fact, your desire to influence your clients' readiness may have prompted you to purchase this book. A few basic concepts about readiness and change are important to review before considering the elements of MI. Many of these elements originate in writings about the transtheoretical model by Prochaska and DiClemente (1984, 1998) but are not tied to that conceptualization of how change occurs.

- *Ambivalence about change is normal.* If changes were so obviously needed and so easily accomplished, they would've happened already, and clients wouldn't need our assistance. But because change is tough, people have mixed thoughts and feelings about it. Instead of viewing this uncertainty as a problem, it is viewed as part of the process and something that we work with the client to resolve.

- *Change is often nonlinear.* That is, clients often do not move in straight lines from non-change to change. In some instances there are initial steps, setbacks, and sometimes a return to old behaviors before change is accomplished. Often clients will have attempted to effect changes without our assistance, with more or less success.

- *Readiness is not static.* We will return to this concept repeatedly throughout the text. While clients may differ in their starting points, it's also become increasingly clear that this is something that we as practitioners can influence up or down. One can imagine many different paths Rick's response might take, based on what I did next in the opening example.

- *Attend to readiness in your work.* Some MI trainers refer to readiness as a vital sign, just as blood pressure, temperature, and pulse are vital signs in health care settings. By attending to readiness levels, the practitioner can direct sessions more effectively. For example, when clients are high in their confidence about making a change but low in their perceived importance of making that change, then attention and energy can be directed to exploring the issue of importance.

Elements of MI

Motivational interviewing contains several important elements. For the sake of clarity, I focus on four: MI principles, OARS (explained a bit later), change talk, and MI spirit. Figure 2.1 provides one way of thinking about how these components fit together and combine to form MI. Before we turn to these elements, it is important to note that many pieces of MI have been present in other systems of therapy, as well as in religious and philosophical thinking through the ages. Unique to MI is how these elements are combined, the timing of how they're used, and their application in an effort to evoke change talk (i.e., statements made by clients, indicating that they are currently considering a positive change in a specific problem behavior, and which are important predictors of change; discussed more fully in Chapter 5).

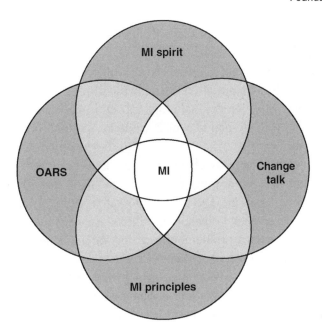

Figure 2.1. MI elements.

Principles of MI

One circle in this diagram reflects the principles upon which MI is built. In 2002 Miller and Rollnick described these principles as expressing empathy, supporting self-efficacy, developing discrepancy and rolling with resistance. More recently, Rollnick et al. (2008) expressed these principles using the acronym RULE:

- R—Resist the righting reflex.
- U—Understand your client's motivation.
- L—Listen to your client.
- E—Empower your client.

These principles, explained more fully below, draw from other therapeutic approaches. For example, the imperative to *listen to your client* relies heavily on the writings and research of Carl Rogers. These principles do not provide explicit strategies for how to do MI, but rather serve as a guiding framework for choosing techniques, strategies, and skills.

Resist the righting reflex refers to the tendency of practitioners to try to actively fix problems in their clients' lives and, by doing so, reduce the likelihood of client change. The goal is to make practitioners aware of this tendency and the trouble it engenders.

The righting reflex begins with our desire to help others. It is a positive motivation that leads us to try to address problems when we see them. We want to help clients change a situation and thereby lead a happier, healthier, more productive life. There is nothing wrong with wanting these outcomes for people. The difficulty of the righting reflex, is that it fails to consider the possibility of ambivalence.

Since clients are naturally ambivalent; there are times when they do not view change as either necessary or possible. This situation is simply the flip side of the coin of change. There may be costs associated with change, including fear and uncertainty, changes to relationships, and monetary and time demands, which argue for maintaining the status quo. All of these costs or factors influence the client to stay with the current behavior.

Resistance is the active process of pushing against reasons for change. Researchers have demonstrated that this active process can be influenced directly, either positively or negatively, by practitioner behavior (Patterson & Forgatch, 1985; Miller & Sovereign, 1989; Moyers et al., 2007). Practitioner behavior that increases resistance includes (1) trying to convince clients that they have a problem, (2) arguing for the benefits of change, (3) telling clients how to change, and (4) warning them of the consequences of not changing. Arguments in favor of change increase resistance, which then reduces the likelihood that any change will occur. In this perspective, then, resistance is a form of energy that practitioners can either intensify or lessen, depending on their behavior. Intensification of client resistance is a signal to practitioners that a change in their behavior is needed. The practitioner's goal is to minimize resistance by not actively fighting against it and to avoid engendering it by trying to fix problems.

Understand your client's motivation is the logical extension of the previous comments about ambivalence. MI takes the position that motivation comes from within the client. That is, we do *not* motivate clients or install motivation in them; rather, we find the motivation that lies within and help them to recognize it. We direct them toward the discrepancies that already exist between what they want and how their behavior impacts these goals. We listen for and often actively seek information about goals, beliefs, and aspirations and then explore how these relate to present circumstances. This directive element is a hallmark of MI and stands in contrast to traditional client-centered work.

The attitude taken in this exploration is one of curiosity about the individual and his or her situation. If practitioners seek this information so that they can use it to convince the clients of their errors, then they are engaging in a subtler form of arguing for change. Our goal, as is discussed later, is to create an environment in which the client tells us why and how change should happen.

Listen to your client may seem obvious, but in practice other imperatives often intrude on this foundational process. If we step back for a moment, the reason why this element of MI is so important becomes clearer.

Clients come to us (sometimes unwillingly) for our expertise. Yet they remain responsible for bringing about any changes in their lives. To assist them with this process, we must create an atmosphere in which they can safely explore conflicts and face difficult realities. We create this situation by being empathetic and communicating that empathy.

Miller and Rollnick (2002, p. 37) described a client-centered, empathic approach to working with people as a "fundamental and defining characteristic" of MI. Clinicians express this principle through the skillful use of reflective listening and an attitude of acceptance of the client's feelings and perspectives. One way to know you're in that empathetic stance is to be able to look at the world from the client's point of view and say truthfully, "That makes sense. I can see why you view it that way." Inherent in this statement is a subtle but important point—acceptance is not agreement or approval. Practitioners can and should disagree with clients at times. The critical element is maintenance of a respectful attitude that tries to understand the person's perspective. This attitude translates into the precept that acceptance facilitates change, whereas attempts to pressure change provoke resistance—a view that research supports (Miller, Benefield, & Tonigan, 1993; Moyers et al., 2007).

Empower your client is the final principle. Rollnick and colleagues (2008) noted that outcomes are better when clients are engaged. This statement is consistent with DiClemente's (2003) assertion that all change is ultimately self-change. Therefore, if change is to occur, our clients will need to actively engage in this process.

In step with these ideas, we support our clients' beliefs that they are capable, have ideas for solutions, and can enact changes if they decide to do so. Miller and Rollnick (2002) referred to this set of qualities as *self-efficacy*; in essence, the client has a "can-do" attitude. Without this belief, awareness of problems triggers defensiveness because clients view change as impossible.

It's important to note that self-efficacy and self-esteem are not the same. *Self-esteem* is a global construct that includes attitudes, beliefs, and behaviors about self and one's value. Low self-esteem is not uncommon for people who have struggled through very difficult life circumstances. *Self-efficacy* is a more targeted perception about one's ability to achieve desired results. Although positive self-esteem is important, it is not required for a client to have high self-efficacy or a can-do attitude about a specific act (e.g., saying "no" to a drink offer, setting the alarm for 30 minutes earlier to allow time for a walk in the morning, calling an office for more information). Building instances of client success does, however, help build more positive self-esteem.

DiClemente (1991, 2003) has described people with whom we work as failed self-changers. That is, clients have tried to change their behavior—in one way or another—prior to our seeing them. As a result, one of the factors we can expect in our clients is a certain amount of demoralization about their lack of success. So, a critical characteristic for practitioners is to be hopeful about the possibility of change for clients. There is a well-established research record attesting to the importance of therapist beliefs and expectancies in facilitating (or impeding) client change (cf. Leake & King, 1977) and how these are communicated—often below our level of awareness—to clients. It is important, therefore, that practitioners actively cultivate a stance of hope and communicate that hope to clients, since they may need to "borrow" some during the change process. Talking about other clients' successes can be one method of accomplishing this aim.

As noted before, these statements should not be taken to mean that we simply agree with our clients. We do not, necessarily. Instead, we offer our views and perspectives without arguing for them. Clients will decide if these ideas fit for them and how they might use them. Again, they are the experts on themselves and should be viewed as reservoirs of information about potential solutions, to which we can add information and ideas.

Foundational Skills

Another circle in this diagram represents counseling skills found in many therapeutic approaches. Here is the overlap between MI and many other types of counseling. Within this circle we find the tools that help build rapport with clients, explore concerns, and convey empathy. These basic skills are conveyed by the acronym OARS: open-ended questions, affirmations, reflective listening, and summaries. The term *basic* should not be taken to mean easy or simple. Each of these skills can be done well or poorly, and training is needed to achieve clinical expertise using them. For some types of counseling, they are all that is ever used. Chapters 3 and 4 discuss these skills in greater depth.

Eliciting Client Change Talk

A third circle represents what is unique to MI: an emphasis on eliciting specific kinds of speech from your client—what we call "change talk." Many of the interventions used in MI are specifically designed to evoke this kind of language and reinforce it when it occurs. This approach is based on the idea that clients will be more likely to do what they have genuinely spoken in favor of during a session. Research by Amrhein (2003) suggests that the trajectory and strength of this change talk predicts commitment, which in turn predicts behavior. A central goal of MI is to help clients articulate their reasons for changing and, in so doing, strengthen their intention to change.

Having your client (rather than you) make the arguments for a particular change is *most* important when the client is ambivalent. Client ambivalence creates a special dilemma: whatever the practitioner argues *for*, the client may argue *against*. The unfortunate result of this ambivalence dilemma is that well-meaning counselors often try to convince clients to move in the direction of a useful change (the righting reflex in action), only to be met with a "yes, but . . . " response. If this dynamic goes on long enough, clients will actually *talk themselves out of changing*, leaving dispirited practitioners behind (or ones who are convinced that clients did not want to change, anyway). Chapter 5 provides more information about change talk, as well as exercises in recognizing, responding to, and eliciting client change talk.

Spirit of MI

The final circle represents the guiding philosophy that informs the principles, the use of "microskills," the application of other interventions and techniques, and the elicitation of change talk. Without this special character, or spirit, MI is not taking place, no matter how skilled the practitioner may be in using OARS. Conversely, when this spirit is present, many, many practitioner interventions can "fit" within an MI framework. MI, then, is not *primarily* a collection of techniques or interventions but a series of specific practitioner behaviors directed by this guiding philosophy.

This guiding philosophy is not unique to MI. Indeed, the elements of MI spirit have appeared in a variety of locations (e.g., religious teachings, psychological treatises).

Recent research (Moyers, Miller, & Hendrickson, 2005) indicates that this spirit is an important predictor of practitioner skill with MI, which in turn predicts client behavior and treatment outcome. Indeed, Miller and Moyers (2006) place such importance on this context that in describing the eight stages of learning MI, they make this the first stage.

Miller and Rollnick (2002) use the metaphor of a song to describe the spirit. Within a song you have the lyrics, which are clearly an important element of that song's interest, attraction, and meaning. Within MI, the lyrics might be OARS and other strategies, as well as change talk—the content of an MI session. The structure of the song—the refrain, the key changes—might be the principles; these things shape the form and the lyrics of the song. Yet, it is the melody—the MI spirit—that creates the music. Melody determines the mood of the song and underscores the lyrics. It is to the melody that we tap our feet and hands, even when the lyrics fail us. It is this "melody" that we bring to encounters with clients, while still recognizing that the other elements are important.

There are three components to the spirit of MI: collaboration, evocation, and autonomy. *Collaboration* refers to the practitioner working in partnership with the client. Although the practitioner brings significant expertise to this relationship, a collaborative stance recognizes that clients are experts on themselves, their histories, their circumstances, and their prior efforts at change. So, the practitioner respects the client's expertise, tries to understand the client's aspirations and goals (as well as his or her own), and creates a positive environment within which change is possible. For example, the practitioner avoids prescriptive and proscriptive advice, even though he or she does offer concerns about certain client decisions.

Evocation, consistent with the comments just made, involves drawing out ideas and solutions from in clients. As experts on themselves, clients have experience with their challenges and the things that help and hinder them in attempting to change. As experts in our fields, we know something about clients with these issues generally, but we don't know what this specific client will need or want. Our goal is to evoke from clients their reasons and potential methods for change and to offer, as appropriate, ideas for clients' consideration. We also acknowledge that there are multiple ways to enact change and that motivation for change comes from within the client.

Recently, Rollnick et al. (2008) likened MI practitioners to guides; that is, someone who does not choose the destination but offers information about the paths the client might choose. *Autonomy* in decision making is left to the client. We may have opinions and even compulsory actions we must take if clients engage in certain behaviors (e.g., continued drinking, abusive parenting), but within MI we recognize that clients are ultimately responsible for choosing their paths. This component of the MI spirit can be especially challenging for practitioners when clients choose paths that negatively affect others who may have few or no options (e.g., children). MI practitioners share this concern and at the same time recognize that they cannot force clients to change. Even within coerced circumstances where we control freedom and reinforcers, clients must choose change. Thus, MI continually emphasizes the need to draw from clients their goals, values, and aspirations so that they—rather than we—argue for why change is required.

Concept Quiz—Test Yourself!

True or false:

1.   T F   MI really is just Carl Rogers with an attitude.

2.   T F   Many MI concepts are drawn from others' theories, writing, and research.

3.   T F   Within MI, practitioners avoid arguing with clients.

4.   T F   Reflective listening is MI.

5.   T F   Evocation means that you're drawing out motivation and resources from within the client.

6.   T F   In MI how you say something is just as important as what you say.

7.   T F   Ambivalence is a sign of denial.

8.   T F   Resistance is an interpersonal process.

9.   T F   Directiveness is a key concept in MI.

10.   T F   Autonomy means that we don't have goals for client's behaviors.

Answers

1.   F   A colleague likes to describe MI in this joking reference. Although MI builds on Rogers's ideas, it adds more than attitude. MI is a combination of directiveness, motivation building, rolling with resistance, attending to change talk, and bringing a particular spirit to the encounter.

2.   T   There have been many sources for the concepts and techniques used in MI. However, this is not the same as saying that MI is simply a new version of an old concept. There are unique elements to MI.

3.   T   We avoid arguing with clients because to do so engenders resistance. This does not mean that we will always agree with everything a client says. MI uses many methods (described in this book) for providing alternative views. However, we begin with a basic stance of curiosity, wherein we try to comprehend how the client understands the world.

4.   F   Reflective listening is a critical skill in MI, but it is *not* MI. Indeed, I have observed practitioners forming very accurate, but MI-inconsistent, reflective listening statements. However, as is noted in Chapter 4, I do not believe that you can do MI well without being able to do reflective listening well.

5.   T   Evocation, a component of MI spirit, refers to a stance of constantly trying to draw out information, wisdom, solutions, etc., from clients. We also use evocation to draw out motivation and then hold this information, as in a mirror, for the client's consideration.

6.   T   The attitude and intent of the practitioner are critical in terms of how communications are received and used. For example, a sarcastic question that asks, "And how is that working for you?" has a very different impact than a question that comes from an attitude of curiosity using the exact same words.

7. F   Although ambivalence can keep people stuck, and its resolution is a central aim of MI, it is not the same as denial. Nor is it a problem. It is a normal part of any change process and should be expected.

8. T   Resistance is not something inherent in a particular disease or disorder. Rather, it is part of an interpersonal process that can be influenced—for better or worse—by the practitioner and should be used as a cue for the practitioner to change strategies.

9. T   Directiveness, a key concept in MI, has two elements: paying attention to parts of conversation that support client change and steering the conversation in productive directions. We will attend to some things and not to others. The practitioner works to build motivation, reduce resistance, and elicit change talk through providing attention and steering the conversation.

10. F   Recognizing client autonomy does not negate practitioner goals. Within MI there are target behaviors for change; if there are no such targets, then this is probably not MI (W. R. Miller, personal communication, June 16, 2008) but more akin to client-centered counseling. Within the MI framework, we (as practitioners) may have an aim we think is important: increasing sexual safety, reducing recidivism, improving diet and exercise, reducing authoritarian and enhancing authoritative parenting, or stopping drug use. Clients will also have goals. We work actively to bring these different agendas into alignment (Steve Rollnick refers to this process as "agenda matching"), while recognizing that clients will and must choose the destination for any change.

In Practice

Let us return to Rick. When we left him, I was annoyed and considering arguing with him. Remember, I was ready to tell him about the data and, in effect, argue for why he was wrong (and I was right). Although this course of action may have felt good to me, it is not MI consistent. Nor would it have benefited Rick or the other trainees who felt likewise. His statements were a form of resistance. So, I needed to return to a more MI-consistent way of responding and roll with it. As is often the case, the easiest route to a more MI-consistent spirit was for me to become more collaborative and to do this by really listening and reflecting. Here is a subsequent dialogue, with commentary.

Statement	*Commentary*
DR: It upsets you that I might be suggesting something that could hurt your clients. You really care about them.	Resists the righting reflex and attempts to communicate understanding of the practitioner's motivation through a reflection.
RICK: Damn right. If I let them scam me, then they aren't going to recover.	Rick responds positively and reasserts his goal.
DR: They don't benefit from your being naive.	Listening.

Statement	*Commentary*
RICK: Right. They'll just take advantage of you.	Resistance begins to drop.
DR: And so sometimes it feels like you really need to get in their face, so they know that you aren't being fooled.	Nonjudgmental stance; trying to communicate understanding of his motivation.
RICK: Yeah. I guess. I mean, that's what I know works. They pay me to do a job and that's what I'm doing.	Rick's response suggests an opening and then a mild up-tick in resistance.
DR: As best as you know how …	Attempt to build a little motivation.
RICK: … with what I know works.	Rick signals that my comment went a little too far; his resistance goes up a little more.
DR: Because you've seen it. Sometimes it works really well.	Affirms trainee's perspective and reopens the door for developing discrepancy.
RICK: Yeah.	Resistance lowers.
DR: … but not always …	Again, this is taking a risk to build motivation by noting a discrepancy, though statements prior to this exchange indicate that this is accurate.
RICK: No. Not always … it's a tough disease.	Resistance drops. The relationship feels more collaborative and less adversarial.
DR: And that's what worries you. You might consider something different, if—and only if—you thought it might work for your clients, and that's the spot you're at now.	Listens to client/trainee and empowers him around doing something different. The relationship is collaborative, and I respect his autonomy to choose.
RICK: Exactly. I'm just not sure.	Rick feels understood and expresses his concern but in less absolute terms.
DR: Well, I am not going to try to convince you that this is the right or only way to work with people, but it sounds like you might be open if you thought it could help.	Reinforces autonomy and continues to build motivation.
RICK: I'll do whatever works.	Rick reasserts his value of wanting to help clients.

Statement	*Commentary*
DR: You're committed to your clients and good practice. It's just now you need some other kind of data—something other than what I've said—to convince you.	Reinforces Rick's value and his need for additional information. Attempts to evoke his understanding of what he needs.
RICK: I'd need to see it work in practice. I need to see it work with some of these meth addicts.	Rick knows what he needs, and it's not research data or my expert opinion.
DR: So, you want to reserve judgment until you've tried it and see how it works.	Respects his autonomy and directs him toward a logical extension of his statements.
RICK: I guess I do need to try it first. I am someone who has to see it firsthand.	Start of change talk.
DR: I wonder if you decided to give it a try, how you might do it.	Reinforces his change talk and autonomy, while also using evocation.
RICK: I've got a follow-up session tonight with a client who had a dirty UA [urinalysis]. I could try it then.	Offers a method, but does not yet commit to doing it.
DR: I'd be curious to hear what happens if you do try it. What, specifically, might you do?	Builds collaborative nature of relationship. Directs Rick toward greater specificity.
RICK: I guess instead of arguing about the accuracy of the UA, which is what usually happens, I'd try to understand this guy's view. Doing more of the reflections and open questions.	Describes a clear goal and specific methods. Although even more detail might help, this is a good start.
DR: You sound pretty clear about your goal and how you'd do it. So, what do you think about tonight?	Empowers clinician. Asks for a commitment, but does not argue for it.
RICK: I'll give it a try. See what happens.	Rick commits to a trial.

This interchange illustrates the components discussed previously, though it's not a perfect interaction. There is the initial annoyance, but then additional work moves the encounter to a more respectful and collaborative approach to this encounter. Rather than attempt to persuade Rick, the collaborative approach I extended valued his stance of wanting to be helpful with clients. There was also a clear directiveness in the encounter as well. Previous information had indicated that Rick's confrontational style with meth addicts was not always effective, and so this point was included as a contrast. This discrepancy allowed

Rick to consider other options, and, eventually, he described a method that would help him decide whether MI fit for him. Throughout this encounter, reflective listening statements were the primary tool.

Try This!

The spirit of MI, noted as critical to doing MI, is better shown than described. Fortunately, most of us have experienced an example of that type of spirit in our lives through either a teacher or a supervisor. Here is an activity, based on the Favorite Teacher Exercise[1] used by trainers of MI, which exemplifies that type of spirit. Subsequent exercises help you recognize MI spirit and help you build the empathy "muscle." Finally, the partner work helps you focus on your strengths and capacities as a person, which in turn you can use to help your clients.

Exercise 2.1. Favorite Teacher or Supervisor

Who was a person that motivated you to learn, inspired you to excel and to try harder than you otherwise would have? You'll be asked to think about this person and then answer some questions. The aim is to draw out characteristics about him or her and how you felt and responded when you were with that person. If you cannot choose one as a favorite, simply choose among your favorites for the purpose of this exercise (and consider yourself fortunate indeed!).

Exercise 2.2. Is It MI Spirit?

It can be very helpful to look at exchanges between clients and practitioners to observe if the MI spirit is present. The worksheet for Exercise 2.2 contains examples of short client statements and practitioner responses. You'll review these exchanges and then decide if the practitioner's response is consistent with the spirit of MI (thumbs up) or not (thumbs down). Then write your reasons so you can compare with the analysis, which follows the items.

Exercise 2.3. Driving in Cars

Sometimes clients are really easy to feel empathy and understanding for, but sometimes they are not. Here are a couple of methods[2] to practice empathy skills while driving in your car. In this exercise you'll take a couple of common events that can occur during commuting and use them as opportunities to build empathy. One involves developing a "back story" for someone who has made a silly or risky driving decision that comes to your attention. If you don't drive, you can also use other opportunities to observe these types of behaviors. The second activity involves listening to a radio and providing reflections.

---

[1] Thanks to Carolina Yahne for this exercise.

[2] Thanks to Dee Dee Stout and Chris Dunn for these exercises.

Exercise 2.4. A Difficult Client

We all have difficult clients. These individuals put us through our paces and may leave us feeling uneasy about our work or even dreading their next visit. Consider your work situation and think about who that client might be. Then complete the worksheet for Exercise 2.4.

Partner Work

Exercises 2.1, 2.2, and 2.4 can all be done as activities with a partner. Exercise 2.3 could also be done as a team activity. In addition you might consider Exercise 2.5.

Exercise 2.5. A Favorite Memory

This activity is based on an exercise called "Reliable Strengths."[3] In this exercise each of you will take turns recalling memories from childhood and describing them to your partner, who will in turn draw ideas about strengths that you demonstrate in these stories.

Other Thoughts . . .

Many MI trainers use ballroom dancing as a metaphor for MI. That is, ballroom dancing can only occur when the two people move together in partnership. When done well, the movement unfolds through a series of subtle presses. This stands in contrast to wrestling, where one grappler attempts to assert his or her will over the opponent. So, one question you might ask yourself in times of frustration and client resistance is, are you dancing or are you wrestling?

A common misconception about MI is that it is a method for manipulating clients into making changes they do not really want to make. Another misconception is that MI is clinically useless, since it works only when clients want to change anyway. I hope that this chapter has illustrated that it is really neither of those things. MI is a series of specific strategies, informed by respect for client autonomy and values, for maximizing the chances that clients will choose adaptive behavior change. MI takes advantage of the natural tendency of human beings to choose what is best for them in the long run by working collaboratively to identify clients' desire for change within apparently destructive behaviors.

Finally, the fact that there is only one brief reference to Prochaska and DiClemente's (1984, 1998) transtheoretical model (TTM) in this chapter on the foundations of MI may surprise some readers. In the 1991 MI edition and earlier writings, TTM figured more prominently, though in the second edition TTM was moved to the second half of the book. It's clear that over time TTM generally and the stages-of-change element of the model particularly have become conflated with MI. These are not MI, as Miller and Rollnick (2009) noted recently, though they share a common heritage. Hence, its deemphasis in a book on learning MI.

---

[3]Thanks to Elaine Christensen for this exercise.

Favorite Teacher or Supervisor

This exercise asks you to think and write about people who may have been significant influences in your life. In particular, consider the role of a favorite supervisor or teacher. During their training, counselors typically have their clinical work reviewed or supervised by more experienced counselors; this may also occur during the early part of their career. This is serious business, because the most important goal of supervision is the protection of the client and oversight of the quality of care he or she receives. Supervisors bear responsibility for ensuring that no harm is done by the fledgling clinician. Still, there is another purpose to supervision: the student should advance in clinical skills and maturity. This advancement usually involves learning something about the specific content important to treating a given client, but it also involves lessons about psychotherapy more generally and the clinician's personal style. Good counselors have usually had more than one influential supervisor.

If you find it hard to identify a favorite supervisor, you might want to write about a *favorite teacher*. This person might have been someone who taught you in elementary school and helped you learn strong habits of mind. Perhaps it was a high school teacher who inspired you to do more. Maybe it was a college or graduate or medical school professor who opened up a new vista on the world. Whoever, whether teacher or supervisor, choose someone who inspired you and helped you grow.

Specifically, who was this person that motivated you to learn, inspired you to excel and to try harder than you otherwise would have? Take a moment to write down this teacher or supervisor's name and jot down the characteristics you remember about that person and how you felt and responded when you were with him or her. If you cannot choose one as a favorite, simply choose among your favorites for the purpose of this exercise (and consider yourself fortunate indeed!). Here is one of my favorite supervisors.

Al

Characteristics: Al expected a lot from me, seemed to have hope for me as a therapist despite my inexperience, encouraged me to show rather than hide my foibles, could be grandfatherly and warm when needed, but was also direct and honest when the situation required. He was thoughtful in his responses to me and to clients, displayed his work in the form of tapes, and provided practical tips about things to consider. My all-time favorite lecture in graduate school was given by Al and was entitled, "What to do when the lawyer calls." He also provided a line I quote often in my training with professionals, "Our clients benefit from neither our naiveté nor our cynicism."

How I responded: I kept trying, despite many mistakes, because I knew he was committed to making me a better therapist and a good psychologist. Over time, I learned to trust my judgment and skills because I knew these were based on a solid foundation. A Rogerian therapist, he taught me the spirit of being a good therapist, as well as the techniques. Specifically, I learned that I couldn't become a good therapist without being truly present in the therapy room myself; this meant including things like my humor in these very serious encounters.

Here is one of my favorite teachers.

Doc

Characteristics: Doc loved to teach high school art. His classroom was a welcome respite from the regimentation of other classes. There was music, independent work and informality. He respected student ideas and choices, encouraging us to be wildly creative rather than doodling at the edges of the usual. He communicated genuine interest in my work and looked carefully at it each day. He provided feedback when asked and suggestions if requested, but never told me

(cont.)

what to do. He held me to account for doing my work and made a clear distinction between sharing ideas and goofing off with friends. It was a relaxed atmosphere in which to explore creativity and abilities, but he also had expectations that you would do the work. He clearly did not believe that there was only one way to paint, draw, sculpt, or be creative. For example, during my senior year, another student and I decided to make an animated movie—an activity that was entirely different from any other student's project and a task that neither of us knew anything about. Doc's response was, "Cool. How are you going to do it?" The movie took the entire year to complete. We wrote scripts, developed animation techniques, learned how to use an editing board, and shot rolls and rolls of film. Doc kept checking on our progress, commiserating with our setbacks and expressing concerns when we didn't complete tasks as promised. He encouraged us to hold a "premiere" for the movie, replete with invited guests, sound system, and popcorn he'd made.

How I responded: I tried things I would never have attempted otherwise. I made mistakes, but I also made discoveries and was not afraid of appearing foolish because I did not know how to do something. When I encountered problems, I didn't hide my inadequacies. I learned what I could overcome and what I could not. Perhaps most importantly, I looked forward to that class and always felt welcome.

Now it's your turn. Think about your favorite teacher or supervisor. Consider, especially, what characteristics he or she had or what he or she did that inspired you to learn and excel. Then answer these questions.

What's his or her name?

What characteristics did he or she have?

What inspired you to do or be your best?

How did you respond to his or her efforts?

After you've completed this exercise, examine the characteristics of this important person and compare them to three MI spirit characteristics: collaboration, autonomy, and evocation. Collaboration is the tendency to work in harmony with others to solve a problem, address an issue, or pursue an idea. Each person may have separate roles, but the process is supportive. Autonomy recognizes the ability and need of the other to choose his or her course, and it reflects faith in the ability of the other to choose wisely. Evocation is the action of one party bringing out the best in the other. The other is not simply left to flounder, but is given just enough direction to succeed. Again, these three elements are the core components of the spirit of MI.

Rating Samples for MI Spirit

Here are examples of short client statements and practitioner responses. Review these exchanges and then decide if the practitioner's response is consistent with the spirit of MI (thumbs up) or not (thumbs down). You might want to jot down a few notes as to why you rated each sample as you did. Then look at the discussion for each example at the end of this exercise.

1. *Sarah's husband (Richard)*: I'm just furious that she lied to me and had this affair behind my back. I can't believe I didn't see it. I feel like such an idiot.

   Practitioner: In retrospect, what signs did you overlook?

   Thumbs up _____   *Thumbs down* _____

   Why?

2. *Arthur*: I know my dad told you I'm depressed, but I'm not. Just because I don't want to play football doesn't mean I'm depressed.

   Practitioner: Your father is worrying needlessly. What do you think he's seeing that makes him worry this way?

   Thumbs up _____   *Thumbs down* _____

   Why?

3. *Tanya*: I need to come up with some sort of plan to help me get back on track now. This health crisis has thrown me for a loop. I can't think about anything else. What do you think I should do?

   Practitioner: Well, I have some ideas about what might help, but first let me hear what you've already considered.

   Thumbs up _____   *Thumbs down* _____

   Why?

4. *Arthur*: I'm not going to keep that stupid thought journal. How does it help me to monitor my "loser" thinking? I'm coming here to feel better, and paying attention to all that makes me feel worse.

   Practitioner: OK, Arthur, you might be right. This works for many folks, but not everyone. Maybe we need to try a different way to approach this. We've talked about other ways to address this issue. What makes sense to you to practice instead?

   Thumbs up _____   *Thumbs down* _____

   Why?

5. *Tanya*: They told me I have to have this surgery right away. But I don't trust them, so I haven't scheduled it yet.

(cont.)

Practitioner: Why take the chance? They're the experts, after all. Let's call from this phone right now—maybe you can get in this week.

Thumbs up _____ *Thumbs down* _____

Why?

6. *Sarah*: I've had it with Richard's guilt mongering. Okay, so I had an affair. I'm ready to end it and start working on our marriage, but I don't think he's ever going to let me forget it. Maybe we should just get a divorce.

   Practitioner: Sarah, you are the only one who can decide if you should stay in this marriage or leave it. I wonder what signs you would need to feel more optimistic about working on things with Richard.

   Thumbs up _____ *Thumbs down* _____

   Why?

7. *Arthur's mother (Peggy)*: They had a little "surprise party" for me. Everyone showed up when I wasn't looking and then spent the next 2 hours telling me how my drinking hurt them. They think I'm an alcoholic! I might have a drinking problem, but I'm damn sure not an alcoholic.

   Practitioner: (gently) Peggy, if it walks like a duck and quacks like a duck, it's probably a duck. I think if all those people are telling you you're an alcoholic, they're probably right. You might be in denial, don't you think?

   Thumbs up _____ *Thumbs down* _____

   Why?

8. *Arthur's father (Lloyd)*: I think Arthur is taking over too many of the household responsibilities. A boy his age ought to be playing sports and chasing girls. Instead, he's worrying about his younger brother and how the house looks. He even does laundry. I can tell you I never did that at his age. But when I try to push him toward more normal things, like football, he just gets mad at me and says I don't understand him. What am I supposed to do?

   Practitioner: In families where alcohol has been a problem, it often works like this. What if you tried the chess club or the school newspaper instead of pushing him toward football? I think he'd be more receptive to that. I don't think you recognize how smart Arthur is. It could be that he will never be all that interested in football.

   Thumbs up _____ *Thumbs down* _____

   Why?

9. *Tanya*: My doctor gave me a long list of all the things I have to do to manage my care. It's overwhelming. I have to take medication three times a day. I can't even remember to feed my dog every single day. I just can't do it. But I'm afraid I'll die if I don't.

   Practitioner: (encouraging) You can do this. You have to.

   Thumbs up _____ *Thumbs down* _____

   Why?

Key for Exercise 2.2

Recognize that MI spirit is typically rated on a continuum, and here we are using a simple dichotomy. We may disagree on the direction of the thumb, so the reasoning becomes far more important. Here are my thoughts ...

1. *Thumbs down.* This is an instance where evocation and collaboration might take the practitioner in different directions. The practitioner might be better served by paying attention to the supportive aspects of collaboration first. More specifically, the practitioner missed the chance to express empathy and instead slipped into information gathering.

2. *Thumbs up.* Again we see collaboration and evocation present, but this time the practitioner attends to the relationship issues first. The practitioner offers a reflection, followed by an open-ended question that encourages exploration in the direction of change.

3. *Thumbs up.* The practitioner avoids the expert role and makes an active attempt to seek collaboration from the client. The practitioner does not dodge the client's request for advice, but ensures that it will occur in the proper context. This practitioner will not miss a chance to hear Tanya's ideas about how to improve her situation.

4. *Thumbs up.* Even the best treatments don't work if clients won't implement them. The practitioner avoids a power struggle and looks for ways to collaborate instead.

5. *Thumbs down.* This practitioner has missed a chance to support the client's autonomy in making a difficult decision fraught with ambivalence. By pushing hard for change, even for compelling reasons, the practitioner will likely elicit the "Yes, but ... " response from this client.

6. *Thumbs up.* The practitioner has acknowledged Sarah's autonomy in making the decision about her marriage, but has also shifted the conversation toward self-exploration and optimism.

7. *Thumbs down.* Confrontation typically leads to increased resistance. This practitioner has violated an important concept in MI: Allow clients to draw conclusions about their own behavior. This approach violates both autonomy and collaboration elements.

8. *Thumbs down.* Even when well meaning (and accurate), advice should be given quite sparingly when using MI, as it may be inconsistent with a spirit of evocation, collaboration, and autonomy. Here there is a quality of arguing for something specific, which will likely engender resistance.

9. *Thumbs down.* Comfort, encouragement, and support are important therapeutic interventions, but always secondary to the importance of MI spirit. In this case, the practitioner's response violates the client's autonomy by indicating that there is no choice. In addition, it fails to recognize that this client's dilemma itself provides the momentum needed for change.

Driving in Cars

These are a couple of exercises for developing empathy while driving in cars.

Imagine you're driving in the heavy Seattle (Washington) traffic, consistently rated as some of the worst in the United States. Here is an opportunity to practice empathy while reducing your stress. The method is essentially this: Wait for a traffic annoyance (e.g., someone cuts you off) that would normally upset you, then create a "back story" for that person.

Example:

> *Wally just cut me off. He's been having a very bad day. He spilled coffee on his pants on the way to work this morning. It hurt. Then he had to go right in—wet pants and all—to give a big presentation that he'd stayed up until very late to make sure was perfect. Next his partner called to say that Cecil the dog had thrown up on the carpet again and maybe it was time to talk about his future. Then, as Wally was packing up his stuff, his new boss dropped off some corrections that had to go out before closing. This little project made him late for his daughter's recital. She is performing third, and he promised that he would be there this morning, so if he just hurries he might make it before she finishes.*

Continue the story until your feelings of antipathy and frustration are replaced by a sense of compassion for the other driver's plight. If you don't drive, consider using this exercise by focusing on annoying people in your life or frustrating situations.

The second approach, while a little less fantasy-based, requires no less creativity. Tune your car or home radio to a talk radio station that you wouldn't normally listen to and may not fit with your beliefs or practices. Your job is to listen to a commentator or caller statement, switch off or turn down the radio, and give a reflection—out loud. Then do it again and again and again, until you feel that you may understand (though perhaps not agree with) this caller's or commentator's point. Alternatively, you could again create back stories, this time for either the commentator or callers.

A Difficult Client

We all have difficult clients. These individuals put us through our paces and may leave us feeling uneasy about our work or even dreading our next encounter. Consider your work situation and think about who that person might be.

Now consider three questions about this person.

Where are you now in your work with him or her?

Where would you like to be?

What's getting in the way of that happening?

Now imagine that you are this client. Really put yourself inside this person's skin.

Where are you now in your work with your practitioner?

Where would you like to be?

What's getting in the way of that happening?

After reviewing both sets of answers, think about the three areas of MI spirit. Then rate where this relationship falls on these three dimensions.

(cont.)

Collaboration

We are working against each other (Wrestling)		We are working in partnership (Dancing)		We are in the room, but not much is happening (Standing)		
1	2	3	4	5	6	7

Autonomy

I struggle with the client's choices and/or press the client to change (Directing)		I recognize and honor client's choices, including no change (Guiding)		I seem indifferent to client's wishes or choices (Observing)		
1	2	3	4	5	6	7

Evocation

I am presenting the reasons for change (Advocating)		I am drawing out the client's views on change (Interviewing)		I just let the session go wherever it will (Following)		
1	2	3	4	5	6	7

What, if anything, do these ratings tell you might need to happen for the relationship to change?

What might you do differently to make that happen?

If you were to try one new approach with this client, what would it be?

A Favorite Memory

Think back to before you were 10 years old and describe a favorite memory:

- Tell lots of specifics, so that your listener can really visualize the memory.
- Listener, your job is to say nothing—just listen.
- After you've both taken your turn, take 2 minutes to jot down a few of the essential elements you heard that were important to this memory. Write those below, but don't share them yet.

For the next task, each of you draws a picture of an event that you feel proud about—something you played a part in.

- Don't worry about your art skills. Stick figures work, but try to add important details.
- Who was there? What was happening?

Make your drawing here:

(cont.)

- When you're both done, show and describe your drawing to your partner.
- When you've each had a turn, spend a couple of minutes writing down two or three essential qualities you heard in this interaction. Write those here.

When you are both done, take a few minutes to identify five strengths that you've heard. Write those below, along with specific examples.

1. Strength:

2. Strength:

3. Strength:

4. Strength:

5. Strength:

Finally, feed back to each other the five strengths that you heard—explicitly or implicitly—in these two activities. Be sure to include specific examples.

Chapter 3

The Use of OARS
Reflective Listening

Opening

Carl is 10 years old. This year is his first year playing baseball. He knows little of the game, but what he lacks in knowledge he makes up for in enthusiasm. He also has attention-deficit/ hyperactivity disorder, which makes it hard for him to focus this energy at practice and in the games. Although he has trouble catching the ball and throwing it consistently to a target, he desperately wants to pitch for his baseball team. His coach, despite reservations about Carl's ability to succeed in the endeavor, assures him that he'll get a chance to pitch; however, he also tells Carl that he needs to practice throwing strikes. Of course, Carl's interest in pitching does not translate into regular practice at home, and so his accuracy doesn't improve much. Still, the coach is true to his word, and one glorious day the moment arrives when Carl pitches an inning for his team. Carl experiences control problems and walks in four runs, the maximum number allowed per inning in this league. Undaunted, he walks into the dugout after his outing, his face beaming, and says, "Pretty good, eh, Coach? I even got one guy out." The coach, standing at the dugout entrance as the team straggles in, says to Carl. . . .

This coach has lots of options of how to respond, depending on what he wants to accomplish. If he thinks the important thing is for the kids to have fun, he might say, "That was pretty exciting, Carl." Or maybe he thinks that kids need encouragement and success, thus leading to more interest and effort, in which case he might say, "You did a nice job getting that guy out. It takes a lot of courage to pitch, but you did it." Or maybe he thinks that setting goals and working toward them are important, in which case he might say, "Yeah, you sure did get the guy out. So, if you wanted to work on getting two more outs, what would you need to work on for next time?" Or maybe the coach is interested in having Carl assess his pitching skills more realistically: "Carl, you did some things very well, and I thought there were some areas that could use some work. What did you think?" Of course, the coach may think that winning is the most critical thing, which may lead to a more confrontative response: "Carl, you sure did get that guy out, and we need to get three outs in each inning for you to be an effective pitcher. So, I want to support your interest in pitching, and I need to see you throw strikes in practice before you pitch again." These examples illustrate how the coach's goal determines the response he selects, which in turn may produce very different reactions from Carl. We can easily see how Carl's motivation to pitch and the direction that motivation takes might be quite different, depending on the coach's response.

In MI we refer to these small responses as "microskills." These skills are fundamental tools that counselors often already have in their clinical repertoire but may tend to overlook as they focus on larger thoughtful interventions. Yet, the strategic use of these skills can have dramatic effects on what happens during the course of an interaction.

OARS is the acronym used to describe these microskills. OARS stand for open-ended questions, affirmations, reflective listening, and summaries. Practitioners use the methods of OARS to intervene intentionally during the course of a session. These skills can be used in the context of larger interventions or as a primary method of intervention. Furthermore, these skills are used strategically and purposefully to address or explore some topics (e.g., change talk) but not others (e.g., sustain talk). Because of the importance of reflective listening in doing MI well, this chapter focuses exclusively on it. Chapter 4 targets the other three microskills.

Reflective listening is *the primary skill* on which MI built. It is the mechanism through which practitioners express their interest, empathy, and understanding of clients. Practitioners can express acceptance of the client and also gently challenge positions; they can encourage greater exploration or a shift away from a problematic statement. Reflective listening is typically used to create momentum, which can then be channeled in directions that are productive.

Reflective listening looks deceptively easy, but it takes hard work and skill to do it well. As a trainer, my experience indicates that this is often the area where practitioners need the most work but are least enthused about spending training time. Yet, without this skill, I don't think it's possible to do MI. In addition, my trainees and clients have taught me humility about reflective listening. Even as an experienced trainer, I encounter times when my biggest problem is that I am not listening to what my client is saying. Thus, I benefit from opportunities at fine-tuning these skills, and I encourage you to spend some time in this area as well, even if this is a skill you already do well.

A Deeper Look

This discussion begins with a consideration of what reflective listening is *not*. Indeed, many of the skills used routinely in clinical work are not reflective listening. Thomas Gordon (1970) grouped many of these activities into 12 areas, which he called "roadblocks" (see Figure 3.1). Gordon called these interventions roadblocks because he felt they obstructed or interfered with a client's forward movement and thus the momentum toward change. Questions—as we'll see in the next chapter—are an important type of microskill, but they cause clients to stop and reflect on the matter queried and thus stop their forward movement. Reflections, meanwhile, generally sustain the forward momentum, even when incorrect.

Thomas Gordon's 12 Roadblocks

1. **Ordering, directing, or commanding**—A direction is given with the force of authority behind it. Authority can be actual or implied.

2. **Warning or threatening**—Similar to directing but carries an implication of consequences, if not followed. This implication can be a threat or a prediction of a bad outcome.

3. **Giving advice, making suggestions, providing solutions**—The therapist uses expertise and experience to recommend a course of action.

4. **Persuading with logic, arguing, lecturing**—The practitioner believes that the client has not adequately reasoned through the problem and needs help in doing so.

5. **Moralizing, preaching, telling clients their duty**—The implicit message is that the person needs instruction in proper morals.

6. **Judging, criticizing, disagreeing, blaming**—The common element among these four is an implication that there is something wrong with the person or with what has been said. Simple disagreement is included in this group.

7. **Agreeing, approving, praising**—This message gives sanction or approval to what is being said. This stops the communication process and may imply an uneven relationship between speaker and listener.

8. **Shaming, ridiculing, name calling**—The disapproval may be overt or covert. Typically, it's directed at correcting a problematic behavior or attitude.

9. **Interpreting, analyzing**—This is a very common and tempting activity for counselors: to seek out the real problem or hidden meaning and give an interpretation.

10. **Reassuring, sympathizing, consoling**—The intent here is to make the person feel better. Like approval, this is a roadblock that interferes with the spontaneous flow of communication.

11. **Questioning, probing**—Questions can be mistaken for good listening. The intent is to probe further, to find out more. A hidden communication is the implication that if enough questions are asked, the questioner will find the solution. Questions can also interfere with the spontaneous flow of communication, directing it in the interests of the questioner but not necessarily the speaker.

12. **Withdrawing, distracting, humoring, changing the subject**—These divert communication and may also imply that what the person is saying is not important or should not be pursued.

Figure 3.1. Thomas Gordon's 12 roadblocks. From *Parent Effectiveness Training* by Thomas Gordon, M.D., copyright © 1970 by Thomas Gordon. Used by permission of McKay, a division of Random House, Inc.

Some roadblocks can be quite useful in working with clients. Indeed, they may be appropriate interventions, but it's important to recognize these are not the same as listening. Praising is a good example. Most of us would agree that there are times and places when praising clients is an important activity and should be encouraged. For example, we ask parents to praise children when they are doing well. Others on this roadblock list may seem less credible. Most of us would forego ridiculing our clients—but we might communicate our belief that they are making bad choices, which has a subtle implication of disapproval. The problem, from the MI perspective, is not that practitioners do these things (though some may be less helpful than others), but rather that we do too many of the roadblocks and too little reflective listening.

So if these things are not reflective listening, what is? To begin it's a way of thinking that includes interest in what the person has to say and respect for his or her wisdom. We start from this rather obvious position that each client knows more about him- or herself than we will ever know. Sure, we can see blind spots that clients cannot, but conversely they know far more about factors that have influenced their personality development, life choices, behaviors, attitudes, and beliefs than we do. If we want to know these things, clients must tell us—and we must listen.

But even if they tell us and we listen, this does not mean that we understand their experience. This lacuna leads to a key element of reflective listening: hypothesis testing. Stated bluntly, what you think the person means may not be what he or she really means. The hypothesis-testing approach corresponds to Gordon's (1970) model of communication (see Figure 3.2).

At point A the speaker has something in mind to say. At point B the speaker actually says it. At C, the listener hears and takes in the statement. Finally at D, the listener perceives the meaning of what the speaker said. Let's look at the example of Arthur, an unhappy young man brought to therapy by his parents. Suppose the practitioner asked Arthur how he felt about coming to therapy.

- At point A Arthur might think, "I'm not sure if I want to be in therapy. It's sort of weird talking to somebody I don't know, especially about *this* stuff. Besides, how can I trust he won't tell my parents what I say? But, if I don't do this, my parents will rag on me even more than they do already. This sucks."
- At point B Arthur might say, "I'm not sure I buy this therapy crap."
- At point C the practitioner might hear, "I'm not sure, but this may be crap."
- At point D the practitioner might understand this to mean several things—"I don't want to waste my time," "I'm not sure I want to be here," "I resent that my parents

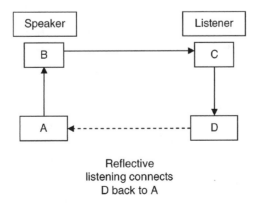

Figure 3.2. Thomas Gordon's communication model. From *Parent Effectiveness Training* by Thomas Gordon, M.D., copyright © 1970 by Thomas Gordon. Used by permission of McKay, a division of Random House, Inc.

made me come," or "I'm not sure I can trust you"—any of which may be more or less accurate.

As the example with Arthur illustrates, at each point in this process communication can break down.

- At point A Arthur may have trouble putting his thoughts together in a comprehensible manner. He may not fully understand all of his thoughts and feelings. Or he may not connect all the elements that are influencing his thoughts and feelings. School may have been tough that day, and then Dad spent the ride to the office badgering him about his future. He doesn't want to think about anything except being somewhere else.
- At point B Arthur may not have the verbal facility needed for this type of communication. He may be someone who is not used to talking with adults. He may be a typical adolescent boy who will use shoulder shrugs and "I don't knows" whenever possible to respond to adult queries. He may know there are multiple pieces, which he can say individually, but finds impossible to put together in an integrated thought. Or, he may be able to express all these things but is not ready to say them to a stranger quite yet. Yet another possibility: He may feel so much resentment about being forced to come for therapy that he communicates things verbally that he may not feel fully (e.g., "I don't buy this therapy crap.").
- At point C the practitioner missed a part of what Arthur said. It may be an insignificant part; it may not. Perhaps the dance studio, on the floor below, is revving up for the evening, and it's a little harder to hear. Maybe the client spoke softly. Or perhaps the practitioner just finished a session with an especially intense client and is still trying to clear his head from that meeting. Maybe the last session went long and the practitioner rushed to check messages, write a note, and review the case materials, so he didn't get a chance to use the bathroom, which he's needed to do for two clients now. Or maybe his back has begun to hurt from sitting all day. And the list goes on.
- At point D the practitioner tries to make sense of what he heard. His experience with adolescents tells him that this young man is likely to be thinking or feeling certain things. Some of these likely thoughts or feelings may be accurate; others may not apply to this young man. He may expect that this young man may be reluctant to be here, since his parents have brought him here. He may read correctly the client's body language and affective tone, but overinterpret its meaning. This client may remind the clinician of another client he found difficult to deal with and didn't particularly like. These assumptions may lead him to choose one understanding versus another of what the client means by his statement.

In Gordon's model the purpose of reflective listening is to address all the various ways communications can go awry by connecting point D back to point A. This connection of D to A is hypothesis testing. That is, "I think Arthur means this, but let me check it out and see if that is accurate." Thus, good reflective listening is meant to close the loop in Gordon's model.

Reflective listening involves making statements, not asking questions. The words may be exactly the same, but the delivery (and effect) is different. For example, say the following two sentences aloud:

"You're not sure you want to be here?"

"You're not sure you want to be here."

Did you notice how your voice turned up at the end of the first sentence and down at the end of the second? This second sentence may feel presumptuous, but it is what reflective listening entails. The listener makes a guess to confirm or deny the meaning of what the speaker said. If not terribly off-target, this statement leads to clarification by the speaker and greater exploration. It creates movement and momentum in the conversation. In contrast, questions interrupt the client's flow. Think about your reasons for buying and reading this book, then respond to the two sentences below.

"Do you want to learn about MI?"

"You want to learn more about MI."

How did you to respond to these two sentences? What thoughts or feelings did they invite or evoke in you?

When using reflective listening, some people find it helpful to use standard phrases:

"So you feel … "

"It sounds like you … "

"You're wondering if … "

"You … "

These phrases can be helpful in getting into the routine of using reflections, but be wary of using them rotely. Clients tire of them and may feel like you are "therapizing" them, if you don't vary your routine. That is, you're using a gimmick rather than truly working to understand them.

This variation in routine should also include changes in the depth of your reflections. There are different depths or levels of reflection, beginning with communications that stay very close to what the client has communicated and moving toward information that moves significantly beyond what the client has said. By varying your depth, you deepen or raise the intimacy level of the session. This change also alters the affective tone of an interaction. Consider these various types of reflections as tools in your therapeutic toolbox, where one tool is not necessarily better than another; it is simply the right tool for the job at hand.

In general, the depth of reflection should match the situation. Early and late in a session, surface-level reflections are typical. In the heart of a session, depth should be increasing. However, with someone struggling to control emotions, more surface-level reflections might be more appropriate. A basic guideline is the less you know what a person means, the shorter should be your jump in levels.

The most common convention used in differentiating types of reflections at present is to distinguish simple from complex reflections. Moyers, Martin, Manuel, and Miller (2003) note that coders (i.e., people trained to code audio/video tapes of therapy sessions) can reliably distinguish between these categories of reflections.

The simple reflection stays very close to what the client has said. The statement adds little beyond what has already been stated, but communicates attention and interest. The practitioner statement uses the same words or very close to the same words the client used. Using Arthur's statement, "I'm not sure I buy this therapy crap," a simple reflection might be, "You're not sure." Moyers et al. (2003) note that a simple reflection may "mark very important or intense client emotions, but do not go far beyond the client's original intent in the statement" (p. 10). Similarly, summaries can be coded as simple reflections if the listener does not "add an additional point or direction." Thus, simple reflections tend to stabilize the client and the communication, as well as keep the conversation alive.

Complex reflections may go well beyond what the client has said. These infer even greater meaning and often cognitively reframe the information. These may also include affect, but must also contain additional depth, movement, or direction. A complex reflection adds to client self-understanding by putting elements in contrast to each other that the client might not have considered. Using Arthur's statement again, a complex reflection might be, "You're frustrated by others making decisions for you." Although this statement is short, it moves well beyond what the client has reported and opens the door to other directions of exploration. In this way complex reflections, when done well, move the conversation forward.

While varying the depth of reflections is important in reflective listening, there are also benefits to overstating and understating a reflection. An overstatement (i.e., an amplified reflection) may cause a person to back away from a position. This tool can be useful when a client takes a near absolute position. The practitioner gently and genuinely presses on the absolute or the resistant element to determine if this is an accurate stance. If the client backs away from the position, then the practitioner has created some space for the client to consider alternatives and subtly reframed the situation. If the client does not move, then it is simply an accurate reflection. For example, with Arthur, an amplified reflection might be, "So, from your perspective, things are going great." The importance of being genuine is clearly evident in this example. Any hint of sarcasm and Arthur will feel it and respond with anger or a counterargument. For this reason, understatement is often preferred by practitioners.

Understatement involves emphasizing statements at, or slightly below, the intensity that the client expresses them. Understatement often leads to continuation and deepening. These concepts are closely aligned with leading and following, though they are not the same. When *following*, the practitioner stays slightly behind the client in terms of conversational direction. This technique typically involves understatement as well as directive intent (i.e., by what is reflected and what is ignored), but it does not seek to lead the client to the next step. *Leading* involves moving slightly ahead of the client and supplying what is unstated, but implied, in the conversation. This technique is known as *continuing the paragraph*. The purpose of this technique is to move the client in a new and perhaps unrecognized direction. If we return to Arthur, a following response might be, "You're annoyed your parents brought you here," whereas a leading response could be, "You're confused about why your parents want you here, and that's information you might be interested in finding out." In the first response, the practitioner follows the client's direction, even as the interaction is deepened by focusing on the client's unstated emotion. In the second response, the practitioner actively leads the conversation in a new direction the client has not articulated. Usually, practitioners will start with following, before moving to leading.

A double-sided reflection highlights the ambivalence in a client's words. It may involve something said in the immediate past or things stated earlier or in prior conversation. The statement can include phrases such as "On the one hand you feel ... and on the other. ... " Whenever I use a double-sided reflection, I inevitably raise my hands like a scale and use them as visual representations of the two sides. I also teach people to start with the element that favors the status quo and end with the dimension that favors change, as this provides a natural stepping-off point for further exploration of change—if appropriate. Also beware of the conjunction you use in this situation. *But* tends to dismiss everything that precedes it, whereas *and* acknowledges both sides as having merit. With Arthur a double-sided reflection might be, "So, on the one hand, you'd rather not be here, and, on the other, you're aware that something may need to change before you can stop coming here."

A final consideration in reflective listening is the use of metaphors. These are regarded as a more complex form of reflection because they typically move well beyond what the client has said, but still contain the essence. The metaphor seems to allow clients to understand their situation in a new way while providing an organizational scheme for incorporating new data. A metaphor for Arthur might be, "So, it's like a game where you are forced to play, but no one has told you the rules or even the point of the game." This metaphor of a game provides a common situation that would make sense to Arthur (organizational element). This new framework then allows Arthur or the practitioner to add ideas about how the situation needs to change (incorporating new data) for Arthur to feel comfortable. The metaphor provides new ways to understand and (potentially) respond to a situation.

Trainees often express concern about "putting words into client's mouths." They feel it is presumptuous and that it should be done with care, if at all. My sense is that MI is based on taking guesses in the spirit of understanding our clients and is therefore necessary. Again, as long as these guesses are not wildly inaccurate, clients will typically respond to an off-target reflection with clarification and more information. Thus, it is my belief that practitioners should not be afraid of taking guesses and being wrong, but instead should add words that clients don't use. It is through this process that practitioners become more refined at guessing, and clients seem to come to a greater understanding of themselves, their needs and their behavior.

The exception to this substitution of language is the use of "hot" words. The nature of these words will vary by the work type and location. However, some words are universally hot (e.g., "manipulated") and, regardless of the situation, will draw clients' ire. It's best to find a different word or phrase as these "hot" words are likely to immediately inflame resistance.

Concept Quiz—Test Yourself!

True or false:

1.   T F   OARS are basic MI skills.

2.   T F   OARS are unique to MI.

3.   T F   Reflective listening is a critical skill in MI.

4.   T F   Reflective listening is a method to check understanding.

5.   T F   Good reflective listening involves repeating only what clients say.

6.   T F   It's important to use a variety of reflection forms.

7.   T F   Amplified reflections gently challenge client absolutes.

8.   T F   You should move quickly into leading clients, if possible.

9.   T F   Accurate reflections can include elements that a client doesn't say.

10.   T F   You should be careful about taking guesses regarding what clients mean.

Answers

1.   T   OARS are referred to as the microskills of MI and are basic to good MI practice.

2.   F   Although a foundation of MI, these skills are *not* unique to MI. Indeed, many practitioners learn these skills in an introduction to interviewing course. What may be unique to MI is the directive use of these skills.

3.   T   Although reflective listening is one of many tools, it is also the backbone of MI. Many trainers believe that you must be proficient in reflective listening to do MI. Preliminary research suggests that not only frequency but depth of reflections distinguish expert from novice MI therapists.

4.   T   This checking is a primary purpose of reflection, and it is why this process is called a hypothesis-testing approach.

5.   F   Although simple reflections may stay very close to what clients say, there is nothing more annoying to clients than a therapist who only keeps repeating back what they said.

6.   T   You should vary the depth of your reflections, as well as under- and overstating and leading and following.

7.   T   The key to offering effective amplified reflections is working gently and genuinely; failure to do so will engender resistance.

8.   F   Leading too quickly is a form of inaccurate listening—the practitioner tries to insert his or her agenda rather than trying to understand the client.

9.   T   Absolutely! Reflections should include information that moves beyond the words the client uses—these additions deepen the reflections.

10.   F   Although you should not be careless or callous, guesses should be made. This process allows the practitioner and the client to deepen their mutual understanding.

In Practice

Note the following interchange with an adolescent client. This young man was brought to treatment because of significant conflict between himself and his father. His father wanted him "fixed," noting that he was a belligerent kid without morals. The young man initially stated that he just wanted to be left alone.

Notice the therapist behaviors and the client's responses. This example is included not because it leads to startling revelations, but rather because it shows how, through subtle therapist behaviors, openings emerge and avenues for further intervention can then be followed. A few microskills that will be discussed in greater detail in the next chapter are also evident.

Statement	*Commentary*
T: How's your week been?	Open-ended question.
C: Pretty good.	Minimal response.
T: Tell me about it.	Another open-ended question.
C: Nothing much's been happening really. Just hanging out and seein' my friends. Well, I guess there was the deal between me and my dad. It was no big deal really. You know—I just don't get him.	More information; slips in data about an event with Dad.
T: So, it was no big deal, but something happened.	Simple reflection.
C: Yeah. He said I couldn't go out one night, but I'd already made plans. It was just this power trip thing. We got in an argument, and he told me to go to my room. I got mad and split instead. When I got home he'd packed up my brothers and taken them to the cabin for the weekend without me. Things have been better since then.	Client continues to reveal more data.
T: So, it was actually an improvement.	Amplified reflection.
C: Well, I guess so. I don't know. I mean, he does this name calling and mocking stuff, and I guess I do it back, which isn't such a good idea—but it pisses me off. It's immature.	He backs away from saying it's better and acknowledges ambivalence about Dad leaving.
T: Maybe it was and maybe it wasn't, but name calling and mocking really bug you.	A rephrase that directs attention to critical element.
C: Yeah, it's so immature—like calling us slobs or losers and being sarcastic. I just can't stand people who are hypocrites—that's a strong word—but that's what it feels like.	He responds with stronger affect.
T: Someone says one thing but does another.	Another rephrase.

Statement	*Commentary*
C: Right. I think my word is my bond. If I say I'm going to do something, I do it. Like, for example, this summer I hit this kid's car with my scooter and put a dent in the door. You're not going to tell my parents this, right?	He deepens the exchange by talking about values and a problematic behavior.
T: Right, not unless there's a danger to you or to someone else.	Clarification.
C: So, I told him I would pay for it. He had to have the door replaced and painted. Well, in the meantime, I wrecked my truck, and I guess his parents felt sorry for me so they said I didn't have to pay them back. But I made a promise so I am going to keep it. I need to get a job and start paying it off. It's about $500, so it's a lot of money.	He gives information about the importance of that value. This is a clue about where a motivating discrepancy may exist.
T: You're willing to keep your word, even if others don't hold you to it and if it costs you something. This is an important value to you. I'm wondering where you got that from. . . .	Affirmation that also explores possible connection to parents.
C: I don't know. My mom, I guess, though my dad can be OK, too.	His position on Dad softens somewhat.
T: OK, so it was probably Mom, though you and your Dad aren't always like this.	Subtle rephrase.
C: Yeah.	
T: So, let me see if I understood all this stuff. You. . . .	Starts to summarize.

The end of this interchange feels hopeful. This young man, whom Dad had described as belligerent and without morals, displays a clear sense of values and behavior that is consistent with these values, even when others may not hold him accountable. This, in addition to the discovery of his ambivalence about his father's departure, suggests possible motivational discrepancies. If you were to provide the summary, with what question would you like to follow it?

Try This!

These exercises will walk you through a series of listening experiences, progressing from the least complex to the subtlest. Although you do not have to start at the beginning, each activity builds on the preceding exercise. The beginning exercise involves spotting what is and is not listening. As was noted in Chapters 1 and 2, MI training now focuses on learning to use your client as a trainer. However, to do this, you must be a good observer of your own and your client's behavior. We begin building this observational skill by watching other people work—specifically, popular TV talk-show hosts. You can watch in real time or a taped version, though I encourage recording because this allows more opportunity to control the speed of the process. The next exercise asks you to practice hypothesis testing. Specifically, you will generate alternative hypotheses to client statements and put these in the form of a reflection. This exercise pushes you to consider more than one way to understand a client's words. The following exercise asks you to take this one step further by generating reflections that are directive. That is, these emphasize different aspects of the same statement and thereby direct where the conversation will move. Next, you are asked to write more complex reflective responses. These statements include greater depth or involve emphasizing different aspects of the communication. Finally, all this written practice leads to an exercise where you have a real conversation and work to be intentional in your use of listening. As with the exercises in the prior chapters, you'll find handouts that match these exercises at the end of the chapter. Although you won't use these exercises with your clients, you will certainly use the skills .

Exercise 3.1. Watching for Roadblocks

Tuning your receptors to detect roadblocks can be a very helpful first step in becoming more conscious of when you use these roadblocks in your interactions. However, it would be impolite to pull out a coding sheet and begin tracking conversations with your friends, neighbors, or family. A better approach is to use TV or radio talk shows on which hosts interview guests. You might choose a program whose host has a reputation for being a "tough" interviewer. You are likely to observe both excellent listening and Gordon's roadblocks. After reviewing Exercise 3.1 (at the end of the chapter), watch an episode of a talk show and note every time hosts use a reflective listening comment and each time they use a roadblock. Keep in mind that roadblocks are not necessarily bad things, and hosts may be quite successful in using these with their guests. However, they do stop forward momentum and can generate resistance. If possible, choose a program where the host is working with someone on a problem. Since programs move quickly, you may consider taping so that you can stop the tape as you think about your answers. Or, you could also put a tape recorder next to your radio and record a show. If you still find that these methods don't work for you (e.g., you're not an auditory learner), you might see if a transcript of a show is available and use this visual format. Tally your scores and answer the questions that follow.

Exercise 3.2. Watching for Listening

This is the second part in tuning your ear for listening. Again, choose a TV or radio program on which a host interviews guests. This time your focus will be on observing and listening. Watch for a few minutes without the sound to see how he or she communicates interest and caring. Then turn the sound on and count reflections. Again, you might consider taping this program so that you can slow down the process. Transcripts may also be helpful if you find that the interaction moves too quickly.

Exercise 3.3. Hypothesis Testing and the Formation of Reflections

Reflective listening involves completing Gordon's (1970) ABCD communication pattern. In the process listeners attempt to ensure that they have understood what the client is trying to communicate by testing hypotheses. Hypotheses can be more or less true and more or less central to the core of the client's communication. In this exercise you will find client statements on the Exercise 3.3 worksheet, to which you respond with guesses about what these statements could mean. You are encouraged to think broadly. This exercise makes explicit a process that will occur implicitly as you begin making more refined reflections.

Exercise 3.4. Directive Reflecting

MI is directive. So, in addition to taking a guess at what is being said by the person, a reflection (in MI) will reflect on certain aspects of a client statement and not others. This process allows the practitioner to focus on motivating pieces of the interchange. However, to be directive, you must first be able to recognize and respond to these parts. This exercise asks you to answer client statements with reflections that use different elements of what is being said. For each client statement, you will generate three reflections—each focusing on a different part of the communication. Notice how what you pay attention to might lead the conversation in a very different direction from what you did not emphasize.

Exercise 3.5. Deepening Reflections

Whereas the previous exercise focused on different parts of the client statement, this exercise asks you to move beyond the immediate content and add greater depth and complexity to the communication. Again, you will make educated guesses at what is implied by the client words.

Exercise 3.6. An Intentional Conversation

This exercise asks you to try out the listening skills you've been developing through written techniques. Put simply: You listen, instead of doing other things, and then observe how this listening affects the interaction. To make this exercise most effective, choose a situation in which you would normally be inclined to give advice. This "pull" to give advice may be hard to ignore, but see what can be accomplished just by listening. It often helps to select the conversation ahead of time (e.g., when my partner and I talk tonight; when my coworker complains about the boss; when my child justifies why homework was not completed). Use the worksheet to prompt your thinking afterward. When I have used this exercise in workshops, people have returned to say that they had found out things they hadn't known in 20 years of marriage. Listening can have profound effects! However, if the exercise doesn't go as well as you like, don't worry. This is practice and can always be repeated.

Partner Work

Many of the exercises described in "Try This!" may also be used as part of partner work, too. For example, you might tape your TV show and code the conversations together. When you get to a difficult-to-code comment, stop the tape and discuss what you are finding problematic. With Exercises 3.3 and 3.4, each of you can fill out the sheets and then give your response, describing your thinking behind it. Or you can watch the tape of the TV show and stop after each "client" statement and generate a reflective response you might use. To increase variety, you could also try generating several reflections of greater depth or complexity.

In an alternative for Exercise 3.3 on hypothesis testing, your partner makes a statement that describes a quality about him- or herself and then you keep using the "You mean … " approach to guess at what this means to your partner. The catch is, your partner can answer only yes or no. Do this until either you can't generate anymore hypotheses or your partner thinks you've got it. Another version is to have your partner respond "warmer" or "colder" as your statements move closer (warmer) or further (colder) from the central idea or ideas your partner had in mind.

You can also practice intentional listening with your partner. Ask your partner to describe a recent weekend and use only reflective listening statements. See if you can go 5 minutes without asking a question. You can also have your partner describe something he or she is struggling to change, but choose only material your partner feels comfortable sharing.

Once you feel comfortable with this type of intentional listening, try it out with clients. If you tend to work in a very different manner, this shift may be noticeable to them and they may ask you about it. You can inform them that as part of professional development, you work to improve your skills and this is part of that process. In this case, you are making sure that you are really being attentive to what the client is telling you. If you have the resources—and approval (client and agency)—you might also tape these sessions for your own review. Use your rating sheets for Exercise 3.2 to code what you are doing. You might also include your partner in this process. Remember, it is easy to focus on the negative when you hear your own work. So, focus your attention on what you are doing well and what you want to do more often in the next encounter. Ask your partner for tips when you get stuck.

Other Thoughts …

This microskill looks easier than it is. Said another way, reflective listening is simple, but that doesn't mean it's easy. If it feels like you get nowhere when using listening only, you're probably sticking too close to what the person said. Make more guesses. There is no substitute for practice in this area.

A few years back, a question was posed to a listserve of MI trainers: "What is it about listening that is helpful?" The answers from fellow trainers ranged from the empirically supported to the theoretical to the phenomenological and are well beyond the scope of this book. Part of my answer to this question is that we help clients organize and understand their experiences. Our job is not just repeating back what we have heard, but rather putting what we have heard into a structure that clients can use to help solve problems and move forward. Some therapists would describe this process as creating a coherent narrative.

There are obviously other important aspects of listening. Rogers (1980) wrote about the power of the experience of having another carefully listen to you. Consider from your own life: When you've been well listened to, has this been helpful? If so, what provided the benefit?

Watching for Roadblocks

Tuning your receptors to detect roadblocks can be a very helpful first step in becoming more conscious of when you use these roadblocks in your interactions. In this exercise you will use TV or radio talk shows where hosts interview guests as your raw material. Consider choosing a program whose host has a reputation for being a "tough" interviewer. You are likely to observe both excellent listening and Gordon's roadblocks. Keep in mind that roadblocks are not necessarily bad things, and hosts may be quite successful in using these with their guests. However, they do stop forward momentum and can generate resistance.

Here are the steps:

- Review the roadblocks listed below.
- Watch an episode of a talk show or listen to a radio show. If possible, choose a program whose host is working with someone on a problem.
- Note every time hosts use a reflective listening comment, and each time they use a roadblock.
- Since programs move quickly, you may consider taping so that you can stop the tape as you think about your answers. Or, you could also put a tape recorder next to your radio and record a show.
- If you still find that these methods don't work for you (e.g., you're not an auditory learner), you might see if a transcript of a show is available and use this visual format.
- Tally your scores and answer the questions that follow.

Thomas Gordon's 12 Roadblocks	*Number*
Ordering, directing, or commanding—A direction is given with the force of authority behind it. Authority can be actual or implied.	
Warning or threatening—Similar to directing but carries an implication of consequences, if not followed. This implication can be a threat or a prediction of a bad outcome.	
Giving advice, making suggestions, providing solutions—The therapist uses expertise and experience to recommend a course of action.	
Persuading with logic, arguing, lecturing—The practitioner believes that the client has not adequately reasoned through the problem and needs help in doing so.	
Moralizing, preaching, telling clients their duty—The implicit communication here is that the person needs instruction in proper morals.	
Judging, criticizing, disagreeing, blaming—The common element among these four is an implication that there is something wrong with the person or with what has been said. Simple disagreement is included in this group.	
Agreeing, approving, praising—This message gives sanction or approval to what is being said. This stops the communication process and may imply an uneven relationship between speaker and listener.	
Shaming, ridiculing, name calling—The disapproval may be overt or covert. Typically, it's directed at correcting a problematic behavior or attitude.	

(cont.)

Interpreting, analyzing—This is a very common and tempting activity for counselors: to seek out the real problem or hidden meaning and give an interpretation.	
Reassuring, sympathizing, consoling—The intent here is to make the person feel better. Like approval, this is a roadblock that interferes with the spontaneous flow of communication.	
Questioning, probing—Questions can be mistaken for good listening. The intent is to probe further, to find out more. A hidden communication is the implication that if enough questions are asked, the questioner will find the solution. Questions can also interfere with the spontaneous flow of communication, directing it in the interests of the questioner but not necessarily the speaker.	
Withdrawing, distracting, humoring, changing the subject—These directly divert communication. They may also imply that what the person is saying is not important or should not be pursued.	
Total Roadblocks	
Reflection	

Here are some questions you might consider as you reflect on this material:

How many roadblocks and reflections did the host use? Are these numbers different? What do you make of that difference?

Where did you have difficulty differentiating reflections from roadblocks?

When did you find yourself agreeing with the host in use of a roadblock?

At what points did you observe guests resisting the host? What was the host doing prior to that resistance?

Watching for Listening

This is the second step in tuning your ear for listening. Again, choose a TV or radio program on which a host interviews guests. This time your focus will be on observing listening.

- Begin by watching the first 3–5 minutes of the host's interaction with a guest without the sound. Notice what he or she does to communicate interest and caring.
- Now turn the sound back on and count the number of reflections used. You can employ the same form as you did for the previous exercise, or you can use the Exercise 3.2 form, which includes different types of reflections.
- Again, you might consider taping this program so that you can slow down the process. Transcripts may also be helpful if you find that the interaction moves too quickly.

Type	Description	Number
Simple	Stays very close to what the person has said; communicates interest and stabilizes the client.	
Complex	Goes well beyond what the person has said and may not use the same words; often cognitively reframes the material, infers greater meaning, and may include affect.	
Amplified	Pushes on an absolute statement by the person; may back the person away from this position.	
Double-sided	Acknowledges both sides of the ambivalence.	
Metaphor	Moves well beyond content to provide a model for understanding.	
Roadblocks		

Questions to consider:

What types of reflections does the host tend to use?

Were some reflections more effective than others? If so, what made them more effective? If not, what do you think got in the way?

When the host doesn't use reflections, what tends to happen with guests?

If you viewed two different shows for Exercises 3.1 and 3.2, how were the hosts the same or different in their use of reflections and roadblocks?

Hypothesis Testing and the Formation of Reflections

For the following statements generate at least five alternate hypotheses for each client statement below. Use the sentence stem "You mean that . . . " to begin each sentence. This phrasing is a beginning form of reflective listening. Here's an example. If you need more examples, check out the answers attached.

I am an organized person.

> You mean that . . . you like to have things orderly.
> You mean that . . . you tend to rely on routines.
> You mean that . . . you don't like when things change unexpectedly.
> You mean that . . . your desk is neat.
> You mean that . . . you think logically.

Notice that several of these statements/hypotheses go well beyond what *organized* might mean. Some may be wrong, though all acknowledge some component of what could be considered organized. This process allows us to find where the boundaries might lie and what is core. Now try this hypothesis testing with the following sentences.

I don't like conflict.

> You mean that . . .

> You mean that . . .

> You mean that . . .

> You mean that . . .

> You mean that . . .

I have a sense of humor.

> You mean that . . .

> You mean that . . .

(cont.)

You mean that . . .

You mean that . . .

You mean that . . .

I let things bother me more than I should.

You mean that . . .

You mean that . . .

You mean that . . .

You mean that . . .

You mean that . . .

I am loyal.

You mean that . . .

You mean that . . .

You mean that . . .

You mean that . . .

You mean that . . .

Sample Responses for Exercise 3.3

I don't like conflict.

> You mean that … it makes you uncomfortable when people disagree.
>
> You mean that … you work hard to resolve differences.
>
> You mean that … you avoid confrontations.
>
> You mean that … you look for ways to work together.
>
> You mean that … anger scares you.

I have a sense of humor.

> You mean that … you like to laugh.
>
> You mean that … you find humor in daily life.
>
> You mean that … humor helps you lighten the load.
>
> You mean that … laughing is something you do easily.
>
> You mean that … you don't take yourself too seriously.

I let things bother me more than I should.

> You mean that … you're somebody who takes pride in the details.
>
> You mean that … you waste energy at times.
>
> You mean that … you're sensitive.
>
> You mean that … you're too sensitive.
>
> You mean that … you wish you didn't worry about what others think.

I am loyal.

> You mean that … you stand by people.
>
> You mean that … you'll stand by people when maybe you shouldn't.
>
> You mean that … if someone makes a mistake, you're forgiving.
>
> You mean that … you value loyalty in others.
>
> You mean that … it makes you angry when others switch allegiances.

Directive Reflecting

Read the sentence stem and write down three different responses to each item. Each should emphasize a different aspect of the statement. Here is an example.

It's been fun, but something has got to give. I just can't go on like this anymore.

1. You've enjoyed yourself.
2. You're worried about what might happen.
3. It's time for a change.

I know I could do some things differently, but if she would just back off, then the situation would be a whole lot less tense; then these things wouldn't happen.

1.

2.

3.

I've been depressed lately. I keep trying things other than drinking to help myself feel better, but nothing seems to work, except having a couple of drinks.

1.

2.

3.

(cont.)

So, I'm not too worried, but it's been over a year since I've had an HIV test.

1.

2.

3.

I know I'm not perfect, but why do they have to always tell me what to do. I'm not 3!

1.

2.

3.

My daughter thinks it's her body and therefore she should be able to do what she wants with it. Hooking up is no big deal to her. She just doesn't get why I won't back off.

1.

2.

3.

Sample Responses for Exercise 3.4

I know I could do some things differently, but if she would just back off, then the situation would be a whole lot less tense; then these things wouldn't happen.

1. You wish she would give you some space.

2. You'd like things to be less tense.

3. You could do some things differently.

I've been depressed lately. I keep trying things other than drinking to help myself feel better, but nothing seems to work, except having a couple of drinks.

1. You've been feeling down.

2. Drinking works in the short-term.

3. You might like if something other than drinking worked.

So, I'm not too worried, but it's been over a year since I've had an HIV test.

1. It's been awhile.

2. You're wondering about your HIV status.

3. You've a little worried.

I know I'm not perfect, but why do they have to always tell me what to do. I'm not 3!

1. Sometimes you make mistakes.

2. It bugs you when they tell you what to do.

3. You feel like you're being treated as a child.

My daughter thinks it's her body and therefore she should be able to do what she wants with it. Hooking up is no big deal to her. She just doesn't get why I won't back off.

1. She's been arguing with you.

2. Her sexual behavior is a concern.

3. She doesn't see how much you care.

Deepening Reflections

Read the sentence stems and write down each of the response types listed. Note that sometimes certain reflections may not fit as well (e.g., amplified reflections). Try to create one anyway. Here is a reminder of each form:

Paraphrase: Moves well beyond the client's words and presents information in a new light.
Amplified: Overstates what the client has said, often increasing the intensity by pressing on the absolute or resistant element.
Double-sided: Reflects both parts of the client's ambivalence.
Affective: Addresses the emotion either expressed or implied.

Here's an example.

It's been fun, but something has got to give. I just can't go on like this anymore.

Paraphrase: So, the fun has come at a cost.
Amplified: You've had a fabulous time.
Double-sided: On the one hand, you've had a good run, and on the other, you can see that it's coming to an end.
Affective: You're a bit worried about where this is taking you.

I know I could do some things differently, but if she would just back off, then the situation would be a whole lot less tense; then these things wouldn't happen.

Paraphrase:

Amplified:

Double-sided:

Affective:

I've been depressed lately. I keep trying things other than drinking to help myself feel better, but nothing seems to work, except having a couple of drinks.

Paraphrase:

Amplified:

Double-sided:

Affective:

(cont.)

So, I'm not too worried, but it's been over a year since I've had an HIV test.

    Paraphrase:

    Amplified:

    Double-sided:

    Affective:

I know I'm not perfect, but why do they have to always tell me what to do. I'm not 3!

    Paraphrase:

    Amplified:

    Double-sided:

    Affective:

My daughter thinks it's her body and therefore she should be able to do what she wants with it. Hooking up is no big deal to her. She just doesn't get why I won't back off.

    Paraphrase:

    Amplified:

    Double-sided:

    Affective:

Sample Responses for Exercise 3.5

I know I could do some things differently, but if she would just back off, then the situation would be a whole lot less tense; then these things wouldn't happen.

Paraphrase: You would like your situation to be different.

Amplified: It feels like she's totally responsible for it; like this is really her fault.

Double-sided: So, she played a part in what happened, and you know there are parts you might want to do differently.

Affective: You're upset about this situation.

I've been depressed lately. I keep trying things other than drinking to help myself feel better, but nothing seems to work, except having a couple of drinks.

Paraphrase: You keep looking, despite the lack of success, for ways other than drinking.

Amplified: Drinking is the only possible way.

Double-sided: Drinking helps in the short-term, and part of you recognizes that this may not be a great long-term strategy.

Affective: You're frustrated by the lack of payoff on your hard work.

So, I'm not too worried, but it's been over a year since I've had an HIV test.

Paraphrase: You've had some risk behavior.

Amplified: It's no concern to you.

Double-sided: You feel you've been pretty safe, while also recognizing there has been some risk.

Affective: It's like there is always a little uncertainty—a little fear—since you've chosen to be sexually active.

I know I'm not perfect, but why do they have to always tell me what to do. I'm not 3!

Paraphrase: They are the parents you don't want to have.

Amplified: They don't let you make any choices.

Double-sided: It feels like they're being pretty bossy, and, at the same time, you know there are some things you could do better.

Affective: And as your anger grows, you may end up feeling like a petulant 3-year-old who wants to pout and say "no."

My daughter thinks it's her body and therefore she should be able to do what she wants with it. Hooking up is no big deal to her. She just doesn't get why I won't back off.

Paraphrase: She doesn't see your concern, only "meddling."

Amplified: You don't feel she's capable of making these types of choices.

Double-sided: On the one hand, you want to help your daughter, and, on the other, you can see that your methods are causing some conflict.

Affective: You're scared to death about what might happen to her.

An Intentional Conversation

Decide that you will practice your listening skills in a conversation with someone. This task is usually best accomplished if you make this decision ahead of time, though it could evolve naturally. In particular, try to choose an interaction in which you would normally be inclined to give advice and try to refrain from this desire. Afterward consider the following questions.

What was it like to listen intentionally instead of using other skills (e.g., questions)?

How did your conversation partner react?

In what ways were you able to vary your type of reflection?

What was hard about doing this type of listening?

What did you learn from this interaction about your own style?

Chapter 4

The Use of OARS
Open-Ended Questions, Affirmations, and Summaries

Opening

Barbara sat down, rubbing her hands, tension etched on her face. She was here for a vocational assessment. The agency asked the practitioner to evaluate her cognitive and academic skills and offer an opinion about whether college was a realistic option for her. A normally developing teen until age 14, she suffered a seizure in school one day. Doctors discovered tumors. Although surgery successfully removed the tumors, it also affected her thinking. Where she had been a hardworking "A" student, she subsequently required special education services to complete high school, including significant tutoring to understand concepts.

On paper, her goal appeared unrealistic to the agency. But she was now 32 and there had been changes since high school. After reviewing the purpose of the evaluation in the waiting room and discussing her questions, she'd signed consent forms.

"You look worried," the examiner began.

"I really want to go to school, and I'm worried you'll tell me I can't."

"Because somebody has given you that message before. . . . "

"Well, yes and no. It's just more like school was a struggle after my tumors, but with a little help I can do it. I also feel more mature."

"The goal is to be successful, and you feel like college is the way to do that. You also feel ready and able to do it."

There are a number of directions we could take now. So far we've done very little, but we learned some important information by doing a couple of reflections. Where would you go from here and how would you get there?

As noted in Chapter 3, MI relies heavily on microskills to move sessions forward. Microskills are basic tools that counselors often already have in their clinical repertoire. These can be remembered by the acronym OARS: open-ended questions, affirmations, reflective listening, and summaries. Whereas Chapter 3 focused exclusively on reflective listening, Chapter 4 targets the other three microskills.

A Deeper Look

Open-Ended Questions

Although short-reply, information-gathering questions are necessary during client contacts, open-ended questions are the backbone of the MI information-gathering process. They set the tone for a nonjudgmental setting in which clients can explore their problem area(s). Open-ended questions are those that ask clients to give more than "yes," "no," or "three times last week" as the answer. So, instead of asking clients "How often and much do you drink?", you might ask "What are your drinking habits like?" Sometimes this wording can be too vague or too broad. Frequently when I ask this question, clients ask what I mean, and I respond with a clarification: "When you decide to drink, tell me about the circumstances." The question creates movement, which then is directed through the use of reflective listening.

Typically, questions early in a session are broad and may sometimes, as in the example above, be too vague. We can always add greater specificity. Our hope, though, is to create sufficient space so that clients can tell us about what is important to them.

Of course, questions often have a purpose and a direction. For clients ready to work, a simple invitation to talk may be enough—for example, "What brings you here?" However, it is common for clients to be ambivalent about making changes. They often need more help in getting underway. However, this does not mean that small talk is needed to make them feel more comfortable. Small talk may delay the business of the session and may postpone what tends to make clients feel most comfortable: the perception that you understand their situation and do not judge them. So, it's often helpful to have some questions at hand that are broad, but not generic, and get the session underway. For an adolescent who has come in via a parent's referral, you might say, "Your dad has some concerns about how things are going for you. What's your sense of why he thinks this is important?" Of course, if a focal problem has been identified, you can always ask directly about that: "So, you've been feeling a bit depressed. What's been happening?" Though, with resistant clients, it can be useful to back away from a specific discussion of the problem area and begin by focusing more broadly on their life before focusing on the area of interest.

There is another category of practitioner behavior that is MI consistent but does not fall easily into the OARS categories. Open-ended statements are a hybrid of a reflection and a question: for example, "I wonder what it would be like if you decided to stop." These are not exactly questions, but act as though they are. The impetus is clearly on the client to respond with more information. In MI research, these statements are considered questions, and generally MI trainers refer to them as such.

> "So, you're here not because you see a particular need but because your probation officer (or husband/wife/partner/teacher/doctor/supervisor, etc.) wanted you to come. I'd like to come back to that in a bit, but first I'd like to find out a little more about you. Tell me a little bit about who you are and what your life is like."

Often with these opening questions a bit of preamble (i.e., a lead-in) can be helpful in establishing the context and building initial rapport. The preamble tells the client what you know and your attitude toward this encounter. In particular, it communicates the nonjudgmental stance noted in Chapter 2 as a component of expressing empathy.

Avoid rhetorical questions for which there is a single, desirable answer. Usually such a question is simply a mask for expressing concern. Consider the question "Wouldn't it be easier if you just agreed to … ?" It is better to express the concern directly and label it as information for the client's consideration. Chapter 9 talks more about how to do this effectively.

There is a ratio that is used to denote good MI practice. MI researchers generally use a two-to-one ratio of reflective listening statements to questions as a standard for expert MI practice (Moyers, Miller, & Hendrickson, 2005). In most instances individuals fall at a level well below this standard when they begin learning MI, usually asking two questions for every reflection. Our research has shown that following a 2-day workshop, we can increase this ratio to a little above one reflection for every question, but this obviously leaves lots of room for practice (Baer et al., 2004, 2009).

You may be wondering why the reflection-to-question ratio is significant. The answer has multiple parts. In MI, as noted earlier, practitioners are attempting to create and then direct momentum. Questions tend to stop momentum in the short-term, which is why Gordon (1970) places them in the roadblock category. Although questioning can be very useful sometimes, it is a method we fall into easily. Practitioners are often very good at asking questions, particularly closed questions that seek small, discrete bits of information (e.g., "How long have you been married?"). Unfortunately, the continued use of questions sets up practitioners for two of the traps the Miller and Rollnick (2002) have identified: the question-and-answer trap and the expert trap.

In the question-and-answer trap the relationship is no longer collaborative but rather an investigative process at the end of which we expect the questioner to provide the correct answer. This trap often occurs in medical settings where patients go in with a set of symptoms, expect the physician or nurse practitioner to ask the correct questions, and then provide the solution. However, it does not happen solely in that instance. It also has the unfortunate side effect of making the client a passive recipient and leaves the practitioner doing all the work.

Related to this trap is the expectation that the examiner is the expert and knows more about the problem than does the client. The relationship is no longer collaborative and evocative, but rather hierarchical, and the cure rests within the practitioner. Although the practitioner indeed may hold the expertise to discern the nature of a problem, the cure often requires active participation from the client—and that's the rub. Obviously, both of these traps are at odds with MI spirit. To sidestep these traps, MI trainers often aim to get practitioners to make one reflection for every question and then when that is happening proficiently, work for two or more.

A third consideration in this area of questions is the differentiation between open-ended and closed questions. In training and in research, there is a clear distinction made between open-ended and closed questions for all the reasons just noted and from the additional perspective that closed questions tend to block momentum even more than open-ended questions. However, in practice these distinctions do not always hold. An open-ended question may bring a single- or two-word response. In adolescents, a well-crafted open-ended query may be met with a shoulder shrug or an "I don't know." Conversely, a closed question may result in a long response, as though it were an open-ended question. The upshot is at times these differentiations may be less important than they appear. So, although in research contexts we track the percentage of open-ended to closed questions as a marker of MI proficiency, it is not evident that this is as strong a predictor of client behavior as is the reflection-to-question ratio. However—and this is the clear caveat—in general, these questions act in the manner described, and this is most evident when working with clients who are actively resistant. The risk in such a situation is that we will fall into the question-and-answer trap. So, in training, the emphasis remains on asking more open-ended questions than closed questions.

Finally, in MI there is a special type of query called the "key question." Miller and Rollnick (2002) divide MI into two phases, as noted previously. The first phase builds motivation for change. The second phase is devoted to developing, implementing, and maintaining a plan for change. The key question lies at the juncture of these two phases and is central by virtue of the timing. That is, within Phase I there comes a point at which the focus of the therapy shifts from building motivation to asking for, or consolidating, commitment. Resistance is lower, the client talks in favor of change even though ambivalence may remain, and he or she may begin asking questions about how to accomplish change. This is a critical juncture when the therapist works to solidify the shift by asking for a commitment. Often a summary is given, and then the key question is asked. The theme of the key question is "What is the next step?", though the specific form can and should vary. Examples of key questions include:

"What do you think you will do now?"

"So, how will you proceed?"

"What do you plan on doing tonight?"

The client response will determine what happens next. As a practitioner, the typical and usually best action is to respond with reflections. The temptation, if the client has come all the way to the precipice of change and then backs away, is to seize the opportunity and argue on behalf of change. Staying consistent with MI, the goal is to avoid this tendency to fix a "wrong" choice. Chapter 10 devotes additional focus to this issue of key questions and Chapter 11 to negotiating change plans.

Affirmations

As noted in Chapter 2, MI attempts to build client feelings of empowerment and self-efficacy. We want to bolster or help build an attitude of "can do." DiClemente (1991, 2003) believes that most individuals who seek help from professionals are unsuccessful self-changers. They've tried to make changes independently, but their efforts have not worked to either their or others' satisfaction. Because of these "failed" attempts, demoralization is a frequent concomitant to individual's seeking help-seeking efforts. Therefore, part of the therapist's role is to instill hope and the belief that the client can indeed change. Affirmations are a way of reorienting the client to the resources he or she has available for this effort.

Affirmations are statements of appreciation for the client and his or her strengths. Although the reflective listening process can be quite affirming, especially when a client feels deeply understood and accepted, affirmations are more than reflective listening. These statements are strategically designed to anchor clients to their strengths and resources as they address their problem behavior.

Affirmations usually take the form of clear and genuine words of understanding and appreciation. For example, for a mother involved with child protective services and fearful of losing her children to the state, the practitioner might say, "You are someone who cares deeply for your children and are willing to fight to keep them." For someone who has repeatedly presented for drug treatment, you might say, "You have great determination, despite setbacks, to make your life be different."

MI trainers have noted that the use of affirmations can be tricky, as clients may react negatively if they feel judged or patronized. They suggest a number of ideas to avoid this problem:

- Focus on specific behaviors instead attitudes, decisions, and goals.
- Avoid using the word "I."
- Focus on descriptions and not evaluations.
- Attend to nonproblem areas rather than problem areas.
- Think of affirmations as attributing interesting qualities to clients.
- Nurture a competent instead of a deficit worldview of clients.

For all of these reasons, I do not teach compliments as affirmations. Compliments typically have an evaluative judgment implicit within them. Many times, though not always, compliments begin with an "I" statement: "I think you care deeply for your children." My approach, which is very *in*consistent with how counselors are typically trained to work or how they teach others to talk, is to use "you" statements: "You are ... ," "You feel ... ," or "You believe. ... " This change in pronouns relocates the affirmation from an external vantage point to rest it squarely on an internal client attribute—which clients find much more difficult to dismiss out of hand. An affirmation communicates a prizing or appreciation of clients for who they are. Though my next assertion awaits empirical data to support it, I believe that this method is a more powerful means of orienting clients to their internal strengths and resources than using compliments or "I" statements.

In practice, affirmations tend to be the least observed microskill. This is unfortunate, as typically clients have often been battered by life experiences and conditioned to expect others to point out their shortcomings, failings, and insufficient efforts. Think of how powerful it can be in your life, as a person working in a helping profession, to have someone recognize the fine work you do. As part of my 2-day training schedule, I often have clinicians give each other affirmations at the end of their first day. It's a required activity, and everyone knows it's expected, and yet there are always lots of smiles during the exercise and a lighter step when people leave the room. When asked about the exercise, invariably someone will say,

"I know this was just an exercise, but … it felt really good." Some practitioners, often those who've struggled to embrace the training, will also say, "It felt artificial," and a response to that comment might be a reflection. Here's one example, "So you know when these feel real and when they don't. And so, if you decide to do this with your clients, you'll want to be really attentive to crafting an affirmation that you know is real."

Consistent with the prior statements, affirmations can be done liberally but beware of overly effusive or forced attempts. Clients recognize a lack of genuineness, and the relationship suffers as a result. Don't affirm folks for breathing—it angers them. But you can often reframe difficulties as a personal strength: "It was very hard to keep going. You must have tremendous internal strength to keep moving forward."

Affirmations do not have a particular structure; however, they should be positively stated. That is, focus on a strength or attribute, not on the lack of something. For example, "You managed to avoid cocaine use" is the start of an affirmation, but it's focused on the avoidance of something. Find the positive element, "Despite serious temptation, you were able to make decisions for yourself—like not using cocaine." Questions, such as those used in solution-focused therapy (e.g., "Given all that, how did you manage to stay sober as long as you did?"), can elicit affirming information. However, this does not replace the active process of holding up the mirror, via reflections or summaries, which show what clients have said about themselves.

There are several methods of generating material for affirmations. For one, the use of other microskills can elicit this information. However, there are specific areas that can be mined for these qualities. For example, probing prior "unsuccessful" change experiences can be useful. There are the usual reasons for probing (e.g., understanding what has been done; evaluating what worked; understanding client's concerns, fears), but in addition, the probings provide opportunities for reorientation to what the client did accomplish. Clients exhibit strengths in these attempts. Note them. Even multiple negative outcomes can be reframed—they suggest persistence and a strong desire for change.

Negativistic or resistant behavior can also be reframed into an affirmation. Clearly, it's not uncommon for clients to be negative about treatment, especially if someone else suggested it. Practitioners can reframe this experience and affirm the client by saying, for example, "You must have a lot of resolve to come today, despite your strong reservations about treatment." Or, "Given your experiences, it makes sense that you might be concerned about coming here today. It must have taken a lot of determination to do it anyway." In both cases, you'll note that an evaluative element has a tendency to slip in. You may not be able to avoid it entirely. Try to be mindful and avoid using this type of element as your primary form of affirmation.

The affirmation is not an endpoint but rather a point on a path where valuable information is mined. Asking for elaboration is helpful in getting clients to move beyond the initial affirmation. For example, this might be a follow-up question to the affirmation in the prior paragraph: "How did you keep that commitment to yourself?" In general, "how" and "what" questions are good ways to do this. "How did you … ?" "What did you do … ?"

Finally, trainees sometimes feel that they're affirming clients just by listening. While this indeed may be the case, I encourage you to be more direct in making affirmations. An analogy might be the love we display for our significant others. Although our actions may communicate this feeling, saying the words "I love you" remains important. Obviously, this is a situation in which an evaluative element and an "I" statement make sense. One could imagine how much more power is added to "I love you" if the speaker also says something like the following: "You make my and others' worlds brighter places when you are present. You see the best in others and by noticing it, help them to embrace it as well. Your humor draws others in rather than comments on their foibles."

Summaries

As my thinking about helping, in general, and psychotherapy and MI, in particular, has developed over the years, I have come to the belief that part of what happens in this helping process is that we assist clients in organizing their experiences. This is not a new notion, and one that is quite consistent with ideas expressed in narrative therapies, but it then requires that we do more than simply hand back to clients what they've told us. That is, reflections should do more than simply repeat what clients have said; they should also enhance their understanding by expressing the element that is less clearly articulated or unexpressed but implicit within the message. This idea of organization comes into clearest focus in the area of summaries.

Miller and Rollnick (2002) describe summaries as a special application of reflective listening. They have described three different types of summaries—collecting, linking, and transitions—that overlap, but often serve different purposes. Each is discussed below, but it's important to note that in each instance the summarizer makes decisions about what to include and exclude and how this information is presented. In my experience as a researcher, trainer, supervisor, and clinician, the best summaries are succinct. Summaries that go on for paragraphs don't help clients organize their experience; rather, these monologues lose clients and therefore lose their power.

Related to the idea of brevity is selectivity. Practitioners should aim to include those elements that will aid the client in moving forward, while keeping in mind the principles of MI. Two important ideas were already noted in Chapter 2: the role of ambivalence in change and the importance of change talk. Specifically, to only focus on the benefits of change with an ambivalent client is to invite counterarguments. Thus, summaries should not focus solely on the pros for change. At the same time, a primary goal of MI is to elicit and reinforce change talk. Thus, practitioners should attend to change talk as clients produce it and then give particular weight to these statements in the summary. A summary for the interchange with Barbara at the beginning of the session might illustrate these ideas:

> "You're here today because the agency asked you to come and not because you're particularly interested in doing this assessment. You worry that this evaluation could interfere with your hopes of going to school, and, at the same time, you recognize that school is a challenge. Finally, you have strengths and you've grown; so part of our task will be to determine how to help you use these to be successful."

This summary, although brief—three sentences—contains multiple ideas and presents them in a manner that is easy to comprehend. These sentences also provide a structure with which to frame Barbara's experience: You don't want to be here, you have some worries, and we share a common goal—for you to be successful. It does not disregard her ambivalence, but it does not dwell there. It has the start of an affirmation and ends with an emphasis on a reshaped goal (i.e., success, which may or may not include college). It is easy to imagine either letting the client respond to the summary or asking a follow-up query regarding how she has grown. It is exactly this approach to summaries that Bill Miller demonstrates on the MI tape for the *Brief Therapy for Addictions* series. His summaries are brief and targeted, so much so that it is easy to get caught in the very interesting client and miss how artfully Bill guides the process forward.

The type of summary described above is what Miller and Rollnick (2002) would call a collecting summary. Its primary purpose is to gather information together, present it back to the client, and to keep the conversation moving forward. Because they are especially useful in reinforcing change talk, summaries are offered periodically during the course of an MI session. Miller and Rollnick (2002) warn against overdoing summaries, though, as this can make the encounter feel artificial. That is, you are performing a technique rather than simply trying to understand the client. I would add that it must feel consistent with your personality and style. As a clinician, I periodically summarize just to ensure that I am retaining and understanding information. Without that bit of behavioral rehearsal, important ideas are lost to me. However, I tend to use very brief summaries—two or three sentences—to accomplish this task.

The border between linking and collecting summaries is fuzzy, but in general linking summaries serve a different purpose. Linking summaries seek to contrast ideas heard in the present moment with information that has been shared previously, with the aim of highlighting either disconnection or relationship between the ideas. This technique is especially useful for developing discrepancy as well as for exploring the client's ambivalence. These ideas are not evaluated by the summarizer but, instead, held in equal position and left to the client to assign meaning. To accomplish this aim, I encourage the use of the conjunction *and* rather than *but*, a position that Rollnick and Miller also hold. The use of *but* negates everything that precedes it—"That is a really good idea, but . . . " or "I like that dress on you, but . . . "—whereas the use of *and* allows both concepts to be held simultaneously, which is the position that the client is experiencing internally: "So, you'd like everyone to just leave you alone, and you're not sure that you want to do the things that might accomplish that." Finally, linking summaries allow the practitioner to integrate outside or collateral information, as well as things the client has said at previous times. For example: "So, you are of the mind now that this relationship thing is not such a big deal. Things have quieted down and there is less conflict. At the same time, you've told me that this is the cycle things tend to go through. Your wife has previously said that if you don't do something differently, she will leave, and you said that you didn't like the way things were going either."

Transitional summaries serve yet another purpose. Practitioners use this type of summary to choose or change the direction in the session. Sometimes this summary is overtly signaled by use of a lead in such as "Let me see if I have understood what you've told me so far" or "Here's what I've heard you tell me about your situation." These tend to be slightly longer summaries and are used as a prelude to an open-ended question that leads in a new direction or can be used to close a session. Transitional summaries typically fall at the juncture between Phase I and Phase II and lead into the key question. Although there is a tendency to cover a lot of terrain with a transitional summary, bear in mind the dual goals just discussed: brevity and organization of client experience. If the client's eyes glaze over or you start losing your way, the summary is too long. Wrap it up, even if you do so abruptly. Too often I observe others, as well as myself, trying to fix an overlong summary and making it more convoluted in the process. It is better to stop, check understanding, and then add to it. An example of a transitional summary might look like this:

> "We are about to finish here, and I just want to make sure I've understood things correctly. You came here today because that's a requirement of parole. You're not sure that you can trust me as a parole officer and this is partly based on some bad experiences from the past. At the same time, you are very clear that you don't want to go back to prison, and so you've been trying to do things differently. You are not hanging out with the same crowd. You are living in a different place. You are trying and making some different decisions, even though it's not easy. One of those decisions is figuring out how to use this time with me, and you haven't made up your mind on that quite yet. What have I missed?"

With a longer summary there is often an invitation to correct or add to what has been said.

In practice, people don't often stop to consider what type of summary they will do next. However, it is helpful to know there are different types and consider the intent of the summary before it unfolds. Do I want to keep the progress moving forward? If so, then a collecting summary makes sense. Do I want to develop discrepancy? Then linking is the ticket. Switch directions or draw to a close? Transitional is the choice.

Concept Quiz—Test Yourself!

True or false:

1. T F OARS are basic skills practitioners often have in their clinical toolbox already.
2. T F OARS are MI.
3. T F Questions tend to stop momentum.
4. T F Closed questions are bad.
5. T F Affirmations are statements that recognize and appreciate client strengths.
6. T F Research supports the use of "you" statements when making affirmations.
7. T F Affirmations are the most frequently occurring element of OARS.
8. T F When doing summaries, it's important to pay attention to ambivalence by placing *but* in the middle of a double-sided statement.
9. T F We use a linking summary to transition from Phase I to Phase II of MI.
10. T F We use OARS to help clients not only see what they've told us, but to also help organize and understand their experience.

Answers

1. T OARS, as noted in Chapters 3 and 4, are not unique to MI and are often already in practitioners' skill repertoire. The unique aspect of OARS in MI is the deployment of those skills in a directive manner.

2. F OARS are not MI, and although knowing these skills is essential to doing MI, other elements are also required. For example, OARS can be done in a manner that is not MI consistent.

3. F This is a tough question, and it could be argued that it is not a clear false. Although open-ended questions help to direct the conversation and lead to new avenues for discussion, in practice questions tend to stop momentum. That is why Thomas Gordon (1970), in his discussion of roadblocks to good communication, includes questions as a roadblock. Typically, practitioners create momentum through the use of an open-ended question and then direct it through the deployment of reflections.

4. F Closed questions are not "bad." They simply are limited as a tool, so we try to avoid using them in favor of open-ended questions. However, there are situations in which closed questions are desirable. In general, the aim is to ask more open-ended than closed questions

5. T The purpose of affirmations is to draw attention to the internal resources that clients bring to the situation. Again, I recommend avoiding compliments (i.e., external evaluations) in favor of recognizing and appreciating internal attributes, qualities, and values. It seems that we are much better served by the statement "You are someone who values honesty" than by "I think you're an honest person."

6. F At this point, there is no empirical support for this position. It is a position based on my experience and observation and should be recognized as a guideline that may sidestep negative client reactions to affirmations. This guideline may need to change as more research is done.

7. F Of the OARS skills, affirmations tend to occur least frequently. It seems that practitioners focus on other areas, and this area is either forgotten or overlooked. Conversely, practitioners can view the whole MI process as affirming and feel it's unnecessary to do so explicitly. Although this may be the case, it seems important to overtly acknowledge and appreciate client strengths because of the demoralization issues noted. Affirmations may also provide some protective benefits when clients encounter value-discrepant information in their own behavior.

8. F Although we've all grown accustomed to using the conjunction *but*, it does have the unfortunate side effect of discounting what precedes it. In contrast, *and* allows both elements to be held in equal standing. Consider how these two statements sound to you:

    "It's a nice haircut, but it's pretty short."
    "It's a nice haircut, and it's pretty short."

    Notice any difference?

9. F OK! This item was just a simple memory test. Linking summaries connect present information with data either heard at prior times or provided by other sources. Transitional summaries are done at the end of Phase I as a lead into a key question and potentially moving into Phase II.

10. T If we simply hold up the mirror, then we aren't helping clients become unstuck. In addition to helping clients hear again what they've told us, we also selectively attend to certain elements and not to others and then present that information back in a manner that helps them attain greater understanding of their situation.

In Practice

Let's return to Barbara and pick up where the dialogue left off.

Statement	*Commentary*
P: The goal is to be successful, and you feel like college is the way to do that. You also feel ready and able to do it.	Complex reflections.
C: That's right. I think I am more mature, and my brain has healed.	Provides additional information.
P: Well, that's probably a really good place to start. You mentioned changing and growing a couple of times. Tell me about those things.	Simple reflection followed by an open-ended question.
C: I've learned more about how my brain does and doesn't work. I know that it takes me longer to understand things. I have to take them slower than other people. I need to ask people to explain things and to use things to help my memory.	Provides a good deal of information and insight.
P: You've really come to know and accept some things about how your brain works.	Affirmation.
C: Yeah. It wasn't always that way. I used to pretend I was the same or fight against it when people told me I had to do things different. I fought with my parents. I guess I didn't want to be different.	Client adds additional depth.
P: Like to admit a change would mean that you'd have to give up on some things you really wanted for your life.	Complex reflection.
C: Yeah. I guess that's true. It's part of what worries me about today.	She ties it back to her concerns.
P: It seems like you're pretty aware of yourself. You're not going to fool yourself about how you're doing. And at the same time there are some things that you want to accomplish, and you're worried about getting there both because of today and some of the struggles you had in school before.	Affirmation as part of a linking summary.
C: I guess that's true. I am worried about today, but I also wonder if I can do it. I think I can, but I'm not sure.	Acknowledges some doubt.

Statement	*Commentary*
P: Part of what you are both worried about and hoping for are some answers that might guide you.	Complex reflection that adds a joining element to the assessment process.
C: That's true.	Confirms accuracy.
P: And the ultimate aim here will to be successful. Tell me a little bit about what your life would look like—college or no college—if you were to be successful with this process.	Continuing the paragraph, followed by a question that moves in a new direction and which frames the discussion.
C: I would have a job that I liked, and I would get paid enough so I could live on it.	Provides a bit of information.
P: Something you liked …	Simple reflection.
C: I mean, it's a job, so I am sure there would be parts that I don't like. When I get up in the morning, though, I wouldn't dread going in and I could feel like it was using some of my brain.	Provides addition information.
P: It wouldn't have to be perfect, but it would value you and the things you bring to it.	Paraphrase.
C: I don't expect perfection.	She broadens the path.
P: And it would have to be enough so that you can make ends meet. What else would tell you that this process was successful?	Reflection acknowledges other information, then asks for additional information.
C: I want to feel productive, like I am contributing something. I also want to be happy.	Offers more information.
P: Right now you don't feel those things.	Continuing the paragraph.
C: Sometimes I do. I mean, I am happy about being a mom. I get along well with my husband—most of the time. Money is an issue sometimes, but mostly I am pretty content. It would just help if we had a little bit more money coming in.	Provides important information about her life more broadly.
P: In some ways, you are not far away from what you want, though you would still like to have a bit more.	Paraphrase.
C: I guess that's true.	Client agreement. Her frame on her situation and goals seems to be both shifting and coming into greater focus.

Statement	*Commentary*
P: What else?	Open-ended question.
C: I'd like to feel like my job was contributing something to the community.	She adds a bit more.
P: It's important to you to make your part of the world a little better place.	Affirmation.
C: A lot of people have helped me over the years, and I would like to give something back.	Provides additional information.
P: Let me see if I have all of this. In many ways, you already have the things you want in your life. You're a mom. You have a loving relationship with your husband. There are some things you'd like to have: a little more money and a job where you felt valued and didn't mind going in the morning. You'd also like to give back to your community, which sounds like a bigger value than even a job—though it would be great if it did. So, what I am wondering is, how does college fit into your definitions for success?	Transitional summary that leads back to a question about college.
C: I guess I always thought that college is what you did if you wanted those things.	Offers some insight into her thinking.
P: Like maybe you had to do it, though now you're wondering.	Complex reflection.
C: I guess I am thinking that maybe I've been a little too locked on to college. Maybe I don't have to, though I am guessing some things would be easier.	She's exploring while offering new information.
P: It may not be the only way.	Paraphrase.
C: It's funny, because I feel less tense now.	She notices her internal reaction.
P: Like maybe a couple of doors have opened. There are more directions to go and a little more room to breathe.	Complex reflection.
C: Yeah. I am not so worried about this testing anymore.	Client offers a changed view.
P: There will be options no matter what.	Continuing the paragraph.

All the microskills are evident in this encounter. It is through careful listening that the openings for affirmations emerge. Questions are used to elicit information and to shift the focus. Summaries helped to organize the client's experience, keep the momentum going, and link ideas. Again, the aim is to create momentum and then direct that process.

This is also an example of a client and practitioner having two different agendas to begin a session. For the client, this agenda was to preserve her self-interest (i.e., attend college) whereas for the practitioner it was to assist the agency in expending its funds wisely (i.e., determine if college was a good option). By spending this time, the practitioner and client were able to identify a broader, mutually agreeable agenda—helping her be successful—which met both parties' goals. The practitioner used OARS to achieve this collaborative relationship. Chapter 7 addresses this topic of agenda setting in greater depth.

Try This!

Exercise 4.1. Converting Closed Questions

We often ask stock questions of our clients. This exercise asks you to convert common closed questions that may or may not be a part of your setting. After completing these questions, think about additional ones used in your work. Write those down and then convert them as well.

Exercise 4.2. Forming Good Questions

It is also useful to practice forming good questions that respond to client material. In this activity you will read a client statement and then form two different questions that might be helpful in response.

Exercise 4.3. Finding Affirmations

In this activity you will read about a client situation, consider the situation, write down the strengths you observe, then form affirmations based on these strengths. Try to use "you" language.

Exercise 4.4. Strengths within my Clients

In this activity you will think about your clients within your work context. You will be asked to consider the challenges your clients encounter in this context and the resources they bring to the session. This exercise can be challenging, since we often focus on deficits rather than strengths. Some examples are provided to help guide you in this work.

Exercise 4.5. Building Summaries

Read the transcript and label the different techniques the practitioner uses. Then place yourself in the practitioner's chair. Write the summary you might find helpful.

Exercise 4.6. Real-Time, Drive-Time Summaries

In Chapter 2 we practiced making reflections in response to talk radio/TV talk shows. This exercise extends that practice to the formation of summaries. If you don't drive then you can do the same technique with a talk show or an advice column.

Partner Work

All of the exercises described under "Try This!" could be done in pairs, including Exercise 4.6. A modified form of this last exercise would be to pick up a local newspaper and find a columnist's article. One party reads the first two or three paragraphs aloud and then stops. The listener should then try to generate one open-ended question, one affirmation, and one summary. The reader should then try to generate a different one of each type. Then switch roles.

Here are some other formats in which you can practice these skills. These are based on questions used in an exercise called Virginia Reel. Choose a listener and a talker (you can alternate turns in these roles). Ask the question and then focus on using each of the four OARS at least once during your conversation about this question. Continue until you've exhausted the area and then switch roles and repeat.

"What's the story behind your name?"

"Describe your first time riding a bike (without training wheels)."

"What was your first date like?"

"What do you like to do on vacation or holiday?"

"If you could do something else for a profession, what would it be?"

"What do you hope to do when you retire?"

"What's the next step in your life that would most support your health and well-being?"

Another approach to practice would be to obtain your free copy of the VASE-R, (see Appendix B, OARS, for ordering information). The VASE-R is an instrument that portrays three different substance-using clients and prompts the viewer to write responses. Watch the DVD together. After each client statement, stop the DVD and write a reflective listening response, an affirmation, and an open-ended question. Then talk about your responses before going on to the next client statement. When you get to the summary items, each of you choose a different kind of summary and try to write that. Then try to write the third type together.

Finally, in working with your clients, you might choose to focus on a single technique in a session. This suggestion does not mean doing only that technique, but rather to consciously look for opportunities to practice that particular technique. For example, you might decide that you want to try to affirm a client at least three times during a session. Pay attention to how the client reacts to your practice and then discuss this with your partner.

Other Thoughts . . .

Leffingwell , Neumann, Babitske, Leedy, and Walters (2006) speculate that social psychology principles can be used to help strengthen the effect of MI. They note the importance of two ideas: defensive bias and self-affirmation theory.

Defensive bias refers to "the tendency of people to minimize the impact of personally threatening information" (Leffingwell et al., 2006, p. 2). Leffingwell and colleagues note that clients engaged in risky behavior tend to downplay the risk, challenge the accuracy of the risk assessment, and generate alternative explanations. This tendency has been found in relation to a number of problem behaviors.

Leffingwell and colleagues (2006) note that self-affirmation theory may be one method to understand this tendency. Specifically, clients have a vested interest in maintaining a positive view of self-worth, which occurs through viewing themselves as competent, responsible, and adaptive (Steele, 1988). When clients engage in behavior at odds with this tendency, they experience a form of cognitive dissonance and thus must react to reduce that psychological discomfort. Specifically, they discount the message. Since MI is often working to bring clients face to face with difficult realities, this defensive bias represents a challenge.

Leffingwell and colleagues (2006) also note that engaging clients in self-affirming activities, prior to encountering these challenges to self-worth, may reduce this defensive bias—even when these prior activities are not directly aimed at the material that follows. For example, having clients explore important personal values seems to provide this protective effect. These conclusions also suggest that having clients engage in an exploration of the positives of a problem area, before asking about the less positive aspects, may help to reduce this defensive tendency by making the behavior less ego threatening. This shift might be expressed in more direct language: "I can see that I get these things out of the behavior, so it's not so odd that I would do it; still, it would be better if I didn't."

Converting Closed Questions

We often ask stock questions of our clients. This exercise asks you to convert common closed questions that may or may not be a part of your setting. After completing these questions, think about additional ones used in your work. Write those down and then convert them as well. Try to identify two alternative questions for each question.

Are you doing OK today?

1.

2.

Are you married?

1.

2.

How much do you drink on a typical drinking occasion?

1.

2.

Did you have a good day in school today?

1.

2.

Sample Responses for Exercise 4.1

Are you doing OK today?

1. What has been good in your day so far?

2. Where would you like to start today?

Are you married?

1. Tell me about the important relationships you have in your life.

2. What's your home situation look like?

How much do you drink on a typical drinking occasion?

1. What's a typical drinking occasion look like for you?

2. Tell me about what a night out looks like.

Did you have a good day in school today?

1. What did you talk about at lunch today?

2. How do kids handle it when they don't understand something?

Forming Good Questions

In addition to having stock questions available, it is also useful to have practice in forming good questions that respond to client material. In this activity you will read a client statement and then write two open-ended questions matched to the content.

1. *So, instead of spanking, I went for walks twice this week and thought about what I wanted to do.*

   Question A:

   Question B:

2. *I don't get what we are supposed to be doing here.*

   Question A:

   Question B:

3. *I love my kids, but sometimes they push me to the edge, and then I do things I shouldn't.*

   Question A:

   Question B:

(cont.)

4. *I am really tired of dealing with all of this crap. I just can't do it anymore. Something has to change.*

    Question A:

    Question B:

5. *My problem is my wife and her constant complaints.*

    Question A:

    Question B:

    BONUS

6. *Here we go again. Same old stuff, just a new version.*

    Question A:

    Question B:

Sample Responses for Exercise 4.2

1. So, instead of spanking, I went for walks twice this week and thought about what I wanted to do.

Sample Question A: How did you keep yourself from spanking?

Sample Question B: What was that like—going for a walk instead of spanking?

2. I don't get what we are supposed to be doing here.

Sample Question A: What's your understanding of why you are here?

Sample Question B: What would need to happen for this meeting to be useful for you?

3. I love my kids, but sometimes they push me to the edge, and then I do things I shouldn't.

Sample Question A: What are the feelings like after one of these episodes when you've felt pushed and then reacted in a way you didn't like?

Sample Question B: Tell me about a time recently when you did something and then afterward felt like you shouldn't have done it.

4. I am really tired of dealing with all of this crap. I just can't do it anymore. Something has to change.

Sample Question A: So, what do you think needs to happen next, if this is to change?

Sample Question B: What have you thought about doing?

5. My problem is my wife and her constant complaints.

Sample Question A: What would need to happen for your wife to quit complaining?

Sample Question B: So your wife is unhappy with some things—how about you?

6. Here we go again. Same old crap, just a new version.

Sample Question A: If you decided to avoid this pattern playing all the way out, what would you need to do differently?

Sample Question B: What don't you like about this stuff?

Finding Affirmations

In this activity you will read about a client situation, consider the situation, write down the strengths you observe, then form affirmations based on these strengths. Try to use "you" language.

A person with diabetes recently switched to using an insulin pump and has been having alternating high and low blood sugar levels. She is checking her blood glucose levels at least eight times daily and is using the pump to deliver extra insulin as she needs it, but this may also be causing the highs and lows as she tries to correct for problems. She is being awakened by low blood sugar in the middle of the night. Her diabetes educator tried to talk with her about this pattern, and she responded by noting that it was their idea that she go on the pump.

   1. Strengths:

   2. Affirmation:

This young man stands before the juvenile justice judge for the third time in less than a year. He was arrested for possession of marijuana. He was hanging out with a group of other homeless young people on the avenue when some college students started hassling them. He jumped in and a brawl ensued. As the police arrived and broke up the fight, his bag of weed fell out of his pocket. He takes an insolent attitude in the courtroom each time he is there.

   1. Strengths:

   2. Affirmation:

A harried executive complains that she is struggling to manage the many tasks in her life. She is always tired and finds it a struggle to get out of bed when the alarm goes off at 5 A.M. She finds herself drinking more than she did a few years ago just to unwind at the end of the night, after the kids are in bed and the last e-mails of the day have been sent. Her husband is worried about her stress, but his attempts to talk about its impact are met with snarling responses about her needing to wear the pants in the family.

   1. Strengths:

   2. Affirmation:

(cont.)

Elmer is 95. He lives alone but now resides in a facility with assisted care available. He attends exercise groups intermittently and enjoys interacting with neighbors. He comes to family gatherings but has trouble hearing in group situations and so often feels isolated. Increasingly forgetful, he requires that things be explained repeatedly. To his son, the recipient of these repeated requests and his father's frequent complaints, these communications feel manipulative.

    1. Strengths:

    2. Affirmation:

Trudy smokes. She knows it isn't good for her and is fed up with people reminding her of it. Over time, she has come to realize that her social habit has moved to a full-fledged addiction. At some point, she will stop, but just not yet. Indeed, with all the other things happening in her life, this is the one area she feels is her own. She feels guilty about and tries to hide it from her son and avoids the topic with her husband. She knows he's right when he brings it up, but it still raises her ire.

    1. Strengths:

    2. Affirmation:

Amos is a "man's man." As he puts it, "I work for a living." He hangs steel on high-rise buildings. He works in an environment where one false step could lead to a very long fall. He doesn't take crap from anyone, including his superiors, and this has cost him at times. His wife complains about his being distant, and he's not even sure he knows what that means. Although he does love her and tells her so, he also is annoyed by her constant nattering and demands that he talk more. He buys flowers for her, watches her programs on TV occasionally, and does his "honey do" list faithfully. He finds himself becoming increasingly ornery when she demands that he go to counseling to learn to communicate better. Last night he swore at her when she again brought up counseling, and now he feels guilty, but he doesn't want to "give in" either.

    1. Strengths:

    2. Affirmation:

Sample Responses for Exercise 4.3

A diabetic is having trouble controlling her A1c (blood glucose).

1. Strengths:
   - Engaged in trying to control her diabetes (checking her glucose 8 times a day, delivering extra insulin to control her glucose).
   - Persistent in checking her bloods.

2. Affirmation:
   - You are quite determined to get this stuff under control, despite some setbacks.

This young man stands before the juvenile justice judge for the third time in less than a year.

1. Strengths:
   - Defends his friends.
   - Willing to stand up for himself, even if it costs him.

2. Affirmation:
   - You are a loyal friend, willing to defend others, even when it causes you trouble.

A harried executive complains that she is struggling to manage the many tasks in her life.

1. Strengths:
   - Willing to work very hard for her family.
   - Continues to rise to the challenge, even though it's getting harder to do.
   - Able to delay her needs until others needs are met (kid's, senders of e-mail).

2. Affirmation:
   - You are someone who is able to work extremely hard, even to the point of delaying your own needs, when you feel that is what is required of you.

Elmer is 95.

1. Strengths:
   - He is independent and sociable.
   - Continues to seek out ways to be active and healthy.
   - He wants to engage with his family and thus asks questions.

2. Affirmation:
   - You are someone who really wants to be engaged with people and especially your family.

Trudy smokes.

1. Strengths:
   - Independently minded.
   - Aware of changes in her behavior and it bothers her.
   - Wants to be more healthy.

(*cont.*)

Sample Responses for Exercise 4.3 (*cont.*)

2. Affirmation:
   - You are somebody who makes up her own mind. You will not simply cave to the desires of others, and in fact you may be quite determined once you've made up your mind.

Amos is a "man's man."

1. Strengths:
   - He loves his wife and tries to express that to her, in his way.
   - He's willing to stand in the face of criticism and disagreement.
   - He recognizes when he's gone too far.

2. Affirmation:
   - You are someone who cares deeply for your wife, and you're willing to show it in ways that make sense to you.

Strengths within My Clients

Think about your clients and your work context. What challenges do your clients encounter in this context? What resources do they bring to the session? For example, in a welfare setting, there is often the perception that clients scheme to gain greater benefits and are not forthcoming in describing their situations. Client strengths within this context might include:

- The ability to observe how systems function.
- The ability to perceive opportunities.
- Awareness of strengths and how to use these to meet needs.
- Creativity in making the system provide what they want and need.
- The ability to make active decisions on their own behalf.
- Determination, fortitude, and *chutzpah*.

Now think about your clients. Don't just stop at the obvious negative evaluations (e.g., "My clients are good at lying"), but find the strength that might underlie this behavior. Once you've made an exhaustive list, consider what resources these strengths bring to your clients and how you might communicate this awareness in a manner that builds momentum for positive change. Here are the steps:

- Make a list of client strengths, then answer each question for that strength.
- How does the client express this strength?
- How does this strength help the client?
- Write an affirmation using a "you" statement.

Worksheet of Client Strengths for Exercise 4.4

Example: *A recent heart attack victim continues to eat high-fat foods.*
Strength: *Determination to make his own decisions.*

> Expression? *Resists changing behavior when his physician tells him that he must change his eating habits or face another heart attack.*
>
> Helps how? *Allows him to maintain some control in a situation that may feel out of control. Provides a sense of integrity. Consistent with values.*
>
> Affirmation? *You're not somebody who does something just because somebody says you must. You have to decide if it is right for you, and sometimes this means standing against some pretty formidable pressure.*

(Copy as needed for different situations.)

Your client's situation:

Strength(s):

    Expression of these strengths?

    Helps how?

    Affirmations?

Strength(s):

    Expression of these strengths?

    Helps how?

    Affirmations?

Building Summaries

Read the transcript and label the different techniques the practitioner uses. Then place yourself in the practitioner's chair. Write the summary you might find helpful. Try to choose one type (collecting, linking, transitional) ahead of time. Remember to be selective. Once you've done one summary, then write another, using a different type.

Practitioner/client statements	*Type of response*
P: Tell me why you are coming to this vocational rehabilitation agency now?	
C: What do you mean?	
P: What is it about right now that made this feel like it was the right time?	
C: I need to get back to work to support my family. My pain is better, so I need to do something.	
P: Feeling better allows you to think about working again.	
C: Yeah. I mean, 2 months ago I would still have worried about the finances, but I was just too uncomfortable to do anything.	
P: You're more comfortable now, and that opens the door to some of these other things you've worried about.	
C: I don't want my wife to work so many hours. She's really had to do extra, and she's got her own health problems. And I just want to take care of my family instead of laying around at home.	
P: You are not someone who likes being idle. You are a provider. It really bothers you that you've been unable to provide, and it hurts even more watching the costs to your wife.	
C: Exactly. I've worked my whole life and then I hurt my back—and all of sudden I can't do anything. I need to be doing something—I just haven't been able to, and that has left me pretty down.	
P: (Write a summary.)	

Key for Exercise 4.5

Practitioner/client statements	*Type of response*
P: Tell me about why you are coming to a vocational rehabilitation agency now?	Open-ended question.
C: What do you mean?	
P: What is it about right now that made this feel like it was the right time?	Open-ended question.
C: I need to get back to work to support my family. My pain is better and so I need to do something.	
P: Feeling better allows you to think about working again.	Reflection.
C: Yeah. I mean, 2 months ago I would still have worried about the finances, but I was just too uncomfortable to do anything.	
P: You're more comfortable now, and that opens the door to some of these other things you've worried about.	Reflection.
C: I don't want my wife to work so many hours. She's really had to do extra, and she's got her own health problems. And I just want to take care of my family instead of laying around at home.	
P: You are not someone who likes being idle. You are a provider. It really bothers you that you've been unable to provide, and it hurts even more watching the costs to your wife.	Affirmation. Brief collecting summary.
C: Exactly. I've worked my whole life and then I hurt my back—and all of sudden I can't do anything. I need to be doing something—I just haven't been able to, and that has left me pretty down.	
P: So you're here now because you can be. Two months ago, you couldn't have done it. But now that you can, it's really important—maybe critical—for you to begin caring for your family and your wife again by working. It's who you are.	Linking summary, which works to solidify motivation.
(Or)	
P: Let me see if I've got this so far. You have been feeling better physically and so you decided it was time to come in. You were feeling pretty down when you weren't working, but now that you can provide for your family, you are ready to do it. What sorts of things have you been considering doing?	Transitional summary that opens a new area of inquiry

Real-Time, Drive-Time Summaries

In Chapter 2 we practiced making reflections in response to talk radio/TV talk shows. This exercise extends that practice to the formation of summaries. Listen for an interchange and then when you've gathered enough information, turn off the radio or TV and create a summary of what you heard. Remember, be succinct, include ambivalence, and reinforce change talk. If you don't drive (or don't want to do it while driving) then you can do the same technique with a talk show and a mute button or by reading a newspaper columnist.

Chapter 5

Recognizing, Reinforcing, and Eliciting Change Talk

Opening

LaDonna, arms crossed, scowl on her face, took a deep breath. She exhaled and her arms relaxed, slipping to her lap. Her eyes became watery and her answer was soft.

"No. I haven't thought about hurting myself since then, but there isn't much keeping me sober either—except my brother will kick me out if I don't." The practitioner sat silently, and she continued, "I've lost most everything else. So, I don't know why I'm doing it."

"So, you're not sure why you're doing it, except that you are."

"It's really hard—I mean, *really* hard—but I keep going to treatment, and I keep going to meetings. Nothing feels any better."

"You must have tremendous commitment. I mean, it's easy to see why you'd do it when there is a lot to lose, but at this point it's hard to see anything, and yet you keep doing it—even when parts of you might want to give up."

"I guess that's true. I hadn't really thought about it that way."

"You hadn't noticed that strength and commitment in yourself."

"No—not really, but … "

"But … "

"Well, I did stay clean and sober for 3 years once."

"So you know how to do it."

"Yeah, I guess I do, but that feeling's a long way away now … if you know what I mean."

"You'd like to get back there, but you're not sure if you can right now."

"Well, I think I can, but I just want to feel better, and I don't."

"Not yet anyway."

"Soon, I hope."

"Yeah, soon. Let me see if I've got this right. It's hard to find external reasons for getting and staying clean, yet some internal reasons seem to be pushing you because you keep doing it—even when it feels really hard. You'd like to feel better and you know you can, you're just not sure how to get there now. The hill you're on feels slippery, but you're determined to climb it."

LaDonna nodded. Forty-five and in her fifth substance abuse treatment program, she wants to return to work, but there are multiple impediments beyond her substance dependence: joint deterioration, chronic pain, learning challenges, and depression/anxiety. She is socially isolated and scared to death about a return to either work or substance use. The interview was for evaluation and documentation of disabilities, yet this exchange shows how issues of motivation can unfold at any moment and how a brief interchange can affect clients powerfully.

When LaDonna made these statements, it was in the context of an inquiry about her current depressive symptomatology and a suicide attempt approximately 6 months prior. As her initial statements indicate, she had very little hope about staying clean, nor a sense of what would maintain that hope. As noted in prior chapters, an attempt to argue for why she should continue to fight would likely elicit, "Yes, but ... " responses. However, implicit in the context was her fingernail-into-rock-face determination to hold on and to have a better life. The practitioner responses are an attempt to draw out what was driving that willingness to hang on. Both parties—client and practitioner—shared a common goal: helping her to stay sober.

Initially, the practitioner's guesses determined the character of the exchange. However, she confirmed and extended these—ever so slightly—as the dialogue continued. She began to make statements in favor of change. At the end, the possibility of change and her capacity for it seemed more in evidence. But, the question remains, is she committed? And, if so, to what? And if not, how do you help her get there?

A Deeper Look

In their original work, Miller and Rollnick (1991) called client arguments in favor of change "self-motivational statements." Although a technically accurate description, this jargon did not fit well for practitioners as they sorted through how clients talked. Over time the phrasing shifted to "change talk"—by which we mean client statements that indicate the person is oriented toward making a positive change in a problem behavior. These are comments we want to listen for, attempt to elicit, and then highlight for the client as they appear to predict changes in behavior.

Over time the concept of change talk has evolved. Presently we think there are four elements in a statement that tell us whether it is truly change talk.

First, change talk represents statements about change. That is, these client statements indicate that they have the desire or ability to change, see the benefits of change, observe the difficulties of their current situation, are committed to change, or are taking steps to change. (It may be that other categories will be added to this list over time.)

Second, these statements are linked to a specific behavior or set of behaviors. This element of specificity is related to the directive component of MI. Each session is focused on a particular goal (e.g., improved health, engaging in prosocial behaviors, avoiding substance use, using safer sex, reducing interpersonal violence, enhancing dental care), and change talk occurs in relationship to that goal.

Third, change talk typically comes from the client, though it does not have to. That is, practitioners reflect what they hear as possible change talk, and if clients endorse this reflection as accurate, it is considered change talk in MI coding systems (e.g., MI Scoring Code [MISC]; MI Treatment Integrity [MITI]). The critical element then is not that the client says the words, but rather that he or she recognizes the accuracy of the statement and acknowledges this to the practitioner.

Fourth, change talk is typically phrased in present tense. That is, clients are referring to things that reflect on their present situations. For example, if a client says, "In the past, drinking caused me some problems," this may or may not be change talk. It's what comes after this statement that determines whether it's change talk. One could imagine this client saying, " ... but, it's not really an issue any more"; this would not be change talk. Or if the client said, " ... and I guess it still is," this would be change talk. Or if the practitioner reflected the original statement, "It caused some problems before and maybe still does," and the client responded with "that's true," then it would be change talk.

In current thinking then, change talk has four elements: content, recognition, a specific target behavior, and present tense. Research by Moyers et al. (2007) indicates that change talk is not specific to MI and that it can predict change in drinking behavior across treatment conditions. This finding supports the idea that eliciting and reinforcing change talk is important, though we have not yet talked about why it is important. For that, we turn to Darryl Bem's self-perception theory (Bem, 1967).

Bem, who offered self-perception theory as an alternative to cognitive dissonance (Festinger, 1957), noted that rather than an innate drive to maintain consonance between beliefs, attitudes, and behaviors, people simply observe their own behavior—as they would observe others—to determine their attitudes. Bem noted that this process occurred in circumstances where beliefs and attitudes were uncertain and external rewards were insufficient to account for the behavior. For example, asking a practitioner who ardently believes in abstinence only to argue for harm reduction is unlikely to cause a change in those beliefs. Having someone with firm beliefs take a position against those beliefs did not result in an attitudinal shift. Nor do individuals necessarily shift attitudes when behavior seems to conform to the demands of an outside authority (e.g., asking an inmate to tell the parole board why they won't reoffend). However, in situations where people are unsure, having them talk in favor of a position causes their attitudes to shift in line with their arguments. In short, we come to believe that for which we argue.

The application of self-perception theory to MI is relatively direct. Because most people are uncertain about how they feel regarding a behavior change (DiClemente [2003] estimates that upwards of two-thirds of people who consider a behavior change feel strongly ambivalent about that change), they are, by definition, uncertain. So, in this circumstance, the practitioner's goal is to help the client identify and articulate reasons for change. Conversely, practitioners avoid situations in which they argue for change, and the client argues against it (i.e., the client argues for why the situation does not need to change).

This theory may also explain why it's important for the client, and not the practitioner, to make the argument in favor of change. If their attitudes are to shift, then clients must hear themselves talk about why the change should occur or acknowledge that a statement is accurate when a practitioner reflects possible change talk.

Although the theoretical underpinnings of change talk have been in place for some time now, there have been no experimental findings to support this mechanism until recently. Data now suggest that (1) natural occurrences of client language during an interview can predict subsequent client behavior (Amrhein et al., 2003; Amrhein, Miller, Yahne, Knupsky, & Hochstein, 2004), (2) therapist behavior predicts the appearance of change talk (Moyers, Miller, et al., 2005; Schoener et al., 2006), (3) change talk early in treatment predicts later drinking outcomes (Moyers et al., 2007), and (4) change talk occurs across treatment modalities and predicts later outcome (Moyers et al., 2007). However, it must be added that only MI seeks to elicit and reinforce change talk.

Amrhein's work suggests that client change talk should be conceptualized in a slightly different manner than Miller and Rollnick (2002) suggest. Amrhein et al. (2004) identifies two broad categories: preparatory language and mobilizing language. Within preparatory language are four components (desire, ability, reason, and need), and mobilizing language includes two components (commitment and taking steps).

Amrhein et al.'s (2003, 2004) work also provided a few other important observations. Preparatory language is important; however, it may exert only limited direct influence on behavior change. Greater effects may occur through increasing the likelihood of commitment language, which predicts client behavior more strongly. Confused? Don't worry about it. What's important for you to know at this point is that preparatory language is important, so the ability to identify, reinforce and increase its occurrence is likewise vital. However, it may not be enough.

In terms of commitment language, it is not the starting point or overall level that appears critical, but rather its trajectory over the course of a session (i.e., Does it increase, stay level, or decrease?) and the timing of it (When does it occur during the session? Does it occur at the end of a session?). Amrhein et al.'s (2003, 2004) research work suggests that change talk that increases over the course of a session, regardless of the initial starting spot, and that occurs at the end of the session predicts changes in substance use behavior.

Finally, as noted before, change talk is viewed through the lens of a specific behavioral goal. That is, change talk is about a specific type of change (e.g., increasing exercise) and not change more generally. For practitioners, this clear division may not be as critical as it is for researchers because behavior is intertwined, so that change in one area may begin to initiate change in others. Thus talk about change—even if not for the specific target behavior—remains important and may signal movement the practitioner can use to aid the client. However, the aim in MI remains to elicit and reinforce change talk in relation to a specific goal.

Preparatory Language

As noted, there are four types of preparatory change statements: those reflecting desire, ability, reasons, and need (DARN). These are presented as discrete types of statements, but for most practitioners (and coders), they overlap quite significantly. So, at times, it can be quite hard to distinguish where one type ends and another begins. For our purposes, the most important distinction is between preparatory and mobilizing language.

Desire to Change

These statements indicate a clear desire for change but stop short of a commitment. Practitioners sometimes can discount this type of statement as idle chatter, but it is an important preparatory step. Making public statements of desire to change can act as powerful springboards to commitment talk and set the stage for discussing plans to change. Examples of desire-to-change statements are:

"I wish things were different."

"I'm hoping things will change."

"This is not the person I want to be."

This desire is evident in a portion of LaDonna's statement, "Well, I think I can, but *I just want to feel better*, and I don't." The problem with differentiating types of change talk is also evident in this statement; there are parts that suggest ability, reason, and need, as well as desire.

Ability to Change (Optimism)

These comments are about self-efficacy ("can-do" attitude) and indicate clients' belief that they can make changes in the problem area. These statements may include knowing what or how to make the change as well as beliefs that they can do it, if they make up their mind to do so. Sometimes these statements come right up to the edge of commitment language. Here are some strong examples.

"I know what I have to do—I just need to do it."

"I can make a change; I just need to commit to it."

"I'm going to prove everybody wrong."

Often, especially early in an encounter, these statements are tentative. As in the example with LaDonna, it may be critical to bolster the client's hope first by using affirmations. Then these types of change statements may follow: "Well, I think I can, but I just want to feel better, and I don't." It is also evident in the sequence of two statements she makes, interspersed by a practitioner comment:

"Well, I did stay clean and sober for 3 years once."

"So you know how to do it."

"Yeah, I guess I do, but that feeling's a long way away now. . . . "

This is tentative change talk and unlikely to be sufficient for a change effort, but it *is* a start.

Reason(s) for Change (Benefits of Change)

These statements indicate that there may be some specific advantage to making shifts in behavior. Clients articulate ways in which life might be better if they decided to make a change. These represent the good things that might come their way if a change happens. For example:

> "My wife might get off my back if I didn't drink quite so much."
>
> "Maybe I would have a little more energy if I was more conscientious about my blood sugars."
>
> "I guess I wouldn't even have to think about it, if I decided to use condoms every time."
>
> "It would be nice if I didn't have to worry quite so much."

In LaDonna's instance, there is the implication that things would be better, but no specific statements about how those areas might improve—or what those areas are. So, this might be a direction to explore further. A reflection, followed by a direct but open-ended question, might work well: "You'd prefer things to be better than they are right now. In what ways have things improved already because you aren't drinking?"

Need to Change (Problems with the Status Quo)

This is a statement that things are not working in the client's life. A basic tenet that flows from the MI spirit of collaboration is that a label ("x is a problem") is *un*necessary for change to occur. However, it is necessary for clients to recognize that aspects of their current situation must change. There may be a general imperative for change, but no specific reasons are articulated. Examples of problem recognition statements are:

> "I've got to make things better."
>
> "I need to get a handle on things."
>
> "My blood sugars can't go on like this."
>
> "I can't go on with the behaviors I've been doing."

It is my belief, but I do not have data to support this assertion, that this is often the first type of change talk to emerge. Practitioners need to be alert for its occurrence, though, as it is often stated in very "soft" terms. In LaDonna's case, it is implied that her substance use has led to difficulties by this statement: "I've lost most everything else." A clarifying reflection might help to solidify this statement: "Your use has cost you almost everything." Again, in this instance, the subtle use of a basic skill—reflective listening—can be employed to great advantage in directing LaDonna's attention and clarifying information, without asking a question. She also indicates a need for change in her statement, "Well, I think I can, but I just want to feel better, and I don't." This statement may actually fit best under the desire category, though need is also present.

Mobilizing Language

Although preparatory language may pave the way for change, it's often not enough. *Commitment statements* are the linchpins in the change talk sequence and are critical predictors of change occurring. These statements contain action words (i.e., verbs) that communicate an intention to take steps. Amrhein (Amrhein et al., 2003) has noted that these verbs can vary in strength from weak to strong, but all contain the goal to act. Desire to change contains tentative (more passive) language that indicates a wish for change but lacks the intentionality of commitment statements. Here are some examples of the more active verbs contained in commitment language.

> "I am going to … "
>
> "I will … "
>
> "I plan to … "
>
> "I intend to … "
>
> "I have already started to … "

The last entry includes the element of taking steps, which is another form of mobilizing language. Taking small, even tentative, steps in the right direction predicts change. This talk describes steps that the client is already making in support of a specific goal:

> "I went to the gym and worked out twice last week."
>
> "I went to the store, bought some vegetables, cleaned and cut them up, and have them in my fridge for snacks."
>
> "I told my boyfriend that he couldn't stay if he was drinking."

LaDonna evidences three of the four forms of preparatory change talk (desire, ability, and need). There is not, however, a firm statement of commitment in this sequence. She talks about continuing to go to treatment, and the practitioner tries to highlight and draw out these statements, but firm commitment is not in evidence yet. Statements about commitment are made by the practitioner, and these do have the effect of drawing her attention to what lies beneath her behavior—and this may be enough to solidify her efforts—but from an MI perspective the goal would be to elicit a firmer statement of commitment. So, how do we get there?

Eliciting Change Talk

As noted in the previous section, OARS can be a very effective method for drawing out this type of language from the client. As evident with LaDonna, this process can include taking guesses about what lies beneath what has been said or done by the client, but it remains a process of noting things within the client. That is, practitioners are not *installing* motivation but rather *drawing it forth* from what the client says and does, and then holding that up for the client to observe. Commitment statements may also emerge spontaneously when a client feels safe and understood. However, sometimes OARS are not enough to elicit this material. Miller and Rollnick (1991, 2002) have provided examples of other methods for drawing forth this crucial form of change talk.

Evocative Questions

These questions ask the client directly for change talk. There was an example of an evocative question displayed earlier in the desire-to-change section. Here are some other examples of evocative questions:

"In what ways does this concern you?"

"If you decided to make a change, what makes you think you could do it?"

"How would you like things to be different?"

"How would things be better if you changed?"

The nature of the question directs the client to a particular form of change talk. As you may have surmised, a particular form of evocative question is the key question. This question asks directly for commitment language.

"So, given all this, what do think you will do next?"

"What's your next step?"

"What, if anything, will you do now?"

Elaboration

Practitioners ask clients for examples of situations that illustrate change talk. That is, the client has already made a change statement, and the practitioner asks him or her to describe an instance of that circumstance:

"Tell me about a recent time when you spent money on gambling that you needed for something else."

"What does that look like when you get too angry with the children? Describe a time when that occurred."

"You said things were better then. Tell me about a time when you and he got along better. Specifically, what was happening?"

The aim with elaboration is to have the client bring into fuller relief what it was like when this circumstance occurred. This instance is shown in contrast with either how things are now or basic values about how clients would like things to be. Sometimes these connections need to be made by the practitioner, but better yet is when the client makes these relationships clear.

Using Extremes

This approach identifies the client's (1) worst imagined outcomes if the behavior continues unabated, and (2) best hoped-for benefits if change occurs. Talking about the worst possibility may make it easier to talk about other, less severe negative consequences:

> "What concerns you the most?"

> "What is the worst thing that could happen?"

The same is true for the other side:

> "What do you hope for the most?"

> "What would a perfect outcome look like?"

The aim is to lay out the client's landscape and then backtrack to explore the less extreme elements. It's as if articulating the worst and then acknowledging that it may not happen allows the client to identify the things that are nearby, could happen, and are more immediately concerning. Conversely, whereas the ultimate benefits may feel very remote, more likely rewards may feel attainable.

Looking Back

This technique asks the client to remember how things were before problems emerged. The practitioner—or better yet the client—then contrasts those descriptions with how things are now.

> "Do you remember a time when things were going well? What has changed?"

> "What are the differences between the LaDonna of 10 (or 20) years ago and the LaDonna of today?"

> "What did you want to be or do when you graduated from high school?"

> "What did you envision for your life when you were young?"

Your clients didn't hope to be drug addicted or homeless or in prison or unable to find a job or in poor health when they were young. They had dreams and aspirations; tapping into these can be helpful in reestablishing client values, enhancing hope for the future, and redefining goals. Looking-back can elicit all four forms of preparatory language.

Looking Forward

As opposed to looking back, this technique asks the client how things might unfold in the future. The focus can be either how things will appear if no change happens or how things might look after a change.

"If nothing changes, what do you see happening in 5 years? If you decide to change, what will it be like?"

"What are your hopes for the near future?"

"How would you like things to turn out?"

"How would you like things to be different?"

The use of looking-forward talk can be very helpful in a circumstance where the client recognizes some concerns, but does not view these as significant. Tone is very important in this type of question. That is, the practitioner cannot assume that he or she knows what will happen, but instead is curious about how the client sees things unfolding. As is evident, these queries overlap with the evocative questions listed earlier.

Exploring Goals

Explore how the target behavior fits in with the values and goals the client holds dearest:

"What things do you regard as most important? How does your drinking fit into this?"

"What sort of person [parent] do you want to be?"

"What sorts of things would you like to accomplish in your life?"

Miller developed a card-sorting activity, based on Rokeach's (1973, 1979) value sorting exercise and available through the MI website (*www.motivationalinterview.org*), that asks clients to review a set of cards, each with a value listed on it. Clients then arrange these values into differing priority levels. After clients have defined the three to five most important values, the clinician explores how these values fit into their life, including their relationship to the behavior in question. In research projects through the University of Washington, we have used a variation of this card-sorting activity in outreach work with homeless cocaine users as well as opiate users awaiting opiate replacement treatment. Again, the attitude of curiosity about clients' values, critical in this process, allows openings for exploration that would not typically appear. For example, in the cocaine users project, a substantial number of people endorsed "Getting right with God" as a top five value. Exploration of spirituality, for these individuals, was often a very powerful method for eliciting change talk.

Assessment Feedback

Many of the research projects involving MI have included personalized feedback—that is, feedback for participants from assessment that is either normatively based or that builds on client goals, values, and perceptions. The aim is to present personalized—not group-based—information and have the person interpret the meaning. For example, norms can be used to indicate a person's drinking level in comparison to peers' use. Here are some other examples:

"Your sexual activity places you at moderate to high risk for possible HIV infection, based on your protection practices. What do you make of that?"

"The testing indicates that your brain is having difficulty processing information efficiently. It looks as though shifting easily between ways of thinking will be hard for you, and so things like multitasking may be very difficult. How does that fit with what you know about yourself?"

"You indicate that independence in decision making is important and that social connections are also important. Tell me about how those things fit together in your life."

Most agencies have some type of intake data that can be a very useful resource in developing feedback. Putting the information on a sheet or form that clients take home can be helpful, but is not necessary to provide feedback. Norms can also be helpful, but again this information needs to be tied to the specific circumstance of this client. For example: "On average, you drink about 28 standard drinks a week. That figure is a bit above the 23 drinks our typical female client drinks when she comes into the program." This type of normative information may be available through your agency. Conversely, this behavior can be contrasted with state or national norms (e.g., "96% of Washington State drivers have one or zero moving violations in a given year"). Drug and alcohol norms are available through national clearinghouse surveys such as the Substance Abuse and Mental Health Services Administration (SAMHSA), the National Institute on Drug Abuse (NIDA), or the National Institute on Alcohol Abuse and Alcoholism (NIAAA).

The purpose of feedback is to place important and sometimes discrepant information in front of the client for consideration. It is not uncommon for resistance to increase in this situation, which is consistent with the defensive bias issue Leffingwell et al. (2006) identified (see Chapter 4). Miller also reports data that support this observation (Miller, Yahne, & Tonigan, 2003). There is a temptation, when clients argue that this information can't be right, to take up the argument for why it is accurate. Instead, a return to reflective listening is often the best response. The aim is for clients to draw meaning and connection. Again, clients—not practitioners—should make the arguments for change. This means that clients decide the data's importance and meaning ultimately.

Finally, it is important to keep in mind that feedback is a tool for eliciting change talk. Feedback is *not* MI, nor is feedback required for a session to be MI. It is simply a tool in the MI clinician's toolbox.

Readiness Rulers

This method combines an assessment of readiness with techniques designed to elicit change talk. After the initial scaling question (below), to which the client responds with an answer, the clinician probes the reason for that answer and then queries why a lower number was not selected. The questions may ask about issues of importance, confidence, and readiness; I typically ask just the first two, as the answers to these provide significant information about readiness and make the last question redundant. The form of the questions is important:

"On a scale of 1–10, how confident are you—if you made a decision to change—that you could change, when *1* represents not at all confident and *10* equals extremely confident?"

"What led you to choose a *6*, versus a *3*?"

"What would it take for you to move from a *6* to a *7* or *8*?"

Too often people, as they learn to use scaling questions, move quickly through the follow-up questions. In fact, it is these probes, and not the actual number elicited by the initial question, which are the critical elements in this process. Note also the relationship of the numbers to each other in the probes. The question about why a *6* and not a *3*? uses a moderate level of discrepancy to ask for change talk. In my experience bigger discrepancies (e.g., why a *6* and not a *1*?) can be off-putting for clients, though this is not supported by any empirical data. Perhaps more important is the one-step-forward aspect of the next probe, "What would it take for you to move from a *6* to a *7* or *8*?" This focus allows for the identification of small, manageable steps. Practitioners should be prepared to listen well, reflect, and explore the answers. Both probes may elicit change talk.

In sum, there are many ways to elicit change talk. At present, there are no data to support one method as more effective than another. In terms of integrating these methods into your practice, one approach is to develop facility with several methods and then choose the method that seems best for a particular client situation. Conversely, a standard method can be developed for your setting that incorporates elements (e.g., a value sort and intake feedback) that typically elicit change talk. Either way, it is important to pay attention to how your client is responding, and to use good-quality OARS.

Concept Quiz—Test Yourself!

True or false:

1.   T F   Self-perception theory holds that having clients argue for a position will change their attitudes about the position, particularly if they are unsure what they believe.

2.   T F   There are six forms of change talk.

3.   T F   Of the different forms of change talk, only commitment language predicts client change.

4.   T F   Creating a safe, supportive environment may be enough to prompt clients to begin talking about change

5.   T F   According to the chapter, one of the ways to elicit change talk is to argue for why a client can*not* change.

6.   T F   If you hear language pointing to a desire, ability, and need for change, then you should try to elicit reasons for change before seeking commitment language.

7.   T F   OARS can be a good method for reinforcing and eliciting change talk.

8.   T F   You must have normative data in order for feedback to be useful.

9.   T F   Clients need our expertise to understand what the feedback means to them.

10.   T F   Follow-up probes and reflective listening are critical elements when doing the scaling questions.

Answers

1. **T**   The basic framework of this statement is true. There is one more element we need to keep track of as well: the lack of an external agent to which clients can attribute their argument. In situations where clients believe strongly in a position or attribute their behavior to an external cause (e.g., "I just did it to please the judge"), then asking them to articulate one side of the argument is unlikely to alter their basic position. In general, however, the fundamental aspects of self-perception theory are present in this statement.

2. **T**   Desire, ability, reason, and need for change, commitment to change, and taking steps are the six forms. Again, distinctions between forms of preparatory language can be difficult to make and are less important than distinguishing this general category from mobilizing language.

3. **F**   This is a tricky question. Although commitment language is critical in the prediction of change, taking steps also predicts change. Furthermore, DARN may predict change as well, though less strongly than commitment language. It is important to note that these two forms are not more important than the other forms. Finally, change *does* occur in the absence of commitment language at times. So, although commitment language is an important predictor of change, other elements (taking steps and DARN, to a lesser extent) also predict change.

4. **T**   Sometimes simply creating situations in which clients don't have to defend themselves has the effect of encouraging them to spontaneously explore the other side of the coin. In this way, listening well can elicit change talk. LaDonna's example at the beginning of this chapter nicely illustrates this point.

5. **F**   Although Miller and Rollnick note that siding with the negative position can elicit change talk, this is different from arguing that a client is *unable* to change. Arguing—regardless of the direction that the practitioner takes—is not MI-consistent behavior. It has the additional concern of being manipulative—like using "reverse psychology" to get someone to do something you want him or her to do. In siding with the negative position, the practitioner is simply saying that perhaps this is not the right time, place, or method by which change can occur. The attitude is one of inquisitiveness, not manipulation.

6. **F**   There is no data to suggest that all, or even most, preparatory language must occur prior to eliciting commitment language. What is clear is that higher levels of DARN predict commitment talk. The choice of what to do next to elicit forms of change talk typically is determined by the client situation, not by a lockstep approach. That is, if the time appears right for a key question, then that is the next correct step. Waiting too long can leave the practitioner lagging behind the client's readiness—rarely an optimal place for a guide to find him- or herself.

7. **T**   As noted above and illustrated in many MI videotapes, OARS often work very effectively in eliciting change talk. However, it is important to have other skills as well.

8. F   Normative feedback can be helpful, but it is not necessary. I have worked on research projects that used feedback forms that were entirely devoid of normative data. Instead, the information provided data about risk categories, risk behaviors, and values.

9. F   Although our expertise can be very helpful, it can also get in the way. As practitioners provide feedback, they should give enough information for clients to understand the information, but then ask and allow clients to decide what it means for them!

10. T   Scaling questions provide useful data, but it is the probes that elicit information about readiness to change and the reflections that allow for further exploration of these topics. So, although the questions are important to launch the topic, the probes are also critical.

In Practice

Let's return to LaDonna. The reason for meeting was to evaluate mental health issues for job readiness. However, the specific goal that emerged was her struggle to remain sober. It is this behavior that is targeted by the practitioner in this example. Here we resume at the end of the previous dialogue.

Statement	*Commentary*
P: Let me see if I've got this right. It's hard to find external reasons for getting and staying clean, yet some internal reasons seem to be pushing you because you keep doing it—even when it feels really hard. You'd like to feel better and you know you can, you're just not sure how to get there now. The hill you're on feels slippery, but you're determined to climb it.	Summary that focuses on her concerns and the change talk.
C: I'm determined, but I don't know if I can do it.	This statement hangs between desire and commitment, but then she adds a concern.
P: There are some real hurdles, and you're determined. I wonder if it would be useful to spend some time talking about that issue.	Simple reflection that acknowledges ambivalence and focuses on her change talk. Then an open-ended statement (question) that attempts to set a mutual agenda and thus a target goal for the MI.
C: Yeah, I guess.	Client agrees, though tentatively.

Statement	*Commentary*
P: You're not sure it would be helpful.	Acknowledges her fears directly by using a complex reflection (i.e., continuing the paragraph).
C: I know I have to stay clean. It's just that I've tried it before and it hasn't worked.	Again, change talk followed by status quo talk.
P: And 3 years clean doesn't feel like success.	Amplified reflection.
C: I guess it did, but it didn't last.	She backs away from the absolute.
P: You were successful for a good chunk of time and then slipped. It seems very important to you now to stop. In fact, it's hard for you to find reasons and yet you're doing it. The confidence side is a little less clear. If you were to rate yourself, on a scale of 1–10, where *1* is not at all confident and *10* is extremely confident, how confident are you that you can remain clean and sober for the next 30 days?	A transitional summary followed by a readiness ruler. The ruler is used not only to assess her level of confidence, but also to elicit change talk in that area of apparent concern.
C: I'd say about a *4*.	She picks a midrange number, higher than might have been predicted based on her prior statements.
P: Interesting, so you're not stuck down there at *1* or *2*. How come?	Practitioner probes further in a manner congruent with the earlier response.
C: Well … even though it's hard, I don't want to go back. I've told myself—even though I don't feel any better—I will keep going to meetings, especially when I feel like using.	Strong commitment language, despite the low confidence score.
P: You just refuse to use.	Reinforces commitment with a light touch.
C: (*Laughs.*) Yeah. I guess that's true. But it feels really hard sometimes.	Accepts and provides additional information about barriers.
P: And that's why you gave it a *4* and not a *7* or *8*.	Complex reflection.
C: Yep. But, I've been through hard times before.	Client accepts reflection and offers information about internal resources.

Statement	*Commentary*
P: You know you're strong.	Affirmation.
C: It's funny, because I didn't feel that way coming in today.	Acknowledges shift in attitude.
P: Recognizing what you've already accomplished, what you know about yourself, and your commitment to yourself has helped you feel more confident. Like maybe your score should be a little higher—like a 5 or 6.	Collecting summary.
C: Probably more like a 6.	Client agrees with greater confidence.
P: Let me ask one more question, and then we probably need to get started on the other parts of the assessment. You're at a 6 now. What would it take for you to move to a 7 or an 8.	Directive element of MI, which asks client to continue to move toward her goal.
C: I need to feel more hopeful.	Client provides a general response.
P: More hopeful. How would you know when that was happening?	Simple reflection followed by an evocative question.
C: I guess I would be happier. I'd have a plan for where I am going in terms of living. I'd have a job.	Client provides a lot of goals, some more distant than others.
P: Wow. That's a lot of stuff for a 1-point step.	Practitioner provides a congruent response.
C: (*Laughs.*) I guess it is. That's part of how I get myself feeling so overwhelmed. OK. One point ... maybe have a plan for my living arrangements.	Client is able to break the goals down into a more manageable task and to acknowledge self-awareness about this process.
P: That feels more doable—like you can accomplish that.	Reinforces change talk.
C: I'm actually in decent shape about that now. I mean, it's not ideal, but I can continue with my brother as long as I stay clean. If I get a job, I can work on saving some money and then start looking for a place.	She describes an initial plan.

Statement	*Commentary*
P: It seems you have a plan already kind of worked out in your head. It's just a matter of saying it aloud, as well as slowing things down—so you don't get ahead of yourself. I wonder if writing it down would help.	Collecting summary and then an open-ended statement (question).
C: I think it would. I'll do that on the bus on the way to my meeting. In fact, I think I'll talk about it at my meeting, because that will help me stick with it.	Commitment and more planning to reinforce it.
P: You really do know a lot about what works for you and what you have to do to support it.	Affirmation.
C: (*Grins.*) Yeah, I do. I just have to remember it.	Client feels empowered and mood is noticeably brighter.

LaDonna did not present for this meeting with an agenda to discuss her substance use recovery plans. However, in the course of the encounter, it became clear that this area was a critical target if she were to succeed in a vocational process. Thus, a focused discussion, directed toward increasing her confidence in maintaining sobriety—without cheerleading by the practitioner—became the shared agenda. This interchange, which would take about 10 minutes or less in real time, illustrates how strategies and OARS can be used to reinforce and elicit preparatory and commitment language generally as well as spontaneously in the context of an encounter designed for other purposes.

Try This!

The development of skills in change talk is a somewhat greater challenge because we need the talker's responses to help shape the counselor's responses. As we move through these exercises, you might think about possibilities for trying out these skills either at work or in opportunistic moments away from work. As with prior chapters, we move from the straightforward to the more complex exercises, in this case beginning with recognizing change talk, then practicing recognizing and reinforcing change talk, and finally ending with eliciting it.

Exercise 5.1. Recognizing Change Talk

You will review transcripts of two exchanges between a practitioner and a client. Read the first transcript and try to identify all of the change talk you hear. When you find change talk, underline it. Jot down the kind of change talk you think it is and your rationale, then compare your answers to the key. Once you've reconciled your answers, repeat the exercise with the next transcript.

Exercise 5.2. Drumming for Change Talk[1]

This training technique tunes your ear for change talk. It involves listening to statements and deciding if they contain preparatory language, mobilizing language, or something else. It is also a kinesthetic activity, with drum rolls and hand rubbing in response to different forms of client talk. The catch is that the "clients" we will be listening to are speaking through the lyrics of their songs.

Exercise 5.3. Reinforcing Change Talk: Treasure Hunt for Change

Read the client statements, then decide if there is change talk. If there is change talk, write a reflective response that would reinforce it; if not, write an evocative question that might elicit it in this situation. For bonus points, write a second evocative question that is different.

Exercise 5.4. Methods for Eliciting Change Talk

In this exercise you'll return to the transcripts used in Exercise 5.1, this time focusing on the work of the practitioner. Review the sequence of practitioner activities and then answer the questions that follow each exchange. Finally, review the commentary, which now focuses on the rationale of the practitioner.

Exercise 5.5. Write a Branching Script

A very interesting research study (Villaume, Berger, & Barker, 2006) involved having students write a script for a branching computer program. The assignment required that the script be MI consistent and reflect multiple pathways that a conversation might travel. The authors found that although there were problems with the software working properly, the process of writing the script helped practitioners become more effective in using MI. This exercise builds on that finding.

There is a basic structure provided in this exercise, and the writer is asked to fill in the practitioner and client responses. The aim is to create interactions that might elicit desired responses. Don't worry about your skill as a playwright or screenwriter. Just imagine your client responses and see where it takes you. Then return to the branching parts of the interchange and play out those as well. Remember, even when you don't get the first response you expected, the goal is to elicit change talk. Use your OARS to help navigate rough patches in the encounter.

Partner Work

In addition to the activities described above, here is another option available when you have a partner.

---

[1] Thanks to Steve Berg-Smith for this exercise.

Exercise 5.6. Drumming for Change

A list of client statements is attached in this exercise. Have your partner read the list aloud. Every time you hear preparatory talk (DARN), drum. This form of change talk is underlined. Mobilizing language (i.e., commitment statements and taking steps), which are italicized, should draw polishing motions (i.e., placing your hands in a praying position and rubbing your palms in a circular motion, as though polishing a pearl). Statements that are neither preparatory nor mobilizing draw silence. If you make a mistake, stop and talk about it with your partner. Figure out where the confusion came from, then continue. Alternate turns drumming and reading.

Other Thoughts ...

Readiness to change and readiness for treatment are independent concepts. This statement is one of the conclusions drawn by researchers Simpson and Joe (1993). This distinction has also been evident in our research (Donovan, Rosengren, Downey, Cox, & Sloan, 2001; Downey, Rosengren, & Donovan, 2000).

Consistent with this finding, some trainers make distinctions between adherence talk and change talk. Adherence is the willingness to engage in treatment as a method for change, whereas change talk is directed toward the behavior in question. The utility of this distinction may lie primarily in (1) preventing practitioners from becoming wedded to the concept of a particular form of treatment as the only method for change and (2) staying attentive to the meaning of client statements. This distinction is also consistent with DiClemente's (2003) assertion that all intentional change is self-change, with treatment representing only one segment in a process that began prior to the client's meeting with a practitioner and continues well after treatment ends.

Finally, MI is more than just a behavioral strategy of eliciting and reinforcing change talk. It is about helping clients lead satisfying lives and choosing activities that support that goal. The goal should not become a series of rote activities toward a preordained end, but the subtle and nuanced exploration of clients' concerns as you assist them in finding the path that leads them to their goals.

Identifying Change Talk

In the next few pages you will find interchanges between a practitioner and a client. In each case read the transcript and then underline what you view as change talk. Keep in mind that the client usually generates change talk, though clinician statements—if affirmed by the client—can also constitute change talk. After you've underlined these sheets, check your answers against the key.

Exercise 5.1, Scenario 1 (Marijuana)

This is a young adult male, coming to treatment for a possible substance abuse issue, at the behest of his parents. The target behavior for change talk is substance use.

P: Let me summarize what we've talked about so far. About 8 months ago you had a pretty serious cancer scare. You took some time off for chemotherapy and for awhile your life plans were put on hold. You're basically doing OK now; the cancer is in remission, and you're trying to get on with your life. Prior to this diagnosis you'd been in school—with kind of mixed results—but you were figuring out what was required of you to be successful, including smoking a little less pot. Your plan is to go back this fall. You also decided that for now you'll stay at home to help cover costs, but this also means that you have to follow your parents' rules, which is causing some friction. Did I miss anything?

C: No.

P: Now, I understand that one of your parents' concerns is pot smoking, and they've laid down the law about that with you. Tell me about that.

C: Well, what do you want to know about it?

P: What's been happening with the pot smoking? What's making your parents concerned? That sort of thing ...

C: Well, I didn't drink or smoke pot until I was a senior in high school. Then I started drinking about halfway through the year—you know, going out on weekends, partying with friends. Then I started smoking some pot. At first, it was the same way—just weekends—but then I started doing it most every day. It was safer than drinking and driving. Pretty soon I decided I'd better start cutting back, so I tried that. Then I decided to stop for awhile, and I did a couple of times for a month or 2, then I tried to smoke just socially, but that didn't work very well. Then I got sick and so I didn't do anything for awhile, but now it started again. So, when my parents said I could smoke once a week I was a little surprised, but I also know it won't work for me. I can't smoke socially. I need to stop entirely, so that's what I'm doing. I haven't smoked in about a week.

P: You're pretty clear that this is something that needs to change and, in fact, you were already picking up on this back in high school.

C: Shortly after high school.

P: How about the drinking? Where do you stand with that now?

(cont.)

C: Well, I plan to continue drinking, but I'm not going to pick up where the smoking left off. My drinking has never been like my pot smoking. I never did it every day or anything. I mean, occasionally we'd go out. And I work at a restaurant and so we have a couple of drinks after work sometimes, and I don't see anything wrong with that.

P: OK. So you are clear that the smoking needs to change—and I'd still like to hear a little more about what led you to that decision—but you're not so sure that the drinking needs to change.

C: Yeah, it's just not that big of a deal.

P: It's not much of a thing.

C: Right.

P: Let me summarize what we've talked about so far. You . . .

Key for Exercise 5.1, Scenario 1 (Marijuana)

P: Let me summarize what we've talked about so far. About 8 months ago you had a pretty serious cancer scare. You took some time off for chemotherapy and for awhile your life plans were put on hold. You're basically doing OK now; the cancer is in remission, and you're trying to get on with your life. Prior to this diagnosis you'd been in school—with kind of mixed results—but you were figuring out what was required of you to be successful, including smoking a little less pot. Your plan is to go back this fall. You also decided that for now you'll stay at home to help cover costs, but this also means that you have to follow your parents' rules, which is causing some friction. Did I miss anything?

C: No.

Commentary: Some issues are noted in the practitioner's summary, but this is not change talk. Remember, change talk in this situation is directed toward substance misuse, and the reference to changes in pot smoking is in the past. However, this summary provides openings to which you could return later.

P: Now, I understand that one of your parents' concerns is pot smoking, and they've laid down the law about that with you. Tell me about that.

C: Well, what do you want to know about it?

Commentary: No change talk here.

P: What's been happening with the pot smoking? What's making your parents concerned? That sort of thing . . .

C: Well, I didn't drink or smoke pot until I was a senior in high school. Then I started drinking about halfway through the year—you know, going out on weekends, partying with friends. Then I started smoking some pot. At first, it was the same way—just weekends—but then I started doing it most every day. It was safer than drinking and driving. Pretty soon I decided I'd better start cutting back, so I tried that. Then I decided to stop for awhile, and I did a couple of times for a month or 2, then I tried to smoke just socially, but that didn't work very well. Then I got sick and so I didn't do anything for awhile, but now it started again. So, when my parents said I could smoke once a week I was a little surprised, but I also know it won't work for me. I can't smoke socially. I need to stop entirely, so that's what I'm doing. I haven't smoked in about a week.

Commentary: Early on the client provides a history without comment on any issues. Beginning with the line "Pretty soon . . . " he begins to articulate events in the past that suggest a possible need to cut back. However, this is not change talk because it remains in the past tense. Without much prodding, he then supplies clear recognition that there is a current issue, and he knows what to do and is doing it. This is need talk and mobilizing language (commitment talk and taking steps); both are worth reinforcing.

P: You're pretty clear that this is something that needs to change and, in fact, you were already picking up on this back in high school.

(cont.)

Key for Exercise 5.1, Scenario 1 (Marijuana) (*cont.*)

C: Shortly after high school.

Commentary: No change talk. Client makes a factual correction.

P: How about the drinking? Where do you stand with that now?

C: Well, I plan to continue drinking, but I'm not going to pick up where the smoking left off. My drinking has never been like my pot smoking. I never did it every day or anything. I mean, occasionally we'd go out. And I work at a restaurant and so we have a couple of drinks after work sometimes and I don't see anything wrong with that.

Commentary: He is quite clear in this area that he does not think there is an issue. No change talk here, but rather support for the status quo.

P: OK. So you are clear that the smoking needs to change—and I'd still like to hear a little more about what led you to that decision—but you're not so sure that the drinking needs to change.

C: Yeah, it's just not that big of a deal.

Commentary: The client shifts his language to suggest there may be more to consider, but not enough to indicate change talk.

P: It's not much of a thing.

C: Right.

Commentary: Still no change talk, but the door is open.

Exercise 5.1, Scenario 2 (Interpersonal Violence)

This middle-aged man is being seen by a child welfare professional after child protective services were called by a neighbor. There was an altercation in the home, and he struck his girlfriend as well as his son. The school has reported previous incidents of bruises, but there has been no formal intervention until now. He's been ordered to treatment and can only have supervised meetings with his two children (8 and 5 years old) until the child welfare professional indicates that it is safe for them to be alone with him. The target behaviors in this instance are making changes in how he manages conflict with his girlfriend and children.

P: I understand that you're not very happy about being here today.

C: Damn straight. The cops didn't listen to my side of the story after the neighbors called them. They just hauled me off to jail, and now they tell me I have to come talk to you if I want to see my kids without a social worker.

P: Nobody has really taken the time to find out how you see the situation. I wonder if we could spend a little time doing that.

C: Whatever.

P: What is concerning you now about your situation with your girlfriend and kids?

C: I can't see them, except with somebody there. My kids don't understand it. They're like, "Why can't you stay at the house, Dad?" I usually help my son with his math homework, and I can't do that now and their mom just isn't very good at that stuff.

P: Being a part of their lives is important to you. You want that and can't do that now—in the way you'd like.

C: Yeah, most of the time. Sometimes they can be annoying, but most of the time it's good.

P: And what about your partner?

C: She's pissed at me. She says I hurt her, but she hit me, too. She says I don't care about her or the kids and that's just not true. She doesn't back off sometimes, though. That's what happened that night. I told her to leave me alone. I left the room and she followed me into another. I went out to the garage and she came out there. It was embarrassing. The neighbors could hear. Finally, I went back inside and told her to knock it off. Then she slapped me, and I guess that was the straw that broke the camel's back. I just kind of swung with my backhand to keep her away and she must have been off balance because she fell. I didn't mean to hit Danny; he just stepped in at the wrong time when she was coming back at me. I was trying to say I was sorry, and she was scratching and hitting and I don't quite know what happened.

P: It seems like you're feeling bad about how things went there. It's not how you want to handle things with your girlfriend. You want to have better control than that.

C: Yeah. I'm not some ogre like these folks are making me out to be. I really tried to avoid a problem there. She just wouldn't back off!

P: That's not the kind of person you are or how you want others to view you.

(cont.)

C: I wish we could talk out our problems, but we seem to get too mad. We need to do something different.

P: Let me see if I have all of this. You're not happy to be here, and at the same time you're not happy about how things went the other night. You want to be able to talk about things, and yet sometimes it feels like there is just no way that can happen. Then you do things you regret. It's clear to you that something has to change.

C: That pretty much sums it up. Something needs to change.

Key for Exercise 5.1, Scenario 2 (Interpersonal Violence)

P: I understand that you're not very happy about being here today.

C: Damn straight. The cops didn't listen to my side of the story after the neighbors called them. They just hauled me off to jail, and now they tell me I have to come talk to you if I want to see my kids without a social worker.

Commentary: No change talk here.

P: Nobody has really taken the time to find out how you see the situation. I wonder if we could spend a little time doing that.

C: Whatever.

Commentary: Practitioner is looking for inroads. No change talk and some clear dissatisfaction.

P: What is concerning you now about your situation with your girlfriend and kids?

C: I can't see them, except with somebody there. My kids don't understand it. They're like, "Why can't you stay at the house, Dad?" I usually help my son with his math homework, and I can't do that now and their mom just isn't very good at that stuff. It stinks.

Commentary: Evocative question designed to elicit change talk. Although he clearly talks about what he doesn't like in this situation, it is not clearly related to the target behavior. There may be the start of change talk—especially "it stinks"—but this is still general dissatisfaction.

P: Being a part of their lives is important to you. You want that and can't do that now—in the way you'd like.

C: Yeah, most of the time. Sometimes they can be annoying, but most of the time it's good.

Commentary: It's still not quite change talk. The practitioner clearly notes problems with the status quo, and the client acknowledges them, but just being dissatisfied with how things are does not imply a need for personal change. Nevertheless, the practitioner is making progress.

P: And what about your partner?

C: She's pissed at me. She says I hurt her, but she hit me, too. She says I don't care about her or the kids and that's just not true. She doesn't back off sometimes, though. That's what happened that night. I told her to leave me alone. I left the room and she followed me into another. I went out to the garage and she came out there. It was embarrassing. The neighbors could hear. Finally, I went back inside and told her to knock it off. Then she slapped me, and I guess that was the straw that broke the camel's back. I just kind of swung with my backhand to keep her away and she must have been off balance because she fell. I didn't mean to hit Danny; he just stepped in at the wrong time when she was coming back at me. I was trying to say I was sorry, and she was scratching and hitting and I don't quite know what happened.

(cont.)

Key for Exercise 5.1, Scenario 2 (Interpersonal Violence) (*cont.*)

Commentary: Again there is clear evidence of his dissatisfaction with the situation and how it turned out. He is leaning more in the direction of a need for change (i.e., his apology), but it's not DARN yet.

P: It seems like you're feeling bad about how things went there. *It's not how you want to handle things with your girlfriend. You want to have better control than that.*

C: <u>Yeah</u>. I'm not some ogre like these folks are making me out to be. I really tried to avoid a problem there. She just wouldn't back off!

Commentary: For the first time, the practitioner offers a reflection that implies change (desire: he wants to have better control), and he acknowledges it.

P: That's not the kind of person you are or how you want others to view you.

C: <u>I wish we could talk out our problems</u>, but we seem to get too mad. <u>We need to do something different.</u>

Commentary: Bingo. Clear need language in the last line, desire in the first.

P: Let me see if I have all of this. You're not happy to be here, and at the same time you're not happy about how things went the other night. *You want to be able to talk about things*, and yet sometimes it feels like there is just no way that can happen. Then you do things you regret. *It's clear to you that something has to change.*

C: That pretty much sums it up. Something needs to change.

Commentary: The practitioner offers a solid MI summary, starting with the man's dissatisfaction with the situation, then emphasizing his desire and need language, which the client endorses and then reinforces.

Drumming for Change Talk[2]

This training technique tunes your ear for change talk. It involves listening to statements and deciding if they contain preparatory language, mobilizing language, or something else. Here are the steps:

- Choose music with lyrics you can understand (ballads often work best). If a song doesn't work, then go on to the next.
- Consider listening to your teen's music.
- If there is preparatory language (DARN—desire, ability, reason, or need), do a drum roll on a tabletop, your knees, or whatever surface is available.
- If there is mobilizing language (commitment talk or taking steps), place your hands together (as though praying) and rub your palms together in circular motions as though polishing a pearl.
- If the statement is neither preparatory nor mobilizing language, sit quietly.

If you do not have music, there are a few other options:

- Listen to a radio advice columnist if you have those in your area.
- Record or watch TV soap operas (or dramas) that deal with relationship conflicts.
- If you feel especially brave, listen to conversations on public transportation (buses, trains) and do small movements for preparatory and mobilizing talk.

---

[2]Thanks to Steve Berg-Smith for this exercise.

Reinforcing Change Talk:
Treasure Hunt for Change (Accident)

This young woman is coming to you because of anxiety. She lives with a roommate and is having trouble venturing away from their house. Her roommate urged her to come see you because of her increasingly constricted world. The woman feels safe at home and the thought of doing exposure therapy is very frightening to her. The target for behavior change is her anxiety about being away from home.

C: *About 8 months ago I was in a pretty serious wreck, and I guess I'm lucky to be alive. I hit my head pretty hard, and the docs said there may be some changes, but basically I think I'm doing OK. Since then I haven't liked going too far from home.*

Change talk?   Yes _____   No _____

If yes, what type?   Desire _____   Ability _____   Reason _____   Need _____   Commitment _____   or Taking Steps _____

If yes, provide a reflective response that would reinforce the change talk.

If no, write an evocative question that might elicit Change Talk.

C: *Since I got out of the hospital, it's been a slow recovery. I'm home most of the time, except when I have to go out. Sometimes my roommate takes me to the corner grocery store, and I can do that, but it's not easy. It seems a bit silly really, but I feel so relieved when I get back home and can close and lock my door.*

Change talk?   Yes _____   No _____

If yes, what type?   Desire _____   Ability _____   Reason, _____   Need _____   Commitment _____   or Taking Steps _____

If yes, provide a reflective response that would reinforce the change talk.

If no, write an evocative question that might elicit change talk.

(cont.)

C: *My sick leave runs out next week, and I have to return to work. I've been avoiding that. I have to take the bus route on which I was injured, and I am pretty worried about that. I don't know if I can do it.*

Change talk?   Yes _____   No _____

If yes, what type?   Desire _____ Ability _____ Reason, _____ Need _____ Commitment _____ or Taking Steps _____

If yes, provide a reflective response that would reinforce the change talk.

If no, write an evocative question that might elicit change talk.

C: *Except that I have to do it. I can't pay my part of the rent. Being off work has eaten up all of my savings, so I have to do it; that is why I am here—I want to figure out some way to cope.*

Change talk?   Yes _____   No _____

If yes, what type?   Desire _____ Ability _____ Reason, _____ Need _____ Commitment _____ or Taking Steps _____

If yes, provide a reflective response that would reinforce the change talk.

If no, write an evocative question that might elicit change talk.

C: *What I would like is for this nervousness to stop. I want my life back. I want to sleep without nightmares.*

Change talk?   Yes _____   No _____

If yes, what type?   Desire _____ Ability _____ Reason, _____ Need _____ Commitment _____ or Taking Steps _____

If yes, provide a reflective response that would reinforce the change talk.

If no, write an evocative question that might elicit change talk.

Key for Exercise 5.3

C: About 8 months ago I was in a pretty serious wreck, and I guess I'm lucky to be alive. I hit my head pretty hard, and the docs said there may be some changes, but basically I think I'm doing OK. Since then I haven't liked going too far from home.

Commentary: This is her description of what led to her more constricted life. It is a factual retelling with no change talk. An evocative question might follow a reflection: "It sounds like you feel tied to home. What is that like for you?"

C: Since I got out of the hospital, it's been a slow recovery. I'm home most of the time, except when I have to go out. Sometimes my roommate takes me to the corner grocery store, and I can do that, but it's not easy. It seems a bit silly really, but I feel so relieved when I get back home and can close and lock my door.

Commentary: The statement's tenor suggests lots of areas where things aren't going well, but she is not explicit. She teeters on the edge of change talk with "It feels a bit silly." You might ask a question, "How have things changed in your desire and ability to leave home, from before your accident until now?"

C: My sick leave runs out next week, and I have to return to work. I've been avoiding that. I have to take the bus route on which I was injured, and I am pretty worried about that. I don't know if I can do it.

Commentary: Yes. She makes clear statements of need, but has low confidence in her ability to meet those needs. A reflection might go like this: "You must find a way to do this, and that's what brought you here today." Or "You're worried and you know that you have to find a way to do it."

C: Except that I have to do it. I can't pay my part of the rent. Being off work has eaten up all of my savings, so I have to do it; that is why I am here—I want to figure out some way to cope.

Commentary: There is more need language and also desire in the last statement. Coming in for a session might also be considered taking steps, but it seems most clearly to be in the area of wanting some skills and coming for help to find them. A reflection might go like this: "You are here to get some tools, because you know the situation requires you do something different."

C: What I would like is for this nervousness to stop. I want my life back. I want to sleep without nightmares.

Commentary: Here is more desire, but no commitment language yet. A reflection might help solidify this change talk and add some commitment to doing something: "You're pretty clear the situation can't go on like this. It's time to do something about it."

Methods for Eliciting Change Talk

This is the same dialogue used in Exercise 5.1. This time focus on the practitioner's behavior. After each practitioner statement, answer the questions. Then write down another response that you might have used instead. Finally, check the key for some commentary.

Exercise 5.4, Scenario 1 (Marijuana)

This is a young adult male, coming to treatment for a possible substance abuse issue, at the behest of his parents.

P: Let me summarize what we've talked about so far. About 8 months ago you had a pretty serious cancer scare. You took some time off for chemotherapy and for awhile your life plans were put on hold. You're basically doing OK now; the cancer is in remission, and you're trying to get on with your life. Prior to this diagnosis you'd been in school—with kind of mixed results—but you were figuring out what was required of you to be successful, including smoking a little less pot. Your plan is to go back this fall. You also decided that for now you'll stay at home to help cover costs, but this also means that you have to follow your parents' rules, which is causing some friction. Did I miss anything?

What potential avenues does the summary open for exploration? If you chose to reconfigure this summary, what would you do? What other approaches might you use?

Example: There are the openings around what was causing trouble at school as well as the friction at home. Also possible is an exploration of fears around the cancer and how smoking may fit with being healthy. Here is one approach:

"It's been a rough few months, especially with your parents. How's pot smoking fit into the rough patch with them?"

C: No.

P: Now, I understand that one of your parents' concerns is pot smoking, and they've laid down the law about that with you. Tell me about that.

(cont.)

What does the practitioner do? What is done that lessens the likelihood of resistance? What would be another way to approach this area?

C: Well, what do you want to know about it?

P: What's been happening with the pot smoking? What's making your parents concerned? That sort of thing . . .

What happens with the client? What does the practitioner do in response? What might have been an alternative approach?

C: Well, I didn't drink or smoke pot until I was a senior in high school. Then I started drinking about halfway through the year—you know, going out on weekends, partying with friends. Then I started smoking some pot. At first, it was the same way—just weekends—but then I started doing it most every day. It was safer than drinking and driving. Pretty soon I decided I'd better start cutting back, so I tried that. Then I decided to stop for awhile, and I did a couple of times for a month or two, then I tried to smoke just socially, but that didn't work very well. Then I got sick and so I didn't do anything for awhile, but now it started again. So, when my parents said I could smoke once a week I was a little surprised, but I also know it won't work for me. I can't smoke socially. I need to stop entirely, so that's what I'm doing. I haven't smoked in about a week.

P: You're pretty clear that this is something that needs to change and, in fact, you were already picking up on this back in high school.

The practitioner chooses a reflective response. Why is that? What's another reflective listening response you might have given?

C: Shortly after high school.

P: How about the drinking? Where do you stand with that now?

What does the practitioner do here? Is this a problem? Why or why not? If you were to choose one of the other strategies for eliciting change talk, what would you choose and why? How would you do it?

C: Well, I plan to continue drinking, but I'm not going to pick up where the smoking left off. My drinking has never been like my pot smoking. I never did it every day or anything. I mean, occasionally we'd go out. And I work at a restaurant and so we have a couple of drinks after work sometimes, and I don't see anything wrong with that.

P: OK. So you are clear that the smoking needs to change—and I'd still like to hear a little more about what led you to that decision—but you're not so sure that the drinking needs to change.

This is a complex reflection. What other strategies might you use in this situation to elicit change talk? Provide an example of what you would say.

C: Yeah, it's just not that big of a deal.

P: It's not much of a thing.

What is the practitioner doing with this reflection? How might you do the same thing, but with different words?

C: Right. Let me summarize what we've talked about so far. You ...

Write a summary that you feel would emphasize his interest in change.

Key for Exercise 5.4, Scenario 1 (Marijuana)

P: Let me summarize what we've talked about so far. About 8 months ago you had a pretty serious cancer scare. You took some time off for chemotherapy and for awhile your life plans were put on hold. You're basically doing OK now; the cancer is in remission, and you're trying to get on with your life. Prior to this diagnosis you'd been in school—with kind of mixed results—but you were figuring out what was required of you to be successful, including smoking a little less pot. Your plan is to go back this fall. You also decided that for now you'll stay at home to help cover costs, but this also means that you have to follow your parents' rules, which is causing some friction. Did I miss anything?

Commentary: The summary provides an overview of what the practitioner has learned at this point. It identifies several possible avenues to explore, including his cancer, his progress in school, what caused his shift in school behavior, and his return home to live. You might begin broadly with the simple reflection and open-ended question noted before, "You also decided to smoke a little less pot. How's that fitting into your life now?" You might ask him to look backwards: "It seems your pot smoking has changed over the past few years. What was it like a few years ago, before it started causing you some troubles in school?" Or you might look forward with a couple of questions: "Where would you like to see yourself in 5 years? How would pot smoking fit into that?"

C: No.

P: Now, I understand that one of your parents' concerns is pot smoking, and they've laid down the law about that with you. Tell me about that.

Commentary: The practitioner places the focus on the area that led the client to treatment. This is done in a matter-of-fact statement, without assumption that there is a problem. The practitioner invites the client to tell more about the situation. The practitioner could also begin with a short statement that acknowledges the situation and the client's responsibility for deciding whether or not an issue exists. For example: "Your parents called because they're quite worried about your pot smoking. However, I don't make assumptions based on parents' statements, because it will really be up to you to decide if there is an issue and what if anything you want to do it. So, what's your take on the situation?"

C: Well, what do you want to know about it?

P: What's been happening with the pot smoking? What's making your parents concerned? That sort of thing . . .

Commentary: There is some reluctance from the client. Although a reflection makes sense, the client is also asking for clarification and a direct response (i.e., a refined question is also appropriate). It may be a simple matter of his needing more direction, so the practitioner addresses that need directly. A reflection might go something like this, "I confused you," or more directly, "Maybe it feels like I put you on the spot."

(cont.)

Key for Exercise 5.4, Scenario 1 (*cont.*)

C: Well, I didn't drink or smoke pot until I was a senior in high school. Then I started drinking about halfway through the year—you know, going out on weekends, partying with friends. Then I started smoking some pot. At first, it was the same way—just weekends—but then I started doing it most every day. It was safer than drinking and driving. Pretty soon I decided I'd better start cutting back, so I tried that. Then I decided to stop for awhile, and I did a couple of times for a month or 2, then I tried to smoke just socially, but that didn't work very well. Then I got sick and so I didn't do anything for awhile, but now it started again. So, when my parents said I could smoke once a week I was a little surprised, but I also know it won't work for me. I can't smoke socially. I need to stop entirely, so that's what I'm doing. I haven't smoked in about a week.

P: You're pretty clear that this is something that needs to change and, in fact, you were already picking up on this back in high school.

Commentary: The client makes change statements, and so the practitioner responds by attending to those statements and emphasizes their importance by referencing back to high school. Alternatively, the practitioner might have reinforced the commitment language by noting, "So you know what needs to be done and you're doing it."

C: Shortly after high school.

P: How about the drinking? Where do you stand with that now?

Commentary: The client makes a factual correction, but rather than attending to this the practitioner moves on to assess the place of alcohol in his substance use. The practitioner's approach is not confrontational, so it's unlikely to elicit direct resistance. However, it shifts the focus from change talk to another area, and so there is a risk of losing momentum. In terms of other approaches, you could ask for his parents' views of his alcohol use. For example: "When your parents called, they expressed concern about your substance use and they mentioned alcohol. What's causing their concern about alcohol?"

C: Well, I plan to continue drinking, but I'm not going to pick up where the smoking left off. My drinking has never been like my pot smoking. I never did it every day or anything. I mean, occasionally we'd go out. And I work at a restaurant and so we have a couple of drinks after work sometimes and I don't see anything wrong with that.

P: OK. So you are clear that the smoking needs to change—and I'd still like to hear a little more about what led you to that decision—but you're not so sure that the drinking needs to change.

Commentary: The practitioner uses a rephrase to subtly change the discussion about drinking in an effort to elicit change talk. You might also try an amplified reflection: "As far as you can see, there are no issues at all." Alternatively, you could also use a reflection followed by an evocative question: "In general, you feel pretty comfortable with your alcohol use. Any elements that you are less happy about?"

Key for Exercise 5.4, Scenario 1 (*cont.*)

C: Yeah, it's just not that big of a deal.

P: It's not much of a thing.

Commentary: The practitioner again directs attention to the part of the client statement that suggests there may be more to understand. Or you might again ask directly about his concerns: "What are the parts that are a little deal?" Or you could use an amplified reflection, such as, "You'll probably drink in this manner for the rest of your life."

C: Right.

P: Let me summarize what we've talked about so far. You . . .

Commentary: The summary might look like this:

This has been a pretty big year in your life. While the cancer is a central element, you also came to some conclusions about your life, and one of them was that your pot smoking had to change. So, you committed yourself to that change and began to do it, even when others might have given you some wiggle room. At this point, you've decided that it's OK to drink, though you're again very clear that this can't just replace the pot smoking. It sounds like you might be planning to keep an eye on that to make sure it doesn't become a problem. I'm wondering, if you decided to, how you might go about monitoring your drinking?

Exercise 5.4, Scenario 2 (Interpersonal Violence)

This middle-aged man is being seen by a child welfare professional after child protective services were called by a neighbor. There was an altercation in the home, and he struck his girlfriend as well as his son. The school has reported previous incidents of bruises, but there has been no formal intervention until now. He's been ordered to treatment and can only have supervised meetings with their two children (8 and 5 years old) until the child welfare professional indicates that it is safe for them to be alone with him. The target behaviors in this instance are making changes in how he manages conflict with his girlfriend and children. As with the last scenario, when you read the dialogue this time, focus on the practitioner's activities and provide alternative responses.

P: I understand that you're not very happy about being here today.

What's another way you might start this conversation about interpersonal violence?

C: Damn straight. The cops didn't listen to my side of the story after the neighbors called them. They just hauled me off to jail, and now they tell me I have to come talk to you if I want to see my kids without a social worker.

P: Nobody has really taken the time to find out how you see the situation. I wonder if we could spend a little time doing that.

If you were to attend to another part of this statement, what would it be? Why? What would you say?

(cont.)

C: Whatever.

P: What is concerning you now about your situation with your girlfriend and kids?

Is this client working with the practitioner? Why or why not? What would you say to help this relationship become more collaborative?

C: I can't see them, except with somebody there. My kids don't understand it. They're like, "Why can't you stay at the house, Dad?" I usually help my son with his math homework, and I can't do that now and their mom just isn't very good at that stuff.

P: Being a part of their lives is important to you. You want that and can't do that now—in the way you'd like.

The practitioner chooses one aspect of the client statement. What other aspects might be productive? How would you address these? Or, if you addressed the same issue, how might you do it differently?

C: Yeah, most of the time. Sometimes they can be annoying, but most of the time it's good.

P: And what about your partner?

The practitioner shifts the focus to the partner. If you were to respond to the client's statement, what would you say?

C: She's pissed at me. She says I hurt her, but she hit me, too. She says I don't care about her or the kids and that's just not true. She doesn't back off sometimes, though. That's what happened that night. I told her to leave me alone. I left the room and she followed me into another. I went out to the garage and she came out there. It was embarrassing. The neighbors could hear. Finally, I went back inside and told her to knock it off. Then she slapped me, and I guess that was the straw that broke the camel's back. I just kind of swung with my backhand to keep her away and she must have been off balance because she fell. I didn't mean to hit Danny; he just stepped in at the wrong time when she was coming back at me. I was trying to say I was sorry, and she was scratching and hitting and I don't quite know what happened.

P: It seems like you're feeling bad about how things went there. It's not how you want to handle things with your girlfriend. You want to have better control than that.

The practitioner takes a pretty big guess. Does it fit for you? Is this a helpful direction? If not, what might you do instead?

C: Yeah. I'm not some ogre like these folks are making me out to be. I really tried to avoid a problem there. She just wouldn't back off!

P: That's not the kind of person you are or how you want others to view you.

The practitioner acknowledges the client's focus on being misunderstood. What's another way you might address that statement?

C: I wish we could talk out our problems, but we seem to get too mad. We need to do something different.

P: Let me see if I have all of this. You're not happy to be here, and at the same time you're not happy about how things went the other night. You want to be able to talk about things, and yet sometimes it feels like there is just no way that can happen. Then you do things you regret. It's clear to you that something has to change.

What would your summary look like?

Key for Exercise 5.4, Scenario 2 (Interpersonal Violence)

P: I understand that you're not very happy about being here today.

Commentary: You might say, "Tell me about your understanding of what this is all about?"

C: Damn straight. The cops didn't listen to my side of the story after the neighbors called them. They just hauled me off to jail, and now they tell me I have to come talk to you if I want to see my kids without a social worker.

P: Nobody has really taken the time to find out how you see the situation. I wonder if we could spend a little time doing that.

Commentary: Here are a couple of alternatives: "And being in jail is something you don't want to repeat." Or, "It feels like you're being treated like a child." Or, "You sound frustrated."

C: Whatever.

P: What is concerning you now about your situation with your girlfriend and kids?

Commentary: It seems like they are not working collaboratively. The client communicates disinterest in the process and asserts that you can't make him do anything. It might be useful to address this directly, though it will keep you focused on the resistant element if you don't use a strategy to move away from that. (This topic is discussed more in Chapter 6.) You might acknowledge the obvious and then ask a question that shifts the focus: "I want to be clear that what happens with these sessions is really up to you. I won't try to force you to do anything. I'm wondering, what would need to happen for this session to feel useful to you?"

C: I can't see them, except with somebody there. My kids don't understand it. They're like, "Why can't you stay at the house, Dad?" I usually help my son with his math homework, and I can't do that now and their mom just isn't very good at that stuff.

P: Being a part of their lives is important to you. You want that and can't do that now—in the way you'd like.

Commentary: You could focus on how he responds to his kids' questions by asking "What is that like for you when your kids ask you those hard questions?" You might also ask what he might be doing now, if he could do what he wanted with his children: "What would you like to be doing with your children, but can't?" You might use a readiness ruler to ascertain how important it is to him to make changes so that he can be with his children in the manner he wants.

C: Yeah, most of the time. Sometimes they can be annoying, but most of the time it's good.

P: And what about your partner?

Commentary: You might say, "It's not perfect, and you really want to get back there."

Key for Exercise 5.4, Scenario 2 (*cont.*)

C: She's pissed at me. She says I hurt her, but she hit me, too. She says I don't care about her or the kids and that's just not true. She doesn't back off sometimes, though. That's what happened that night. I told her to leave me alone. I left the room and she followed me into another. I went out to the garage and she came out there. It was embarrassing. The neighbors could hear. Finally, I went back inside and told her to knock it off. Then she slapped me, and I guess that was the straw that broke the camel's back. I just kind of swung with my backhand to keep her away and she must have been off balance because she fell. I didn't mean to hit Danny; he just stepped in at the wrong time when she was coming back at me. I was trying to say I was sorry, and she was scratching and hitting and I don't quite know what happened.

P: It seems like you're feeling bad about how things went there. It's not how you want to handle things with your girlfriend. You want to have better control than that.

Commentary: This practitioner response seems on target and helpful. It might also be useful to focus on his feelings afterward: "She was bugging you, and you knew right away that what you did was not right. Then it got worse when Danny was hit. It sounds like you don't want to end up back there again."

C: Yeah. I'm not some ogre like these folks are making me out to be. I really tried to avoid a problem there. She just wouldn't back off!

P: That's not the kind of person you are or how you want others to view you.

Commentary: A double-sided reflection might work well: "You're not an ogre, and you know that you're not happy with how you responded. Nobody has to tell you that." Or you could use a looking-forward technique: "If you look forward 5 years and nothing changes, what do you see happening in your family?" Or, "If you were able to make some changes in what you do, what would your family look like in 5 years?"

C: I wish we could talk out our problems, but we seem to get too mad. We need to do something different.

P: Let me see if I have all of this. You're not happy to be here, and at the same time you're not happy about how things went the other night. You want to be able to talk about things, and yet sometimes it feels like there is just no way that can happen. Then you do things you regret. It's clear to you that something has to change.

Commentary: Here is an alternative:

You'd like things to be different; you're just not sure how to get there. You know that you have a part in all of this, and you really tried to avoid a problem. You're still a little annoyed at having to do all of this, and you'd like some tools so you don't have to do it again. What's the next step look like?

Write a Branching Script

In this exercise you will write a script that branches in various directions. The codes for those directions are preestablished, and you will have to decide client and practitioner statements that fit each box.

Begin by looking over the following sample to see how practitioner behaviors and client statements lead down different paths. A white box indicates that the client responded positively to the practitioner intervention. A gray response would be neutral. A diagonally lined response indicates that the client is not moving with the practitioner. Notice how the statements in the sample match the different client codes.

Once you feel clear about the codes, decide what the focus of this discussion is and what the circumstances are. On the diagram, write in what the practitioner would say. Then use the pattern to determine what type of client response to write. Again, a white response would indicate that the client responded positively to the practitioner intervention. A gray response would be neutral. A diagonally lined response indicates that the client is not moving with the practitioner. Then write a practitioner response that might follow. Note that at the fourth level the client responses branch again, so write a practitioner response in each box that might result in the type of response observed.

The reason for doing this exercise is not to generate the perfect script, but rather to understand what types of practitioner statements might lead to specific client statements. When the client box indicates client change talk, make sure that you include the type of response that would elicit this type of response.

You can try to work in some of the strategies for eliciting change talk, though you may need to go a few iterations beyond what is drawn to make these work sensibly. You can always draw rectangles and lines on a blank sheet to create these extra spaces.

Example for Exercise 5.5

Area of Concern: Diabetes

Practitioner: I understand your blood glucose levels have been running high.

Branch 1:

C: Much higher than these usually are. That's not good.

P: You're a little worried about these.

C: I know I can do better. I just need to get refocused.

P: You know what you need to do.

C: Yeah. I've had pretty good control in the past. Things just got out of balance.

P: What would it take for you to begin this process?

C: I guess just putting a plan together and then starting.

C: I'm not sure that I'd say *worried*.

P: Worried is a little too strong.

C: A little.

P: Maybe not worried, but you are paying attention. What about it has your attention?

C: I know the long-term risks if I don't take care of it.

Branch 2:

C: Yeah, my doc is a little worried.

P: And maybe you are too.

C: Yeah, a little I guess.

P: What do you think you might do about this?

C: At this point, I have no clue.

P: You might like to do something; you're just not sure how to start.

C: Exactly. I'm feeling a little adrift.

C: I'm not worried.

P: You wouldn't go so far as to say *worried*.

C: More like taking notice.

P: And being serious about it.

C: I guess I am taking it seriously or I wouldn't have come.

Branch 3:

C: I think the doc overreacted.

P: He's making too much out of it.

C: A little, but I appreciate his concern.

P: So, you're glad he's looking out for you.

C: I don't know that in this case I'm so glad.

P: But here you are. Given our time here, what would you like to do with it?

C: I don't know. I've never been in this situation before.

C: He didn't even bother to find out why.

P: And you think he should have.

C: Damn right, before he sends me off to talk to you.

P: You sound pretty annoyed.

C: Yeah. I guess I am.

Worksheet for Exercise 5.5

Area of Concern: _____

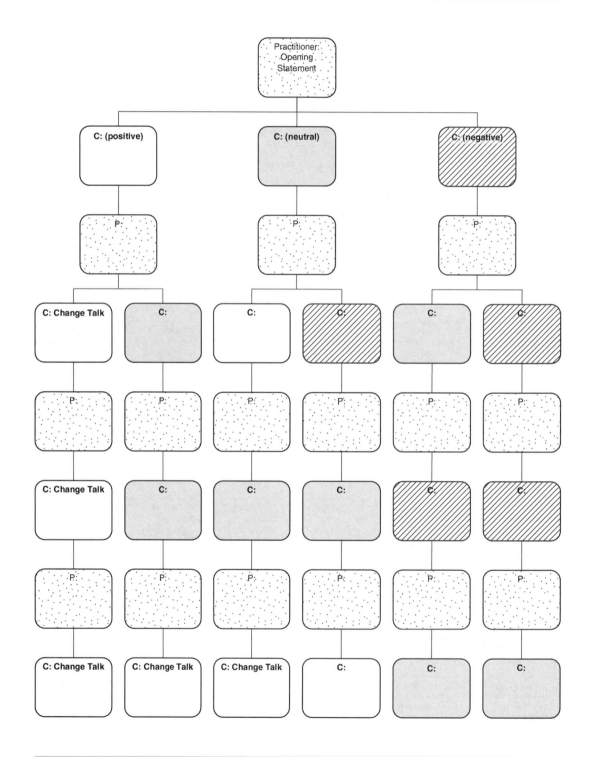

Drumming for Change[3]

This activity requires a partner. Below is a list of client statements about behaviors related to diabetes management. Most behaviors that improve health (e.g., weight loss, healthy and moderate eating, exercise, stopping smoking, moderate to no drinking) also assist in glycemic control (i.e., keeping blood sugars within a specific, healthy range). Have your partner read the list aloud. Every time you hear preparatory talk about making changes in health (DARN), drum. This form of change talk is underlined. Mobilizing language (commitment talk or taking steps), which is *italicized*, should draw polishing motions (i.e., hands together as though praying and rubbing your palms together in circular motions, as though polishing a pearl). Statements that are neither preparatory nor mobilizing draw no response. If you disagree, stop and talk about it with your partner. Figure out where the confusion came from, then go on. Alternate turns drumming and reading.

I hate all the poking for blood I have to do.

I want to be like everybody else.

Some folks are worried about my eating, but I don't think it's a big deal.

I am tired of all the trouble my high blood sugars are causing.

If my partner would stop nagging me about it, I would eat better.

I brought out the rowing machine and rowed while watching TV.

I'm doing the best I can.

I've lost 2.4 pounds this week.

When I reach 10 pounds, it will be time for celebration.

I need to eat more fruits and vegetables.

I'm doing just fine.

I checked my blood sugars before every meal yesterday.

I'd like to quit smoking.

I am not giving up ice cream.

I hate having to inject myself in restaurant bathrooms.

My doctor is monitoring my eyes for glaucoma.

My feet are tingling more, and I've lost sensation in part of my right foot.

Starting tomorrow, I will get up at 5 A.M. to walk.

I think I can eat better, it's just a matter of making up my mind.

I was just out dancing.

The hardest part is starting. Once I'm going, I'm OK.

I want to be a healthy role model for my kids.

I passed up seconds and had fruit for dessert.

---

[3]Thanks to Steve Berg-Smith for this exercise.

(*cont.*)

I want to get a simple meal plan together.

I know I've lost a lot of weight, but I needed to.

I'm good.

My A1c is at 7.9, and I like to keep it below 7.0.

I'd like to fix better meals, but I don't have enough time to even think sometimes.

A little treat every once in a while is no big deal.

I don't like taking medications.

I hate doing it, but I know I just have to get up earlier if I'm going to exercise.

I started using a salad plate, instead of a dinner plate, to limit my meal size.

I tried eating vegetable and fruit snacks in the morning and afternoon.

At this point, smoking is all I've got.

I know I should quit drinking, because it will help my control, but I just love a cold beer after a tough day.

I suppose I could take the dog for a little longer walk in the evening.

I think my husband would support it.

I checked my blood glucose four times yesterday.

I drank five beers last night and watched a movie.

You only live once. *C'est la vie!*

I made an appointment to see my doc.

I guess I just like watching TV.

I love real cheese.

I went to the gym three times last week.

I told my friends it was none of their business how much I ate.

I went for a run instead.

I'd like the house to be cleaner.

It just feels so pointless trying to make changes now.

I can't wait until the kids are older, then I can really focus on getting healthier.

Even if my partner won't do it, I'm going to start dishing out smaller portions.

I know how to lose the weight, it's just keeping it off that's hard.

So, I set up a schedule for the meals, and it's been a lot easier to eat right.

Sometimes I think it's not possible, but then I stop myself and remind myself I can eat better.

Tomorrow's the day I start running.

Help!

Chapter 6

Managing Resistance

Opening

Sean sat in the conference room with his head hanging. The school principal, directly and not unkindly, presented the reasons for the meeting: to understand what had happened and find an appropriate course of action. In addition to Sean and the administrator, present were his mother, two police detectives, his academic advisor, and a counselor. A gifted athlete with a capable intellect, Sean had struggled to find his way at this school and now had been accused of possible criminal behavior on campus. His youthful bravado was crumbling beneath his mother's withering glare. Clearly at a crossroads, growth still seemed possible as he mumbled through a cursory review of what had happened. The detective, unhappy with Sean's degree of disclosure, decided more pressure was required to force open the small crack beginning to show on Sean's face. The detective recited the possible charges and accompanying sentences, if Sean didn't come clean and were tried as an adult. His mother's disappointment and anger, emblazoned on her face only moments early, shifted to a worried furrow. Concerned for her son's freedom, she wondered aloud about needing an attorney. The detective, acknowledging her right to make that choice, pressed on.

Then, it happened. Barely discernible, but there it was. Sean flexed his jaw muscle. Where there had been uncertainty only a moment before, there was resolution now. The harder the detective pushed, the tighter he clamped. His mother, furious with him only moments before, now turned her anger on the school and the detective. The principal, walking a tightrope between the safety needs of the school and a learning opportunity for this student, was knocked free of his line by the mother's request to adjourn to consult an attorney. The other detective, perhaps waiting to play good cop, never said a word.

The practitioner followed Sean and his mother into the hall and asked to speak to them briefly. It was fairly clear that Sean had engaged in the alleged behavior. The evidence, including his statements to peers, was overwhelming as to his culpability. It was also new behavior, according to other students. He was a hurt and troubled young man from a single-parent family in which his mother struggled to fulfill all roles and make ends meet. In previous chats with Sean, it had become clear that trust was a central issue. It was also evident that this would be the practitioner's last chance to talk to him, given what had just transpired. At 17, it might also be Sean's last chance to look inward at his choices and his life direction, before incurring adult consequences.

After informing them that this was a clinical discussion and would not be shared with the people in the conference room, the practitioner apologized for the direction the meeting had gone. It was not the intent of the principal for this meeting to have been so adversarial. Then the practitioner empathized with Sean and his mother: "You both must be scared to death about what might happen." The shift was immediate. Sean's jaw relaxed, his mother's shoulders dropped. Then the practitioner asked permission to offer a word of advice. They agreed and so the practitioner said, "Sean, people make mistakes, but those mistakes don't have to define who they are and what they become. From what you've told me before, this behavior is not the person you want to be. You've told me about other, bigger hopes and dreams. Regardless of what happens in there, you still have an opportunity to choose the type of person you become. What do you think about that?" Sean mumbled a noncommittal, "I don't know." Time was up. Sean's mother was dialing the attorney as the practitioner walked away; Sean was looking out the window. They returned shortly to tell the group that the meeting was over, and all future meetings would happen only with an attorney present. Sean, already suspended, withdrew from school a few days later.

Clearly, this meeting didn't go as anyone had hoped. What might have been done differently?

A Deeper Look

In Chapter 5 we focused on indicators that change might occur. In this chapter our attention shifts to markers that indicate change is *unlikely* to occur. Miller and Rollnick (2002) have struggled to define what these markers reflect. Originally, they used the term *resistance* but over time have become dissatisfied with this label. Most recently, they and other MI trainers have begun to differentiate between statements that reflect active resistance to interventions and those that express acceptance or benefits of the status quo.

Miller, Moyers, Amrhein, and Rollnick (2006) suggest that this type of client language should be referred to as *sustain talk* and note parallels with forms of change talk. Specifically, the client expresses (1) a desire to sustain the status quo, (2) an inability to change, (3) the benefits of the current situation, or (4) a need for the status quo. They also note that commitment talk for the status quo also occurs.

A desire for things to stay the same is not an uncommon experience. Graduation each year is a reminder of children growing up and venturing into the world. As much as parents nurture and encourage growth, development, and independence, there may also be a part of us that will miss them terribly and therefore wishes it wouldn't occur. Similarly, when clients have change thrust upon them by others or by circumstances, they may lament the possibility of losing the status quo. Even when this is not the case, clients might still wish they didn't have to give up all aspects of a particular behavior. In the realm of addictions, this idea is expressed in the quip that clients don't want to give up their addictions, just the consequences of them. This connection to the status quo is the expression of the other side of ambivalence.

There are many reasons why clients might not want to give up the current situation. They may believe that their strengths, skills, and abilities lie within these domains only. For example, they know how to function within a substance-abusing world. They may know how to get money, how to acquire drugs, and how to maintain relative safety while doing so. In contrast, they may know little about functioning in other parts of the world or without substances. Their knowledge and skills lie within a world they know, even as they may recognize that it does not serve them well.

Clients may have little hope that things could improve. Either change is not possible or even, if possible, unlikely to result in a better situation. Salespeople, for example, may stay in a job with an overbearing boss because their experience indicates that bosses are always this way. There is no reason to expect that a job change would lead to a better situation. Better the devil you know. …

There may be things that the client receives from their situation as currently configured. Homebound individuals with agoraphobia do not have to face the fear-inducing situations as long as they stay home. The immediate benefits of staying home seem to far outweigh the long-term benefits of greater freedom and choice.

Clients might also observe the disadvantages of change. After all, *risks* are associated with changing. If jobless clients decide to return to work, they may trade financial benefits as well as considerable free time for what may be a low-paying, high-effort, and minimum-respect job. Risks might also be intrapersonal in nature. The effects of trying and failing may be much worse to the client's sense of self-competence and self-esteem than is the self-derogation that accompanies the current situation.

These types of client views would indicate that they are thinking about or committed to things as these currently stand. Although they might consider making a change, change is unlikely to occur as long as these status quo factors outweigh the benefits or needs for change. These client statements represent one aspect that weighs down the "against change" side of the ambivalence scale. In contrast, resistance involves an active *pushing against* the practitioner personally, even in its apparently passive form. For example, what appears to be compliance can be a form of resistance. Let's look at my personal interactions with a health care provider as a case example.

She was a well-meaning, dedicated individual who, I'm sure, was very frustrated with my diabetes management at times. She would praise me for my efforts at improved self-care, but also scold me for areas that needed improvement. While my A1c control was generally good, there was room for improvement. At first I tried to explain to her why her suggestions were difficult for me to implement. I'm sure that my behavior looked like active resistance. My frequent "Yes, but … " responding she knew well. Her response was to reemphasize the importance to my long-term health and to warn me of possible dire consequences (all of which were true, and I was well aware of them). Over time, I learned that she really did not understand my situation, and although her heart was good, her aim was bad. It was just easier to agree to her suggestions and state that I would try, rather than endure extended lectures. So, that's what I did. On the surface our interactions were friendly, and although I listened to her suggestions without argument, I rarely implemented them in the manner she specified.

A more active form of resistance occurs when the client directly argues with the practitioner. He may argue that the "driving under the influence" (DUI) results are wrong. She may contend that the practitioner doesn't know about this type of child, who needs a firm hand (bolstered by a hard smack) to show that you mean business. He may believe that playing video games and instant messaging have no direct influence on his study habits and resent your implication that these are linked. She may talk over you, contending that "hooking up really" is a low-risk activity. He may believe that every fall most people become more irritable and moody as they're forced to spend time indoors and refuse to talk about seasonal depression. She may discount your expression of concern and contend that everything is fine as she juggles three children, a full-time job, multiple volunteer activities, and seeing friends regularly, even as her partner complains about the pace and their lack of couple time. Not only have we heard these things, we've probably done them as well.

Unfortunately with clients, we've tended to label these behaviors as expressions of denial. The reality seems evident to us, but the other person just doesn't see it that way. In contrast, when it's our own denial under review we readily see the reality of the environmental pressures that influence our behavior. Social psychologists have labeled this phenomenon the *fundamental attribution error* (as well as the correspondence bias or overattribution effect; Jones & Harris, 1967; Ross, 1977). That is, when we observe others, we tend to give greater weight to internal attributes leading to behavior and underestimate the effects of the environment. In contrast, when we observe our own behavior, we give much greater weight to environmental influences and less to our characteristics.

It's not much of a surprise, then, that clients may discount or ignore practitioners. We just don't understand from their point of view. I once watched a young man, forced to see me, spin in his chair for an entire 50 minutes without talking. Clearly, he wished to communicate that even though he had to be there, I couldn't make him talk. I had gotten the message pretty clearly after about 10 minutes, but he sized me up as a slow learner and decided I needed the whole hour to get the message straight. During the next session, we left the therapy room and shot baskets on a nearby playground; then he was quite willing to talk. Apparently having set the ground rules, and with a change in venue, he was ready to chat.

Clients may also interrupt or talk over practitioners. This situation is often evident in classrooms where teachers are struggling to maintain control. The more the teacher tries to clamp down on this kind of behavior, the stronger becomes the response. Another common example is discounting the counselor. The client may say, "What do you know? How could you understand me?" An adolescent client once asked me, "What are you, my rent-a-friend?" Resistance may also present as a filibuster: The client takes the floor and refuses to yield. This can happen in groups where one member monopolizes the time, and others simply cede the control or actively look to their peer to take the focus from themselves.

Finally, clients can simply change the subject. My youngest child, a preschooler, is a master at this activity.

"OK. Your 5 minutes are up. It's bath time."

"Five more minutes."

"No, we already did 5 minutes."

"Have you seen my stick pony?"

"No, and it's bath time. I gave you the extra 5 minutes, so let's hit the tub."

"My pony's name is Cotton Candy."

"Yeah. I know. Hi, Cotton Candy. Why don't you ride her up to the tub?"

"I love you, Dad. I want to give you a big kiss … and now a hug. … "

"Thank you. It's still bath time."

"Five more minutes."

Clearly, I am overmatched. Which leads us to the question, so what do you do with sustain talk and resistance? While it may be tempting to try to bust through it, such a strategy is rarely helpful from an MI perspective. Instead, the recommendations involve returning to familiar skills and adding a few strategies.

In training, I focus on three reflective listening skills. First, use simple reflections. These skills keep the conversation in motion and allow you to direct it, depending on the elements you address. Simple reflections can be helpful with sustain talk, and they are particularly useful with strong resistance that leaves you temporarily flustered or even discombobulated. When a client hits you with a jolting statement, a simple reflection can buy you some time as you figure out how you might proceed more effectively. For example, a client who says "I'm going to drink myself to death" may leave you very uncertain of how to proceed; a safe response might be, "You are going to drink till you die." This response does not change meaning and stays close to the client's words. Even a minor shift in the simple reflection focus may alter client perspective, "At this point, you are going to drink till you die." The phrase *at this point* opens the door to other possible futures.

Amplified reflections are also very helpful in responding to statements endorsing the status quo. These skills allow you to "press" on sustain talk to determine the degree of commitment to the statement, as well as to explore the person's intent. For our client who says "I'm going to drink myself to death," an amplified response might be "You can't see any purpose in living." This statement presses the client to see if there is really no reason or simply to see if the preponderance of evidence is falling in one direction. It may also point to aspects that are more ambivalent.

A final reflective skill is the double-sided reflection that contrasts the status quo with other elements clients have shared, might possibly consider, or are implied within their statements. Again, to our client intent on drinking until she dies, we might say "So at this point you're feeling this way, and you haven't always felt this way." An alternative response is "For now, you expect to die drinking, and on the other hand, you recognize that you might change your mind."

A number of strategic elements can be used to respond to resistance and sustain talk. I most commonly teach two: recognizing personal choice and control and shifting focus. Both approaches may utilize OARS microskills, but they also include a strategic choice to alter the interaction pattern.

I have always found it helpful to make the obvious *obvious*.[1] That is, name whatever is happening or is influencing the situation but has not been acknowledged so that it can

---

[1] Thanks to Dennis Donovan for teaching me this pearl of wisdom.

be addressed directly. In this instance, making the obvious obvious involves reminding clients that only they can choose to change their behavior. In the end, it is entirely up to each individual to decide if a change is needed and how that change will happen. Even in situations where people appear to have little choice, they still choose—even if passively. For example, the alleged DUI driver may choose to go to jail rather than accept treatment. Some clients will grumble that they don't have a choice. They must do this—whatever *this* is—or else some unwanted consequence will befall them. The temptation is to argue that it's still a choice (I certainly have done so). You are served much better, however, by using your OARS:

"It feels like a really crummy choice to you. What do you think you'll do?"

"I guess I'll do it."

"You don't really want to."

"Isn't that obvious?"

"It really makes you mad that you're in this circumstance."

"It pisses me off when people tell me what to do."

"And that's how it feels now, even though you know that only you can decide if you'll go along with the treatment or not."

This type of interchange is not uncommon, and although the client is unsatisfied with the direction he chooses, this approach allows the practitioner to come alongside the client as he faces this unwanted decision. This position is better suited, from a MI perspective, for helping the client move forward than an adversarial position wherein the practitioner continues to assert a limit.

The second strategy is one of shifting the focus. This approach acknowledges that we've run into an area that doesn't feel like it will be productive. So, as a result, we shift focus to an area that may be more helpful or productive for the client. This shift is typically accomplished by either a reflection or a summary, followed by a question. Continuing the dialogue from the last example, a shift in focus might go like this.

"And that's how it feels now, even though you know that only you can decide if you'll go along with the treatment or not."

"Yeah, I guess."

"So, you're not crazy about the choice, but it seems like for now you've decided to hang with this—at least for awhile longer. I wonder what *for you* would be helpful to spend time on today. What would need to happen for you to leave today and feel like you got something from this?"

Bill Miller, in a video demonstration of the use of MI with a man talking about how cigarette and alcohol use affect his life (i.e., the soccer guy), uses a simple question to shift focus (i.e., "What would you like to be different?"). Terri Moyers, in her video with a man presenting for a DUI evaluation (i.e., "the Rounder"), asks, "What would you like to do here today?" Steve Rollnick uses a prop—an agenda menu—from which clients can choose an area of focus. This menu includes blank items where the client determines what should be inserted. Contained within these queries is a joining process wherein clients are asked to choose a direction and the practitioner respects clients' ability to decide what they need.

Some practitioners might worry that clients will take a totally inappropriate focus to avoid dealing with "the problem." When clients choose a direction that seems off-task, clinicians may feel compelled to redirect the conversation to the problem area. We'll address this concern in more depth in Chapter 7 when the issue of agenda setting is discussed, and Chapter 9, when expressing a concern is a focus. For now, suffice it to say that MI respects that clients make the choices and that it must be *their* agenda, not ours, if change is to occur. If we insist on this session focus or on a particular change, we are more likely to get, at most, temporary compliance than true change.

Other strategies for managing resistance or sustain talk—reframing, agreement with a twist, and siding with the negative—represent skillful forms of reflective listening. These approaches require that practitioners employ reflections deftly and on demand so that when the need arises, these can be done naturally, with empathy. The goal is not to make clients comfortable but instead to bring them face to face with difficulty realities (which may be at odds with their position) without engendering more resistance. These techniques require considerable skillfulness and are the reason that I typically reserve them for more advanced MI training. In practice, these strategies tend to emerge more spontaneously and without intention from the practitioner, perhaps with the exception of siding with the negative.

The first strategy is reframing. A reframe places a client's statement in a new light, a new perspective. This approach often involves taking the resistant or the sustain talk element and recasting it. Holding one's liquor, for example, is addressed as tolerance and the risks associated with that condition made explicit. Or reluctance to come to a session is recast as strength in pushing forward despite concerns. Or multiple past failures in changing behavior are reframed as continued commitment to making life better. In the context of the prior dialogue, reframing might look like this:

"It feels like a really crummy choice to you. What do you think you'll do?"

"I guess I'll do it."

"You don't really want to."

"Isn't that obvious?"

"So, you're the kind of guy who can decide what needs to be done and do it—even when you don't like it. That seems like a real strength that probably has served you well over your life."

Agreement with a twist typically involves a simple reflection followed by a reframe. It might also be a complex reflection or might not even be a reflection at all, but just agreement, "I think you're right." Regardless of specific form, the interaction begins with a statement that appears very consistent with what the client has just said and then, by virtue of the reframe, the client "lands" in a totally unexpected direction. The original metaphor that Miller and Rollnick (1991) used to explain this technique was jujitsu (a martial art) wherein an aggressor's energy is not opposed but instead redirected. However, concerned with the power dynamics inherent in this analogy, Miller and Rollnick (2002) moved away from it and toward the image of ballroom dancing wherein the slight presses and pulls by the lead dancer direct the pair to move in new directions. Regardless of the analogy, the underlying idea is the same: Do not oppose energy; instead, gently redirect it in productive ways. An example of an agreement with a twist might look like this in our prior exchange:

"It pisses me off when people tell me what to do."

"It makes you mad, particularly because you know when you are making good choices and when you aren't—you don't need anyone to tell you that."

The first sentence is a simple reflection, whereas the second inserts an element not directly expressed but implicit in the client's statements. The result: The client's energy is now focused in a new direction—making good choices.

As can be seen in this repeated exchange, multiple directions can be used to respond to sustain talk or resistance. As noted earlier, when resistance is particularly strong or unbalances the practitioner, it's usually easiest to begin with a simple reflection that allows time to regain footing. It is also typically true that a single exchange does not entirely drain resistance of its power; instead, a series of exchanges is needed. So the first response does not have to be perfect but rather sets a beginning course. Finally, if not already evident, it should be noted that resistance takes considerable energy to sustain. If the practitioner does not push against this energy, the resistance often drops—sometimes relatively quickly. Or as my mother liked to say, when my brother and I would fight and then blame each other for the scrap, "It takes two to tango."

Finally, there is siding with the negative or coming alongside. This is not reverse psychology, as noted in Chapter 5. Rather, it is a simple acknowledgment that this may not be the right time, place, or circumstance for change. I teach this technique only in advanced trainings because it can leave practitioners and clients in the unfortunate position of feeling stuck. Although sometimes feeling stuck can be quite helpful—to fully experience the discomfort of current circumstances in order to mobilize client resources for change—it can also leave new practitioners unsure of what to do next. For example, an exchange might go like this:

"It's hopeless. Seems like there's no point in changing now."

"So maybe that train has left the station."

The hope in providing this type of reflection is that the client will more fully explore the situation and determine if the conclusion drawn is a correct one. This requires that the practitioner be able to sit with this discomfort—which can be quite challenging. In the Edinburgh interview (see Appendix B), we observe an MI clinician sitting with a client who says that he expects to drink himself to death, just as his father before him did. Through the process of accepting this position and then exploring it further, we observe this practitioner and client move to a much more hopeful position. In an accompanying commentary, we learn about how uncomfortable this process was for the clinician, even as she maintained her MI-consistent stance.

This approach does not have to be dramatic, however. Returning to our now familiar dialogue, the exchange might go like this.

"It feels like a really crummy choice to you. What do you think you'll do?"

"I guess I'll do it."

"Well, you could. On the other hand, you might decide you're willing to pay the price because it's that important to you to *not* feel pressured into a choice."

Again, attitude is critically important. Any sense of sarcasm or manipulation on the part of the practitioner and the client will react strongly. The practitioner must be genuine.

Concept Quiz—Test Yourself!

True or false:

1. T F   Self-perception theory holds that having clients argue against a position will change their attitudes about the position, if they're ambivalent and don't feel compelled to make this argument by someone.

2. T F   Sustain talk and resistance are the same thing.

3. T F   There are parallel forms of change and sustain talk.

4. T F   More sustain talk than change talk suggests change is unlikely to happen.

5. T F   Creating a safe, supportive environment may be enough to encourage clients to begin talking about change when you have a lot of time, but it doesn't work when people could die from their behavior. Then you must bust through their denial and talk reality about the situation.

6. T F   Reflections alone may be enough to reduce client resistance.

7. T F   Amplified reflections may be especially helpful when clients talk in absolutes.

8. T F   Simple reflections are often very helpful with an angry client.

9. T F   Emphasizing personal choice involves directing the client's attention to the truth: Only he or she can make the decision to change.

10. T F   Siding with the negative and an amplified reflection both press clients to step away from an absolute position.

Answers

1. T   This is a continuation of the issues noted in Chapter 5. It points out why we don't wish to strengthen resistance but instead "roll with it." Rather than engaging in an argument, we find another approach—including understanding the client's position.

2. F   Increasingly, MI experts differentiate these two types of behavior. In a consensus statement about change talk, Miller, Moyers, et al. (2006) recommend that trainers use sustain talk to identify client statements that favor maintaining the status quo and use resistance to describe client behavior that signals "dissonance" in the clinical relationship itself.

3. T   Desire, ability, reason, and need for things to stay the same, as well as commitment to sustaining current behavior, may all describe client statements about sustaining the status quo, according to the change talk consensus statement (Miller, Moyers, et al., 2006).

4. T   This is generally true. However, it may not be the exact amounts of each that matter, but rather their trajectory over the course of a session. If there is a lot of sustain talk and very little change talk, at the beginning, but then sustain talk diminishes while change talk rises then change is more likely. Further research is needed to confirm this trajectory, though initial data from Amrhein and colleagues (Amrhein et al., 2003) suggests this might be so. Nevertheless, in general, more sustain than change talk indicates that change is less likely.

5. F   Sometimes clinicians can see the benefits of MI in "counseling" situations but feel that it may not be enough when there is great risk. Although Miller and Rollnick might agree that a more advice-giving, directive role may be needed in some situations, this would not lead them to endorse an aggressive denial-busting approach. Instead, they would argue that advising can be done in a variety of ways, some of which will be more effective than others. A denial-busting mode, in contrast, is likely to engender resistance, and resistance is likely to lead to worse outcomes. Sean's example, from the beginning of the chapter, illustrates the peril in this approach. Miller (personal communication, July 25, 2008) notes, "If you have very little time in which to evoke behavior change, you don't have time *not* to listen!"

6. T   Skillful reflections often have the effect of reducing resistance. Remember, it is tough to sustain resistance without someone pushing against it. If the practitioner's reflections do not push against the resistance, then the energy is likely to dissipate.

7. T   Amplified reflections can be very useful when clients take a particularly strong stance. The amplified reflection often "presses against" the resistant element in a client statement. Many times (though not always) this approach will cause the client to back away from the absolute. If the person does not, it means that your reflection was simply accurate. It may be time to shift focus.

8. T   Simple reflections are a helpful place to start with angry clients. Typically, the practitioner will move on to other types of reflections as the interchange progresses, but this is a very good place to begin. Remember, *simple* is not the same as *easy*, and there is skill required in what the practitioner decides to attend to.

9. T   We are just making the obvious obvious. Although there may be contingencies present, it is still be up to clients to decide if they will go with the reinforcements or press against the consequences.

10. T   Amplified reflections involve pushing on the resistance or sustain element with the intent of moving a client away from an absolute position. Siding with the negative involves agreeing that this may not be the right time, place, or method for change, again with the intent of nudging the client to explore this idea more fully.

In Practice

Arthur is a 15-year-old adolescent who had recently broken up with his girlfriend. He came not because of his interest or need, but because of his parents' concern. Let's look at this initial encounter in light of the issues and techniques just discussed.

Statement	*Commentary*
P: Thanks for spending that time reviewing the consent with your dad in the room. I can see from your face, you're not too keen on being here.	Begins with a brief acknowledgment, then an affective reflection of facial expression. Notice how the emotion is understated.
C: You got that right. This is my parents' idea. I don't need to be here.	Client agrees and adds a bit more information.
P: So you didn't have much choice.	Rephrase.
C: More like *any* choice. They told me I had to come.	Affect is still high, but the client is engaging with the practitioner.
P: Or else ...	Continuing the paragraph.
C: I would lose my drums, which would really piss me off.	Client reveals something he values.
P: So you weren't happy about coming, and you also didn't want to lose your drums.	Double-sided reflection.
C: Exactly.	He feels understood, and his affect is beginning to lessen. Notice, no questions have been asked yet.
P: I wonder if you had some thoughts about what this might be like—coming to talk to a shrink.	This is an open-ended statement that asks clients to say more, but doesn't pose a question directly. The use of "shrink" is often a good leveling comment with teens. It lets them know you don't take yourself too seriously and that you *might* understand what they're thinking about.
C: I had no clue. I've never done this before. I was wondering if you were going to make me lie down on a couch.	He responds with an affective shift and is now joining with the practitioner.
P: So this was all a mystery.	Rephrase.
C: Yeah.	He is no longer challenging the practitioner and will be more receptive to information about treatment.
P: Is it OK if I share a little information about what happens here?	Closed question that asks for permission to share information.
C: Sure.	Affect may take a tick back up, but he's still following.

Statement	*Commentary*
P: Well, as you can see, I have a couch and you are welcome to lie on it if you like, but that's not usually how I work. More importantly, I want you to know that I will not make you do anything. It's really up to you to decide if this can be useful to you.	Information exchange follows, then a focus on client choice and responsibility.
C: So, I don't have to come here if I don't want to?	As many teens do, he goes to the heart of his concern.
P: From my perspective, you don't. But based on your dad's statements and what you've told me, I am guessing your parents might feel otherwise. I can see that puts you in a dilemma.	Client asked for information and it was provided directly and honestly. This was followed by a reflection based on observation.
C: Yeah. I was not happy about coming, but I also don't want to lose my drums. Can you tell my parents that I don't need to be there?	Client, also honest and direct, asks for what he wants.
P: Well, I can't really do that because at this point, I don't know if you do or don't. Let me ask you a question. What would you need to do or say in order for your parents to no longer think you needed to be here?	Again, direct answer to a direct question. Although a reflection might also work, teens often perceive that strategy as avoiding their question, and this perception damages the rapport. A question then shifts the onus back to the client and in the process shifts the session focus.
C: I don't really know. Maybe be less bummed out around the house.	He supplies the information that he doesn't really know what his parents want, but also admits that some things aren't going as well as he'd like. This is a weak form of change talk.
P: Because you've been feeling pretty sad about the breakup.	Affective reflection that guesses at the reason for the young man's dysphoria and focuses on the change talk. The attention could also have been directed toward finding out what he needed to learn from his parents.

Statement	*Commentary*
C: I mean, it's not as big a deal as my parents think, but we had been going out for quite awhile.	Ambivalence creeps in, but he also acknowledges a loss.
P: So there's a void.	Rephrase.
C: Yeah, and everything is just sort of weird—at school. She's in a bunch of my classes.	More information revealed. He is working with the practitioner now.
P: And you don't know quite how to act around her.	Continuing the paragraph.
C: It feels really awkward …	

Once again, there is interplay between practitioner behaviors and client responses. The effect of doing mostly reflections is an affective shift and a joining together of practitioner and client activity. Although ambivalence still appears, it is not directed toward the practitioner. By the end of this sequence the client has given tacit approval to explore this area further. More information can be collected later, and his parents' expectation can be clarified.

The client presents questions and challenges in this encounter, even when the initial affect had lessened. The practitioner addresses these directly. Often clients ask for things as a way to test the practitioner. I find that direct response followed by some other practitioner activity is the least complicated, easiest, and most respectful way to manage these concerns, especially with teens.

Try This!

Real-time practice—although always important—becomes especially so when dealing with clients who are angry. However, we'll work our way to that point. We begin with a series of exercises in which you will use the same prompts but will be asked to create different responses. Maintaining the same prompts may seem redundant, but it is intentional. Part of the goal here is not only to practice but also demonstrate how there are typically many responses for any client statement. The ability to move easily and fluidly between different types of responses will enhance your ability to work effectively with clients.

After the first three exercises, you will manufacture a list of resistance statements you've heard in your work situation and try to create as many response types as you can. Next, you will generate responses to people's comments on TV or radio talk shows. Finally, you will practice finding the nuggets of possible change within client resistance and status quo statements. This practice will prepare you for that angry encounter, but you will also need to try these techniques in situations where you might have responded to provocation differently.

Since we are all human and therefore err, these opportunities should present themselves with some regularity. Embrace them!

Exercise 6.1. Simple Reflections in Response to Resistance and Status Quo Talk

We'll begin by generating simple reflections to client statements. Write two responses to each, and try to vary the focus.

Exercise 6.2. Double-Sided and Amplified Reflections in Response to Resistance and Status Quo Talk

Using the same prompts as those in Exercise 6.1, try to write one double-sided and one amplified reflection for each prompt.

Exercise 6.3. Other Responses to Resistance and Status Quo Talk

Using the same prompts a third time, try to employ one of the other forms of reflections, as well as personal choice and shifting focus. It may not be possible to use the latter two categories each time without sounding redundant, but try your best.

Exercise 6.4. Your Clients' Resistance and Status Quo Statements

Make a list of status quo or resistance statements you've heard from your clients. Try to fill the sheet provided. Then write as many resistance-lowering responses as you can think of, but do at least three for each statement.

Exercise 6.5. Radio Resistance and Talk Show Hubris

This exercise is a little harder because you have to find a show on which callers or guests tend to be resistant. If you have political debates occurring in your area, you might try to watch, listen, or tape these encounters for practice purposes. Use all of the response types done in the earlier exercises to respond to resistance statements. Once you're well practiced, try listening to people who hold strong but different views from your own. Political talk shows can be a rich source for this kind of material—but, remember, avoid being sarcastic (most of the time).

Exercise 6.6. Practicing with a Client

We all have clients who feel stuck. Spend some time using reflections to understand why they feel stuck. Begin with a preamble: "We've been working for a time now, and it feels as though we are struggling to make headway. It seems like a good time to step back and get a sense of the big picture of your situation. Most often there are reasons why people do things. So, what are the good parts of where you are right now?" Practice the different forms of reflection. Since you don't want to reinforce the status quo only, you should also ask about the less good parts. Remember to use elaboration with the less good parts.

Partner Work

The initial four exercises can be done with your partner as a verbal exercise. That is, one partner says the prompts (use a little Thespian zest here), and the other responds. Begin with simple reflections; once one partner has worked through the form, switch roles. Continue through the sheet a second and a third time practicing the skills described. On the fourth exercise, you should each complete your sheets independently and then take turns providing responses to each other's prompts. Don't forget to try to generate three reflections for each prompt. In all of these exercises the speaker should repeat the prompt between each response.

Exercise 6.7. The Client from Hell—Maybe

Choose someone with whom you have really struggled in your treatment situation, then play this person with your partner so that he or she can practice. Unlike the client from hell, please throw your partner a bone when he or she deserves it. That is, if his or her work begins to soften your resistance or status quo resolve, then go ahead and say so. Also, since this is practice, throw your partner some bones even if his or her attempt is less than perfect. Remember, this is practice! You're trying to learn, not prove something.

Other Thoughts ...

Some MI writers have noted that it is sometimes quite difficult to differentiate sustain talk from early forms of change talk. That is, in statements like, "I can't stand that my PO [probation officer] is making me come here," there might be the start of change talk: "I might come here if my PO didn't make me." These are nuances that MI writers have articulated.

For example, Barth (2006) notes that sustain talk can be a step in the right direction. Specifically, when clients regard a behavior as something that just *is*, not something that is causing them trouble or about which there is any choice; there is no reason to defend it. Our aim is to help them see the problem. Barth indicates it may not be possible to elicit change talk initially, but instead the practitioner may need to aim for developing client openness to ambivalence. Thus, when a client says, "Well, it never occurred to me that it might be an issue, and I don't really see that it is," this may be the beginning of a change process.

This intermixing of concepts (i.e., resistance, sustain, and change talk) can create great difficulties for researchers who wish to parse out the effects of a particular variable, but it is a boon to practitioners. It suggests again that the subtle application of listening skills is extremely important. Practitioners must train their ears to hear these nuances and respond to the change-directed element contained within the resistance or sustain talk statements.

For example, buried within the client response "I've tried everything already, and nothing works" is a clear statement of a desire for change. The person continues to try to change, despite repeated failures. This statement implies that change is very important to this person, even as he or she dismisses the practitioner's statement.

Finally, Allison (2006) notes that engaging in behavior that maintains the status quo can be every bit as heroic as changing, not in terms of the outcome, but in the effort. He suggests that people who engage in resistance are often attempting to sustain what they know is unsustainable. They know their predicament must change, and yet they cling desperately to measures to maintain it—against all odds. Thus, a client says, "I know smoking is killing me, but it feels like my little bit of peace and quiet when I light up and have that first drag." Allison suggests that this type of effort, however misguided we may view it, deserves respect and not a nomenclature that demeans or diminishes it. Labeling something as bad, problematic, or denial does not give clients the full respect of knowing that their position is unsustainable. In Allison's view, labeling this behavior as resistance does not reflect the fact that the client knows it is damaging and that it takes tremendous effort to continue to fight for this bit of "peace and quite." I would add that it implies that we know better, and our job is to help them see their folly. Allison suggests that a more neutral terminology—such as sustain talk—is not only more respectful, but also hopeful. It acknowledges the client's capacities and strengths. So, once again, words matter.

Techniques for Responding to Resistance

You will use this handout for most of the exercises that follow.

Simple reflections stay close in content but keep the conversation moving. Remember to consider carefully on which elements you wish to focus.

Double-sided reflections include both sides of the ambivalence.

Amplified reflections add some intensity to the resistant part of the statement.

Agreement-with-a-twist involves either a reflection or a statement of agreement, followed by a reframe.

Reframing places a client's statement in a new light, a new perspective. This approach often involves recasting the resistant or sustain talk element.

Siding with the negative or **coming alongside** responses acknowledge that this may not be the right time, place, or circumstance for change.

Emphasizing personal choice and control responses make the obvious obvious. Such a response reminds clients that only they can choose to change their behavior. In the end, it is entirely up to them to decide if a change is needed and how that change will happen.

Shifting focus responses acknowledge that the current area feels unproductive and shift to an area that may be more helpful or productive for the client. This shift may be accomplished by a reflection, summary, question, or a combination of these.

Simple Reflections in Response to Resistance and Status Quo Talk

Generate simple reflections in response to client statements of resistance or status quo. Begin by writing two responses to each, and try to vary the focus on each. Use the handout, Techniques for Responding to Resistance, as a reminder if needed.

I thought red wine was supposed to be good for your heart. That's why I drink it each night.

1.

2.

I know it would be good for me, but it's just too hard to exercise regularly. I'm too busy.

1.

2.

I think everyone is blowing this out of proportion. So I drank a little too much at the holiday party.

1.

2.

I agree, it's not perfect, but you don't understand what it's like. It's different now.

1.

2.

(cont.)

OK, so there are some costs. I'm not someone who wants to spend the rest of my life coloring inside the lines. I want to have a little fun and spend a little money.

1.

2.

I don't think the meds helped all that much, and I really didn't like the way they made me feel.

1.

2.

Listen, I know my boss is mad. Still, I'm not going to take any crap from anybody. You show weakness here, and you'll get eaten alive.

1.

2.

I tried all of those things, and none of them worked. Don't you get it?

1.

2.

Why do I have to be here? I know things aren't perfect, but I am doing better. There have been no incidents with my kids, so why do you still make me come?

1.

2.

Double-Sided and Amplified Reflections in Response to Resistance and Status Quo Talk

Now use a double-sided (DS) or amplified (A) reflection. Remember, double-sided reflections include both sides of the ambivalence, whereas amplified reflections add some zing to the resistant part of the statement. Try to write one of each type. Use the handout, Techniques for Responding to Resistance, as a reminder if you need it.

I thought red wine was supposed to be good for your heart. That's why I drink it each night.

1. DS—

2. A—

I know it would be good for me, but it's just too hard to exercise regularly. I'm too busy.

1. DS—

2. A—

I think everyone is blowing this out of proportion. So I drank a little too much at the holiday party.

1. DS—

2. A—

I agree it's not perfect, but you don't understand what it's like. It's different now.

1. DS—

2. A—

(cont.)

OK, so there are some costs. I'm not someone who wants to spend the rest of my life coloring inside the lines. I want to have a little fun and spend a little money.

1. DS—

2. A—

I don't think the meds helped all that much, and I really didn't like the way they made me feel.

1. DS—

2. A—

Listen, I know my boss is mad. Still, I'm not going to take any crap from anybody. You show weakness here, and you'll get eaten alive.

1. DS—

2. A—

I tried all of those things, and none of them worked. Don't you get it?

1. DS—

2. A—

Why do I have to be here? I know things aren't perfect, but I am doing better. There have been no incidents with my kids, so why do you still make me come?

1. DS—

2. A—

Other Responses to Resistance and Status Quo Talk

Now using the same prompts a third time, try to use one of the other forms of response (i.e., reframing, agreement with a twist, siding with the negative, personal choice, and shifting focus). It may not be possible to use the last two categories each time without sounding redundant, but try your best. Use the handout, Techniques for Responding to Resistance, as a reminder if you need it.

I thought red wine was supposed to be good for your heart. That's why I drink it each night.

1.

2.

3.

I know it would be good for me, but it's just too hard to exercise regularly. I'm too busy.

1.

2.

3.

I think everyone is blowing this out of proportion. So I drank a little too much at the holiday party.

1.

2.

3.

(cont.)

I agree it's not perfect, but you don't understand what it's like. It's different now.

1.

2.

3.

OK, so there are some costs. I'm not someone who wants to spend the rest of my life coloring inside the lines. I want to have a little fun and spend a little money.

1.

2.

3.

I don't think the meds helped all that much, and I really didn't like the way they made me feel.

1.

2.

3.

Listen, I know my boss is mad. Still, I'm not going to take any crap from anybody. You show weakness here, and you'll get eaten alive.

1.

2.

3.

I tried all of those things, and none of them worked. Don't you get it?

1.

2.

3.

Why do I have to be here? I know things aren't perfect, but I am doing better. There have been no incidents with my kids, so why do you still make me come?

1.

2.

3.

Sample Responses for Exercises 6.1, 6.2, and 6.3

I thought red wine was supposed to be good for your heart. That's why I drink it each night.

1. This is confusing to you. You thought you were doing something good for your heart. (Simple)

2. And you're right—it does look like there is some health benefit to red wine, along with the risks. (Agreement with a twist)

3. You drink wine to be healthy. What else do you do to be healthy? (Shifting focus)

I know it would be good for me, but it's just too hard to exercise regularly. I'm too busy.

1. You're really busy. (Simple)

2. You couldn't possibly exercise, given everything that's on your plate. (Amplified)

3. It's hard to know where health fits into all these other competing demands, and yet you know it's important. (Double-sided reflection)

I think everyone is blowing this out of proportion. So I drank a little too much at the holiday party.

1. You had a little too much. (Simple)

2. On the one hand, it feels like people are overreacting and, on the other, you know that you drank a little more than you would've liked to. (Double-sided)

3. So what you thought would be fun has become something else—all because of a little alcohol. (Reframe)

I agree it's not perfect, but you don't understand what it's like. It's different now.

1. Things have changed. (Simple)

2. This may not be an area where you can change right now. (Siding with the negative)

3. I don't understand. If I did, I might see how hard it is for you to consider a change. (Agreement with a twist)

OK, so there are some costs. I'm not someone who wants to spend the rest of my life coloring inside the lines. I want to have a little fun and spend a little money.

1. You want to enjoy your life. (Simple)

2. You want to enjoy your life and are willing to take on the costs that might bring. (Double-sided reflection)

3. And it feels like an either–or choice. You can't have both. (Reframe)

(cont.)

Sample Responses for Exercises 6.1, 6.2, and 6.3 (*cont.*)

I don't think the meds helped all that much, and I really didn't like the way they made me feel.

1. The meds didn't make much difference. (Simple)

2. The meds didn't help you at all. (Amplified)

3. You may be willing to put up with how you feel because the meds are too problematic. (Siding with the Negative)

Listen, I know my boss is mad. Still, I'm not going to take any crap from anybody. You show weakness here, and you'll get eaten alive.

1. You're not going to show weakness. (Simple)

2. Even though you know you're tough enough to take it, you wonder what it may cost you with the boss. (Double-sided reflection)

3. And that's the struggle. Because you know that by fighting, it gives them power to decide what you will do. (Agreement with a twist)

I tried all of those things, and none of them worked. Don't you get it?

1. It feels like I don't understand. (Simple)

2. Nothing worked at all, not even a little bit. (Amplified)

3. Despite the fact that things haven't changed, you keep trying. (Reframe)

Why do I have to be here? I know things aren't perfect, but I am doing better. There have been no incidents with my kids, so why do you still make me come?

1. You're ready to be done. (Simple)

2. Things are better, and maybe there are still a few troublesome spots. (Double-sided reflection)

3. It feels like I'm making you come, rather than you making that choice yourself. I think there are some things we might still work on, and yet you're the one who has to decide about whether those are worth the hassle of coming. On the flip side is the court stuff, but I can't decide that for you. It really is your call. (Emphasizing personal choice)

Your Clients' Resistance and Status Quo Statements

Make a list of status quo or resistance statements you've heard from your clients. Try to fill the sheet provided. Then write as many resistance-lowering responses as you can think of, but do at least three for each statement. Use the handout, Techniques for Responding to Resistance, as a reminder if you need it.

Client Statement:

1.

2.

3.

Client Statement:

1.

2.

3.

Client Statement:

1.

2.

3.

(cont.)

Client Statement:

1.

2.

3.

Client Statement:

1.

2.

3.

.

Radio Resistance and Talk Show Hubris

We continue to use radio and TV shows as source material. This exercise is a little harder because you have to find a show on which callers or guests tend to be resistant. If you have political debates occurring in your area, you might try to watch, listen, or tape these encounters for practice purposes. In the United States, Sunday morning political shows might be a good resource. Begin with shows that are closer to your views or values.

As before, listen to a statement and then turn the sound off and offer one of the types of responses listed. Work on altering your response type. Like Tiger Woods hitting practice balls, you should practice all of the shots you will need—not just those at which you are good already. Use the handout, Techniques for Responding to Resistance, as a reminder if you need it.

Once you're well practiced, try listening to people who hold strong but different views from your own. Again, political talk shows can be a rich source for this kind of material—but, remember, avoid being sarcastic (most of the time).

Practicing with a Client

This is a real-time practice opportunity. Most practitioners have clients who feel stuck. Identify an upcoming appointment about which you have some sense of unease. If you are hoping for a no-show by this person, this is probably the right individual with whom to do this activity.

Your goal will be to use the techniques discussed in this chapter, as well as the other microskills, to understand why the client feels stuck. Begin with a preamble: "We've been working for a time now, and it feels as though we are struggling to make headway. It seems like a good time to step back and get a sense of the big picture of your situation. Most often there are reasons why people do things. So, what are the good parts of where you are right now?" Practice the different forms of reflection. Since we don't want to reinforce the status quo only, you should also ask about the less-good parts. Remember to use elaboration with the less-good parts.

When you hear resistance, attempt to use the different skills that have been discussed. Use the handout, Techniques for Responding to Resistance, as a reminder if you need it.

The Client from Hell—Maybe

Choose someone with whom you have really struggled in your treatment situation, then play this person with your partner so that he or she can practice. Unlike the client from hell, please throw your partner a bone when he or she deserves it. That is, if his or her work begins to soften your resistance or status quo resolve, then go ahead and say so. Also, since this is practice, throw your partner some bones even if his or her attempt is less than perfect. Remember, this is practice! You're trying to learn, not prove something.

Here are some questions for the debriefing:

What did your listener do well?

What techniques seemed to lessen your resistance?

Were there any times when your resistance or adherence to the status quo went up?

Were there any things the listener could have done to help bring that resistance or adherence back down?

What did you learn about your client, through role-playing this person?

Chapter 7

Opening a Session or Topic

Opening

Laurie was struggling academically and socially in this private, college-preparatory school. Concerns were present in many spheres. Each year of high school an event or health concern had impeded her ability to succeed. She was also struggling to fit in socially. Now rumors had begun to surface about her possible drug and alcohol involvement. These concerns were passed along to the school counselor for further assessment. The counselor contacted Laurie via e-mail, and she agreed to come by for a visit.

"Thanks for coming in today. I bet you're wondering why I asked you to check in with me."

"Yeah. Your e-mail was pretty cryptic."

"I wanted to check in. I know from your advisor that the first couple of years have been a bit bumpy for you, and I wanted to see where things stood. I also had a couple of things I wanted to ask you about. Before we do that, let me say a couple of things. This is a private conversation between you and me. I will not share this information with the school or your parents, unless you give me permission to do so or if I have reason to believe that you're a danger to yourself or someone else. Does that make sense to you?"

"Yeah, but it also sounds pretty ominous."

"Like maybe you're in trouble."

"Or could get in trouble."

"Not exactly an invitation to share more."

"Now I really am wondering what this is about."

"Sorry about that. It sounds like you feel more worried."

Laurie is now sitting with legs crossed and foot bouncing. The issues of privacy and disclosure have been covered briefly. The dynamic is not collaborative at this point, though the practitioner has used MI reflections to deal with Laurie's affect. So, where would you go from here? How would you rearrange this introduction to go more smoothly? What if Laurie were 45, overweight, presenting with hypertension and a chronic cough from smoking? Would it be different if she were 35 and you were a child support worker asked to come into her home because of rumors about her meth use and her children being quite thin, wearing dirty clothes, and being observed outside, alone late at night?

A Deeper Look

Practitioners are often asked or required to discuss difficult topics with clients who are, or seem to be, less than motivated to provide a full answer. This conundrum may be what piqued your interest in MI. The central problem is that the clinician or provider has a concern, but the client has not identified that concern as a personal issue. So, how does the practitioner raise the issue without building resistance?

In Chapter 6 we discussed the importance of keeping resistance low and noted that many of the skills (e.g., reflections) and strategies (e.g., emphasizing personal choice and responsibility, shifting focus) can aid in reducing resistance or status quo talk. However, in the example just provided, these skills may not deflate the concerns—at least, initially. Indeed, the nature of the topic seems to override the impact of these skills.

In Chapter 2 we discussed the spirit of MI, one component of which was collaboration. In this instance, the practitioner may be working in a manner that is MI consistent, but the collaboration is not yet evident. Although knowledge of these three components (evocation, autonomy, and collaboration) may aid us at a conceptual level as to what needs to happen, it does not provide the skills or strategies to manage this situation.

Here is the bad news. There is no magic wand that can be waved to make these issues suddenly less "itchy"—a term that Steve Rollnick likes to use in discussing difficult topics. The good news is that there are some key points, techniques, and skills that can aid us in moving forward with the itchy topics. Although none is likely to work all the time, and it does take practice to become more proficient, these are skills that can be learned, refined, and used effectively. Here are some key points to keep in mind when using these strategies.

Key Points

We have touched on some of these concepts previously—which is no surprise, since they build on the spirit, principles, and microskills already discussed. However, the concepts do take on special significance for this situation.

Begin with an attitude of curiosity and a goal of trying to understand more. Your object is not to gain a confession or an acknowledgment of a problem, but rather learn how this behavior or concern fits into this person's situation and worldview. Avoid beginning with a prejudgment that there is a problem. My belief is that language is critically important in this regard and that transparency will serve the practitioner best. So, communicate your intentions and agenda, remembering that how you do this is important.

Match your strategies to the client's readiness to change. If the client has not identified the area of concern as an issue before now, then it is unlikely that he or she will spring immediately into action. Your intervention goal would be to move the client further along on the readiness continuum.

Remember that highly confrontational approaches are likely to engender resistance. You might expect that clients will downplay the significance of an area initially, especially if they feel that their character, judgment, or behavior is being questioned. As has been noted repeatedly, the practitioner should work to create an atmosphere wherein the client can explore issues safely.

One way to accomplish this aim is to elicit clients' view of the situation and to try to understand the behavior, issue, or concern in the broader context of their life. Find out about this context, their values, and then ask them to describe how the behavior fits with those values. If they decide that change is needed, then ask them for possible remedies. This last point is noted at several points in this book because of its centrality. Our clients simply know far more about their lives, their abilities, and their willingness to do an activity than we know. This awareness does not diminish our expertise and the value of our knowledge in identifying what works, but it requires that we remain vigilant to how our suggestions might or might not fit for a particular client.

Finally, when you explore an issue with clients don't gather evidence in support of your position. Remember, the important element is that they provide the change talk and develop the argument for why change must occur. At the same time, if you have a concern, then share it directly. We discuss how to do this below, and Chapter 9 also provides suggestions in this area.

Keeping in mind these key points, here are four strategies for opening a difficult discussion or topic.

Strategies

Agenda Setting

Steve Rollnick and colleagues (e.g., Rollnick, Heather, & Bell, 1992) have talked about the importance of establishing an agenda for many years. Although this may seem very basic, it's surprising how often the need to cover many topics in a session allows us to meander without aim. Agenda setting, which is not unique to MI, can be accomplished in several ways, all having the final outcome of balancing client desires and practitioner needs while providing a session focus. One method to accomplish agenda setting is to address the matter directly. For example:

"We have about 15 minutes to talk today. I have a couple of things I need to talk with you about, but I also want to make sure we get to your concerns as well. So, what is uppermost in your mind today?"

The goal in this process, especially when time is limited, is to identify one or two topics as the session focus. You might prepare yourself for the client who says it is not enough time, there are too many issues, or the issues are too intertwined. These are all excellent opportunities for reframing and brief information exchange. For example:

"You're right. It is not much time, so if we are going to be effective, we need to get really focused. The good news is that since things are so intertwined, if we start making changes in one area then this will begin to affect these other areas as well. So, if you look at all of these areas and can only choose one, which one really jumps out at you?"

Often clients agree with this rationale and identify a single issue. If they don't, then move on—your rationale should not be a point of argument, and you can return to it later if things bog down. Similarly, it is not uncommon for clients to raise another area of concern as this discussion unfolds. In response you can point out that this new topic is important and a different agenda than the one identified originally. Ask if they would like to shift the agenda, with the prompt that staying focused is often helpful for clients in accomplishing more in a short period. For example:

"So, we've moved into talking about your parents and away from the pot. It seems like this is an important area to you as well. I'm wondering if you'd like to switch your agenda to that or to stay with the original agenda. It's your call. Again, I bring it up because people often find it helpful to choose one thing they will work on."

Intermixed within these discussions is the insertion of the practitioner's agenda, though the introduction of it should typically be done after clients negotiate their agenda. If we return to Laurie, this portion of the interchange might look something like this:

"So, my agenda is, I would like to spend a few minutes hearing how school is going and then I also have a couple of questions about how substance use may or may not fit into that picture for you. But I also want to hear about what is on your mind. What would be helpful, from your perspective, for us to spend some time on today?"

For many years Rollnick has (e.g., Rollnick, Mason, & Butler, 1999) used a menu method to aid in agenda setting, as noted previously, employing a variety of props to accomplish this strategy. The basic idea is to create a visual menu (e.g., using a dinner plate or a sheet of paper with circles on it) that contains frequent topics for discussion in that treatment realm. In a probation setting, the circles might include topics such as: managing free time, old friends, the old neighborhood, job finding, stigma, money, family, living situation, and substance use. For cardiac care, the menu items might include medication management, weight loss, diet, exercise, smoking, and alcohol use. The sheet should include a couple of blank circles or blank spots in which clients insert the topics important to them but not listed on the sheet. The introduction of this agenda-setting task might go like this in a parole office:

"There are a number of different ways we could spend our time today. On this sheet are some areas that we could talk about—things like 'the old neighborhood,' 'stigma,' or 'finding a job.' You'll also notice that some areas are blank. That's because there may be things that feel really important to you today but aren't listed here. As you look at this sheet, what jumps out at you as an area on which we should spend some time?"

After a selection, you can also insert your agenda:

"In addition to talking about 'stigma,' I also need—as part of my job—to check in to see how 'the job finding' and 'living situation' areas are going. OK, let's make sure we reserve a few minutes for that. Let's start with stigma. What's been happening in that area?"

Again, renegotiation of focus should always be an option. As with all of these strategies, a liberal dose of OARS is used after the initial strategy is implemented.

A Typical Day

This strategy asks clients to describe what a typical day is like in their life. It begins with breakfast and ends with bed. This technique is bolstered by displaying a curious attitude. Ask for details (but don't spend an hour doing so).

"I know something about how your life works, based on some of the things you've already told me. Still, I don't know what a typical day in your life would look like, and that seems pretty important. So I was hoping you could fill me in, starting with when you get up in the morning. What's your morning routine like?"

You will typically need to provide prompts for details (e.g., "What time do you roll out of bed?", "What happens then?", "What's breakfast like?"). If the client does not identify the problematic behavior as part of a typical day, then ask about it directly.

"On days when the kids are more challenging and you feel a little less in control, tell me about how that's different."

There are a few other ideas to keep in mind. Once again, avoid the use of the word *problem* (unless the client uses it) to sidestep the risk of engendering resistance unnecessarily. You can also use this approach to segue into days when things go particularly well and the accompanying issues or difficulties are absent. This focus on positive exceptions is consistent with many treatment approaches (e.g., solution-focused therapy) and facilitates identification of client strengths.

Normalize the Behavior

This approach involves a couple of different components. One is to embed an inquiry in a series of questions that have a natural flow, so the question doesn't feel as intrusive. For example, when I do evaluations, I always ask about substance use initiation immediately after inquiring about education in primary and secondary school:

"Junior high or high school is often a time when folks first try alcohol. How about you? Tell me about when you first used alcohol?"

This process of normalizing can also extend to providing a range or bracket for response, within which clients can provide an acceptable answer. This bracketing allows people to endorse responses within the range and not underreport, especially around sensitive topics. However, normalizing does not mean that the behavior is acceptable, only that it occurs within a range of behavior in which people engage and that you won't be shocked if they endorse it. For example:

> "Couples handle disagreements and fights in a variety of ways. Some talk it through. Some yell and scream. Some don't talk to each other. Some break things or put holes in the wall. Some get physical. Some slap. Some punch. Some kick. Some pull hair. There is a whole range of responses couples use. When you two get angry, how do you fight?"

This method can also be streamlined.

> "On days when people drink, some drink 1 beer; others drink 24 beers. What is your drinking like?"

Of course, critical in this process is your ability to hear all responses with equanimity. If the client feels judged, then the conversation will end. You can always come back and express a concern, but your initial response should be to simply accept what the client offers. However, at this juncture, clients are often very afraid of being labeled. OARS can be a very helpful adjunct when hearing difficult information.

Offering a Concern

Practitioners should feel empowered to offer concerns about a client's decisions or positions, but they should also be thoughtful about how they approach such a communication. Instead of telling clients they are wrong, the MI practitioner offers a different vantage point or view. Clients are left to make the final decision about the accuracy and meaning of the practitioner's statement.

Offering a concern is also helpful in situations when there is a topic that needs to be discussed but no easy path leading to that domain. As we observed with Laurie, this does not mean that using this approach will avoid dissonance (i.e., the client and practitioner are out of tune). Indeed, dissonance in the relationship might be expected as practitioners work to understand the "tunes" that clients "sing." Instead, the practitioner should be prepared to work within the general strategy and to use OARS to bring the relationship back into harmony (consonance). For example, if we were concerned about a parolee engaging in risky situations with old substance-using friends, we might say:

> "I'm concerned about your decision to hang out with your old friends in your old haunts. My concern is that this puts you at risk for a return to old ways of doing things, including getting high, and you've told me that's what led you into prison last time. You've also told me that you don't want to go back to prison. Of course, it's you who will decide

about doing something, or anything, about that. What do you think about those concerns?"

This statement contains three elements. First, there is a direct report of the practitioner's concerns. The statement is made without judgment and uses prior client statements when possible. Then there is a statement about the client's responsibility for choice and change. Finally, the client's view is solicited.

The temptation is to argue on behalf of the position just stated. This is a persuasion trap and should be avoided. Even when subtle, it tends to engage resistance. A more helpful approach is to use OARS to understand the client's view. Offering a concern is discussed more fully in Chapter 9.

Concept Quiz—Test Yourself!

True or false:

1. T F A common practitioner problem is the requirement to raise difficult topics with clients.

2. T F Avoiding "itchy" topics is a core characteristic of MI.

3. T F When raising a difficult topic, you should maintain a curious attitude about how the area fits into the person's life.

4. T F Language doesn't matter, as long as you maintain an MI-consistent approach.

5. T F Your goal in raising a difficult topic is to move the person forward in readiness, not necessarily to change immediately.

6. T F Clients are often not honest, especially around problem areas, so you need to be skeptical of their views about a situation.

7. T F OARS are important skills in opening difficult discussions.

8. T F Many times you just need to get in somebody's face to get his or her attention.

9. T F Once you set an agenda, you shouldn't renegotiate.

10. T F Normalizing the behavior means that the behavior is OK.

Answers

1. T Although not all practitioners face this dilemma, it is a challenge for the many who must raise and address problematic behaviors without increasing client resistance. Whereas this challenge is most evident in areas such as criminal justice and child welfare investigation, it is also present in health care situations where lifestyle issues and treatment compliance are often critical elements in improving client health.

2. F Although MI seeks to avoid raising resistance levels and may at times encourage shifting focus away from a resistance-increasing discussion, MI also addresses itchy topics directly, encouraging frank interchanges but in circumstances wherein clients feel safe.

3. T   This is a key point. The attitude of curiosity communicates concern for the welfare of clients and helps the practitioner maintain an approach of discovery and appreciation rather than one of gathering ammunition for a later confrontation. We are not laying a trap; rather, we are endeavoring to understand clients. Later, this information will help us offer ideas that match their needs and desires.

4. F   Although attitude is critical, language can also be very important. Thus, using words such as *problem*, even with MI spirit present, can lead to defensiveness in clients who have not used that term. Labels are sticking points for many clients. For this reason, MI suggests the use of more neutral language (e.g., *issue, concern, hitch, less good*) until the client endorses *problem* and does not feel the need for a client to "accept" a diagnosis in order for change to occur.

5. T   Although you might want the person to jump into action, especially if the behavior impacts others significantly, this desire fails to accommodate the process of how people change. Helping someone move from "there isn't a problem" to "maybe I need to think about this" may be a significant change.

6. F   There may be both external and internal sources of motivation to be less than forthcoming in any situation where change is needed. This dynamic is not specific to one class of people or disorders (e.g., people with alcohol dependence). There may also be fundamental differences in how observers and the individual in the situation interpret a situation (see Fundamental Attribution Error, Chapter 6), but this is different from being dishonest. The issue is, *Does practitioner skepticism help the client become more honest?* From an MI perspective, the answer is no. The MI practitioner works to create a safe environment in which the client can come face to face and explore difficult realities (Miller & Rollnick, 2002). Skepticism interferes with this effort. As noted in prior chapters, this position does not mean that we agree with clients' views—only that we accept that what they are saying represents their view of reality.

7. T   Without OARS and MI spirit, the techniques described above can be wooden and unsuccessful. At worst, the techniques become nothing more than efforts to manipulate clients into self-revelation and then using that information against them. Such an approach is tantamount to interrogation, which is entirely at odds with MI spirit.

8. F   This item seems like a "no brainer," based on all that has been said, yet trainees still sometimes feel that for really tough clients, they need to get their attention with some confrontation first. Although such an approach may work on occasion, typically it serves to increase resistance—and that usually produces worse outcomes.

9. F   It is very helpful to have an agenda that guides and focuses the session. As noted previously, part of our task may be to help clients organize their experience, and focusing the session may help in this manner. However, agenda setting is a tool, and it should be open to alteration as the client and session dictate. Bottom line: if clients opt to change the focus of their agenda, that is not a problem.

10. F   *Normalizing* means that you place the behavior within a range of previously observed behaviors. Few people would agree that drinking a gallon of vodka a day, gambling away the family house, or punching your children are generally accepted behaviors. Nevertheless these behaviors occur, and communicating to the client that you've heard this all before allows them to admit to their experience of the behavior and opens the door for additional discussion (the goal of raising the topic).

In Practice

We left our practitioner and Laurie in the beginning of a conversation. The groundwork has been laid for a private discussion, but there is also an up-tick in apprehension and concern for Laurie. We'll start with the practitioner's response to her last statement.

Statement	*Commentary*
P: Sorry about that. It sounds like you feel more worried.	Apology followed by a reflection.
C: Yeah. So what's the story?	Tired of reflections, she wants answers.
P: Well, the things I wanted to check in with you about have to do with some rumors—specifically, the rumors about you smoking pot and that maybe that's giving you some grief.	A direct statement that is likely to engender more affect rather than less. It also addresses the client's request to get on with it.
C: About me? Smoking pot? Are you kidding me? Who?	As expected, concern goes up and collaboration goes way down.
P: Well, if it's OK I'd like to back up just a bit. It's clear this is pretty surprising news and a bit upsetting. It's also only a small part of why I wanted to chat with you today. We'll get back to it after a bit, but first I was hoping we could just spend some time talking about the big picture.	Practitioner recognizes the increase in affect and shifts focus away from the resistance.
C: Big picture?	Affect is still high and client is wary.
P: Yeah. Let's start with here. What's been happening with school?	Practitioner continues in a new direction.
C: Well, school is hard. I work all the time and all I get are B's.	Client follows and offers a glimpse of her struggles.
P: So, there is only a little reward for your work.	Simple reflection that offers a subtle shift.
C: Before I came here, I was getting all A's and not working nearly so hard.	Client continues to provide information.
P: Sometimes you wonder if it's worth it.	Practitioner continues the paragraph with some amplification.

Statement	*Commentary*
C: I know I'm getting a good education, but sometimes I do wonder, what if I went somewhere else? It would be a whole lot easier, and I'd have more time for friends.	Client adds more detail and provides some other avenues for exploration.
P: And friends are important to you.	Practitioner chooses one.
C: Well, yes and no. They are important, but I haven't made that many friends since I came.	Client acknowledges the area is a concern for her.
P: It sounds a little lonely.	Affective reflection.
C: I don't know. I guess.	Language may have been too strong, though there is some agreement.
P: Maybe a little.	Practitioner softens language with a simple reflection.
C: A little.	Client endorses it.
P: What about family? How do they fit into all of this?	Practitioner inquires about another area that could be important.
C: My parents are pretty intense. They think I should be getting better grades. They just don't get how hard it is here.	Client is clearly engaged with practitioner.
P: They're nudging you to do more.	Practitioner chooses softer, but still evocative, language in reflection.
C: Always … maybe more than nudging, too.	Client adds to it.
P: It feels pretty intense for you and not many places where it feels good. When does it feel good?	Practitioner asks for other side. This may or may not be an entrance into substance use.
C: In my room—when I can just chill.	Client follows, but is circumspect.
P: I want to hear more about that, but I also want to get a sense of how all of this fits together. Tell me a little bit about a typical day for you, starting with when you get up in the morning and ending when you go to be at night.	Practitioner could follow up on "chilling" directly, but instead decides to get a broader picture and then see where chilling and substance use may fit in.

(Fast-forward to the end of the typical day.)

P: So, I noticed you didn't mention chilling in your room during a typical day.	Practitioner returns to the opening the client created.

Statement	*Commentary*
C: That's because it doesn't happen on a typical day.	Clarification.
P: On a day when it does happen, where does it fit in and what are you doing?	Open-ended question that asks for the information.
C: It's usually late at night—mostly the weekends, but sometimes during the week. I've got my iPod on, and I'm either just zoning out, lying on my bed, or checking Facebook.	Client responds.
P: So, you really are out of the usual routine. Earlier I brought up pot smoking. How does that fit into chilling?	The question now has a context and may feel less intrusive.
C: Sometimes I smoke a little weed to help me relax.	Client tests the waters.
P: And the weed helps you chill.	Practitioner stays close to client information and uses language she already used.
C: Yeah. It does, but it's not like I do it all the time. Only sometimes.	Client acknowledges the behavior and then has some reservations.
P: And you're kind of worried I might misunderstand what you're saying.	Practitioner addresses client concern directly.
C: And then you would go running to my parents.	Client surfaces her fear.
P: That's your big worry—that your parents would find out and then there'd be trouble.	Practitioner again responds, using a reframe.

This clinical encounter takes a little longer than asking directly about substance use. For practitioners strapped for time, this interchange may feel too long. Yet, by taking this time, the likelihood of meaningful discussion appears to have increased dramatically, given where the discussion began. The aim is not just to obtain information but for that information be accurate and useful.

Try This!

Practice opportunities in this realm may be a little more direct than in prior chapters. That is, although there is value in rehearsing the prompts to be used when agenda setting or inquiring about a typical day, this practice can also be done in interactions with clients. These exercises ask you to identify how and when the four strategies discussed in this chapter—agenda setting, typical day, normalizing, and offering a concern—might be used with your clients and then trying them out.

Exercise 7.1. Agenda Setting

Create a menu for your workplace of common issues that your clients must manage. Although this could be a simple, bulleted list, spending a little extra time to create a visually interesting menu may be worth the effort. The worksheet for Exercise 7.1 contains an example. This document was created by using MS Word and can be replicated and modified to fit your work needs. Once you've created a menu that might fit your setting and your client issues, you'll develop the preamble (i.e., lead-in) you would use to introduce it; then try it out.

Exercise 7.2. A Typical Day

You can begin your practice of opening difficult conversations by asking about a typical day. We start this activity by having you write a preamble that you might use with a client. Then you'll modify it for use with a friend. For example, you might ask him or her about a typical day at work. Once you've practiced it there, then you can try it out with a client.

Exercise 7.3. Normalizing the Behavior

Many areas can be sensitive to inquiry. Consider this list: anger, eating, exercise, alcohol use, drug use, sexual activity, criminal activity, parenting, finances, medication use, self-care, and sexual identity. Two methods often used to normalize behavior are *bracketing* and *embedding the inquiry in a sequence*. In this exercise you'll practice using these techniques to talk about sensitive areas.

Exercise 7.4. Normalizing Your Clients' Behaviors

Think about all the sensitive areas about which you have to inquire in your work setting. Make a list. If there are more than five, choose the five most frequent. Then develop a bracketing question or a sequence of queries or both that you could use for asking about these behaviors. Think clearly about your setting and style and ask questions that match how you work. Once you've done this task, give one set a try in your next client encounter, then revise it based on your experience. We are rarely perfect on the first try at something, so expect that some aspects will need tweaking.

Exercise 7.5. Offering a Concern

On this task you will practice formulating how to offer a concern. As part of this exercise, try to anticipate the client's likely response and then write a follow-up prompt. Once you have completed this written exercise, you might try offering a concern to a client.

Partner Work

Several of the exercises described previously could be tried with your partner pretending to be a client. This type of practice would allow you to experiment with and refine the language. Do the sequence all the way through and then discuss, from the "client's" perspective, what did and did not work. Now reverse roles and try it again.

Exercise 7.6. Lightning Round

This game should be a source of some laughs as you practice thinking on your feet. Take the list of issues provided, cut them into slips (one issue per slip), fold them, and place them in a hat. Then you take turns drawing a slip. You have 30 seconds from the time you draw a slip until you must address the behavior in question by using any of the methods discussed in this chapter: agenda setting, a typical day, normalizing the behavior, or offering a concern. Some exchanges may be over very quickly, whereas others will take more time. **Have some fun with this one and remember: do not tell your partner the issue on your paper**—until after he or she has expended all effort to guess it.

Other Thoughts . . .

Here is a reminder. Introduce yourself to your clients. If you are the person with the chart, file, or clipboard, there is an often an inherent power differential. The simple action of greeting a person makes him or her feel more welcome. It's also a leveling activity. My endocrinologist always shakes my hand. You can also use this moment to indicate the parameters of the meeting (e.g., how much time you have).

Consider how you construct your workplace. You may or may not have ways to personalize where you work, but these ways can provide clues to the client about who you are. In the office where I worked with adolescents, I kept a cookie jar stocked with treats and had a retro radio/CD player. I also had various toys and gizmos that people could pick up and play with as we began talking. My office was painted "sea foam," which, believe it or not, is very soothing. My art was evocative. All of these things allowed me to create an environment conducive to people feeling safe. It also allowed clients to know something of me, before they were asked to talk about themselves. So, consider what your workplace says about you. How would you feel coming into your space? Is your space MI consistent, or does it say "EXPERT"?

Opening a difficult topic or discussion is an area in which MI is misunderstood at times. Among some trainees, the feeling is that MI does *not* address problems directly and instead "soft-soaps" the issues. For trainees from a confrontational tradition, the MI model can be difficult to embrace in this respect. These individuals are often concerned with life-threatening issues or problems that affect others; failing to confront might feel unethical to them. Thus, their difficulty comes from a place of genuine concern for clients and fear of allowing a behavior to go unaddressed.

In one sense, MI is actually quite confrontative, if you think of confrontation in its original meaning of "coming face to face." In this sense, confrontation is a *goal* of these encounters, rather than the *technique*. Then the question becomes, "Which approach will best accomplish this goal?" Whereas a confrontational technique of "speaking truth" may help practitioners feel that they discharged their duty, it may not accomplish the goal of helping the person come face to face with his or her difficult reality. It may instead inflame resistance.

The methods in this chapter are the start of a confrontation. Their aim is to raise issues for discussion as a first step. Even in the direst of situations—"If you do not change this behavior immediately, you will die"—we cannot force clients to make that change. We can voice our concerns directly, but clients will decide ultimately—and that fundamental reality can be either disheartening or empowering to practitioners and clients alike.

Agenda Setting

Using the menu below as a model, design a Menu of Options for your workplace. It should include the most common challenges presented by your clients, as well as blank spaces for client-generated issues or concerns. This menu can be done either free hand or with a word-processing program. There is also a blank form for you to use, though I would encourage you to consider making a form using your own word processor. This little extra effort allows you to create a form that is easily modified and might include additions such as clip art.

Once you've made a menu that fits your setting and client issues, develop the preamble you would use to introduce it. Write this down initially to help you organize your thoughts and to refine your message. This should be brief but provide enough information so that the client understands the task. Write your introduction to the menu here:

Once you've done that, imagine that your client balks at choosing one item only. Provide an explanation (either written or aloud) that you would offer in response. Remember, your goal is not to persuade but rather to offer information about why it would be helpful to focus.

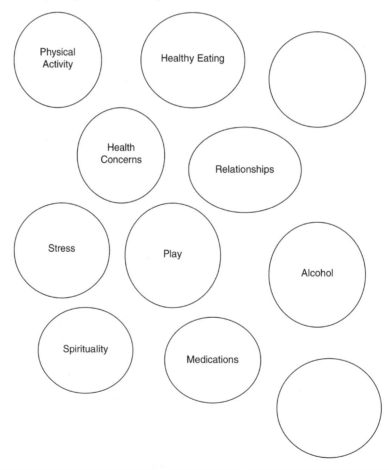

Worksheet for Exercise 7.1

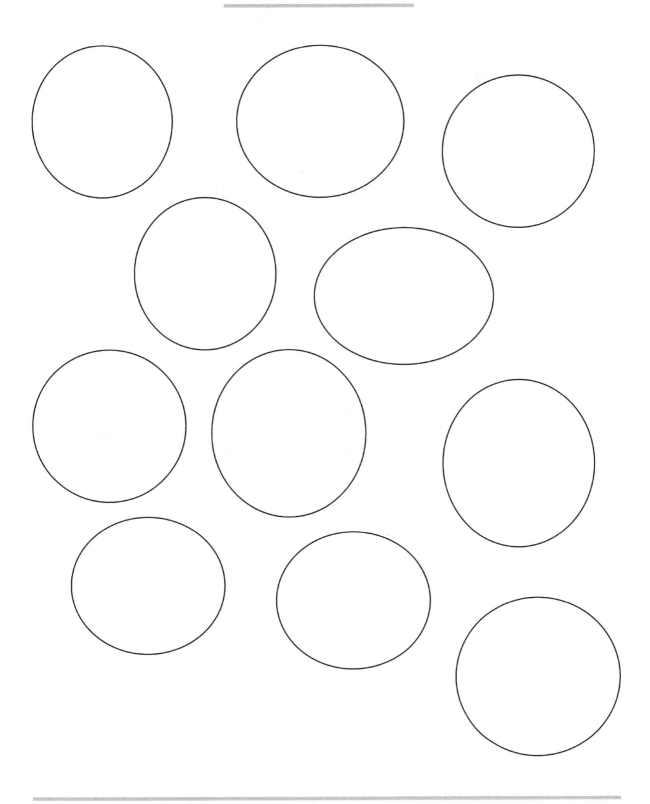

This exercise asks clients to describe what they do across the course of the day—from the time they rise until they retire for the night. The purpose of the activity is to understand more about a client's life and, when appropriate, where a problem behavior fits into it.

To begin this exercise, write the preamble (i.e., the lead-in) you would use to introduce this query to clients. Here is an example:

> "I know we've talked a lot about your life, but I also realize there is still a lot I do not know. For example, I don't know what happens during a typical day for you. If you don't mind, I would like to take a few minutes and hear about what a usual day in your life is like."

Write this statement below. Remember, it doesn't have to be long, but it should contain enough information so that the client knows what you are asking and why. The wording should fit you and your style as well as convey curiosity.

Preamble:

Once you've polished this preamble, think about how you might modify it to ask about a friend's life at work, your spouse/partner's day, or someone else whom you know but don't necessarily know the details of his or her daily life. (By the way, I have done this with my wife, and I'm always fascinated by what I don't know about her day!) Once you've got this revision firmly in mind, give it a try.

Normalizing the Behavior

Below is a list of topics that can be delicate to bring up in a session. For this list devise a method to bracket the behavior in an inquiry or to place the inquiry within a natural sequence of questions so that it becomes less sensitive. Here are two examples:

1. Bracketing—"People show a range of drinking habits. Some drink none or 1 beer in a typical day; others may have 24. What are your drinking habits like?"
2. Sequencing questions—"What kind of student were you in high school?"; "Tell me about the areas in which you excelled"; "What sorts of struggles did you have in school?"; "Junior high, high school—this is often a time when kids experiment with alcohol. What was your first experience with alcohol? Tell me about the last time you had anything to drink at all—a beer, a wine cooler, a drink?"

For each of the behaviors listed below, provide either bracketing or sequencing responses to normalize the behavior. You can also do both if you want more practice. As you do this activity, take your time and really craft your queries or sequences.

Anger management

Eating habits

Exercise

Alcohol use

Drug use

Sexual activity

Criminal activity

Parenting/discipline

Sample Responses for Exercise 7.3

Anger management

So, there are a variety of different ways in which people express anger. Some people give others the cold shoulder. Some yell. Others threaten. Some people break things or put holes in the wall. Others hit or kick or pull hair. There is a whole range. How about you: how do you express your anger?

In everyday life there are always things that will go wrong and annoy us. What are the little things that annoy you and how do you respond to them? There are also things that push a button a little more for us then they do for other people. What kinds of things do that for you? How do you handle those? Then there are times when we are just flat out steamed. How do manage that, when you are really, really angry? During those times, sometimes people go a little further than they would have liked to, or regret what they did later. How about for you?

Eating habits

There are all sorts of ways people manage their eating. Some people eat whatever they want whenever they want it. Others watch every single thing that goes into their mouth and sometimes deny themselves things they might really like. How do you manage your eating?

There are all sorts of tasks we have in daily living; cleaning up in the morning, taking care of our household, managing meals. What do you do when you get up in the morning? What about breakfast? What happens after breakfast? What do you typically do for lunch and dinner? How about when you're eating more than you usually do? How about when you're restricting what you eat? What about when you think you need to lose a few pounds; how do you manage that?

Exercise

People really vary in how much exercise they get. For some people the only exercise they get is pressing the TV remote control. Others run all night ultra-marathons. Then there are all sorts of people in between. What does the exercise regimen in your life look like?

People take care of themselves in lots of different ways. One of these ways is sleep. What does a typical night's sleep look like for you? Then there is also rest and relaxation. How do you work that into your life? Fun is also an important part. How do you work fun into your life? Exercise can be another piece. In what sorts of ways does exercise fit in your life?

Alcohol use

(See examples at the beginning of the exercise.)

Drug use

In terms of drug use, there are lots of ways people go. Some folks try a few things and then decide that it's not for them. Others dive in head first and try all sorts of stuff. Some people have a period where they used a lot then stopped. Others built up to things and have used sort of steadily over the years. Some start and stop. What has your drug use looked like?

Sample Responses for Exercise 7.3 (*cont.*)

Junior high, high school—this is often a time when kids experiment with alcohol. What was your first experience with alcohol? Tell me about the last time you had anything to drink at all—a beer, a wine cooler, a drink? What about weed—when was the first time you tried it? Tell me about the last time. There are other drugs people try as well. Let me just run through the categories. What about opiates, things like heroin, methadone, Percodan, Percocet, Dilaudid, Oxycontin . . .

Sexual activity

There is a whole range of ways in which people express themselves sexually, from choosing to abstain to being very active with different partners. Some people like erotica, while others view it as pornography and dislike it. Some people are clear in their sexual identity and others are still sorting that out. There are lots of way sexuality is expressed. How does sexual activity fit into your life?

As with alcohol and drugs, the early teen years is often a time when people begin to experience themselves as sexual beings. Sometimes it's earlier. Sometimes it's later. Sometimes it's wanted. Sometimes it's not. What was your situation when you first became aware of yourself in this way? How about when you first became sexually active? There are times when people have been approached or touched in a way they didn't like. What's your experience been like with that?

Criminal activity

There is a broad horizon for people in terms of their relationship with the police and criminal justice system. Some folks have never talked with a police officer. Other people have picked up a few tickets along the way. Some others seem to always have police showing up at the house for one reason or another. Others had some trouble at some point and did some time as a result. What about for you? How has the law figured into your life?

So, even good folks get into trouble sometimes. Some kids get into disciplinary trouble at school. They do things like talk back to teachers, skip classes, or come to school drunk or high. What about you? How about getting into fights either during or after school? Sometimes people get into trouble with the law. Ever been arrested? (Note that this is a closed question with a purpose.)

Parenting/discipline

There is a whole range of how people discipline their kids. Some people try to simply focus on the positive and ignore bad behavior. Others feel like if you spare the rod, you spoil the child. Some people use time outs. Some people give kids a swat on their behind or cuff them on the back of their head. Sometimes people end up getting more angry then they mean to and do things they might otherwise not do, like yelling, swearing, hitting, kicking. What ways do you use when you discipline your children?

Raising kids can be a tough business, because even good kids get into trouble once in awhile. When your kids get into trouble, how do you get them back onto the straight and narrow?

Normalizing Your Clients' Behaviors

Think about all the sensitive areas about which you have to inquire in your work setting. Make a list below.

1. _____   6. _____

2. _____   7. _____

3. _____   8. _____

4. _____   9. _____

5. _____   10. _____

If there are more than five, choose the five most frequent. Now list those in the spaces provided on the next page and then develop a bracketing question or a sequence of queries or both for these behaviors. Think clearly about your setting and style and ask questions that match how you work.

Once you've done this task, give one set a try in your next client encounter, then revise it based on your experience. We are rarely perfect on the first try at something, so expect that some aspects will need tweaking.

Normalizing Your Clients' Behaviors

1. Behavior: _____

   Strategy: _____

   How you would do it:

2. Behavior: _____

   Strategy: _____

   How you would do it:

3. Behavior: _____

   Strategy: _____

   How you would do it:

4. Behavior: _____

   Strategy: _____

   How you would do it:

5. Behavior: _____

   Strategy: _____

   How you would do it:

Offering a Concern

On this task you will practice formulating how to offer a concern. Brief scenarios are included below; these will not provide the entire context, nor will they match your work circumstance. Simply try to imagine yourself as either a helper or a concerned friend. Begin by writing a statement that expresses concern in response to each of the issues noted below. Then write what you think the client might say in response to your statement. Finally, write your follow-up to this client statement. Once you have completed this exercise, try offering a concern to a client. (Remember to use OARS!) If you don't feel ready quite yet, try moving through these exercises again, offering a concern with a different focus.

Issue: *The client was caught driving at twice the legal limit for blood alcohol, but she doesn't feel that she was impaired. The court has ordered her to receive treatment, but she feels that it was just bad luck and that she does not have a problem with alcohol. Failure to go to treatment would result in 12 months jail time and loss of her license.*

Your concern:

Client's likely response:

Your follow-up:

Issue: *The client just had a heart attack. He continues to smoke, eat red meat, and consume at least three drinks a night. He is 40 pounds overweight and has a history of high blood pressure and high cholesterol.*

Your concern:

Client's likely response:

Your follow-up:

(*cont.*)

Issue: *The client feels that her son is being disrespectful and has taken to giving increasingly onerous punishments, including whipping him with an electrical cord. The son, now 13, hit her back after the last punishment. She loves her son but is struggling with her solo parenting.*

Your concern:

Client's likely response:

Your follow-up:

Issue: *The client has been failing to floss his teeth regularly. His dental hygienist has previously indicated that although his brushing is very good, his failure to floss is causing decay in a number of areas. He is not yet at risk for tooth loss, but there are a number of sensitive areas, and his risk is increasing.*

Your concern:

Client's likely response:

Your follow-up:

Issue: *This 16-year-old girl, a junior in high school, dresses in extremely tight-fitting clothes with plunging necklines. A buxom girl, her shirt almost always reveals cleavage. She sees no problem with her dress, viewing it as consistent with her peers. You've noticed that many boys ogle her and that most of her peers dress in a more conservative style.*

Your concern:

Client's likely response:

Your follow-up:

Sample Responses for Exercise 7.5

Issue: *The client was caught driving at twice the legal limit for blood alcohol, but she doesn't feel that she was impaired.*

Your concern:

Is it okay if I share with you a concern I have about this situation? You've said this just feels like bad luck, and at the same time, you were at a level where you were twice the legal limit. I worry about that last piece and that it might get lost in your being angry with the courts and the cops.

Client's likely response:

It wasn't like I hit anybody or was weaving all over the road. I just got caught in a trap. They're just making too big a deal out of it.

Your follow-up:

So, it was a bit of bad luck and maybe it's a little bit of a deal.

Issue: *The client just had a heart attack.*

Your concern:

If it's alright, I'd like to share a little concern about your situation. I know you want to live your life in your own way, and I worry that you may be making some risky choices to affirm that nobody can make you do anything you don't want to. What do you think?

Client's likely response:

I don't think I'm trying to prove anything to anybody. I just don't want to have to deal with all of this non-sense.

Your follow-up:

It's not about control; it just feels like too much to deal with.

Issue: *The client feels that her son is being disrespectful and has taken to giving increasingly onerous punishments, including whipping him with an electrical cord.*

Your concern:

It is clear you love your son, and at the same time you can feel how your attempts to parent are resulting in push back. I am worried that if things continue down this path you might have more trouble, not less. What do you think?

(*cont.*)

Sample Responses for Exercise 7.5 (*cont.*)

Client's likely response:

I think kids need discipline and they need to respect limits.

Your follow-up:

And if you were not to address this it would be sending the wrong message. So, for you, it's about how can I address this in an effective manner.

Issue: *The client has been failing to floss his teeth regularly.*

Your concern:

So, I have a concern; is it okay if I share it with you? I know taking care of your teeth is important to you. Your coming today reinforces that, as does your flossing when you come. So, my concern is that you're starting to show some sensitivity, and this suggests that your risk for some problems is increasing. Of course, you have to decide what that means for you, but it does concern me.

Client's likely response:

Well, it's not like I have gum disease or my teeth are rotting out.

Your follow-up:

And those would be a clearer signal that it's time for a change.

Issue: *This 16-year-old girl dresses in extremely tight-fitting clothes with plunging necklines, revealing cleavage. She sees no problem it, but you've noticed that boys ogle her and that her peers dress more conservatively.*

Your concern:

This may seem a bit odd, but I've been noticing how the boys have been noticing you. It is okay if I share that with you? I am a bit concerned that the boys may be interpreting how you look in a sexual way that may not be what you had in mind. I'm wondering what you've noticed.

Client's likely response:

I don't know. I prefer the attention to no attention at all.

Your follow-up:

So, the attention feels good, and you're not particularly worried that they may be interpreting your dress in a sexual manner.

Lightning Round

This game should be a source of some laughs as you practice thinking on your feet. On the next page you will find a list of client issues. Remove it from the book and cut it up so that there is only one issue per slip. Then fold the slips and place them in a hat or some other receptacle. One person is the contestant, the other is the "client." With eyes closed, the contestant draws out a slip of paper and reads the issue silently. The contestant has 30 seconds to begin using one of the four methods discussed in this chapter: agenda setting, a typical day, normalizing the behavior, or offering a concern.

The "client" does the timing. <u>Do not tell the client what is on the paper</u>. Remember, the contestant's response should fit the issue. The interaction should continue until your partner guesses the behavior. Some exchanges may be over very quickly, whereas others will take more time. Again, do not tell your partner the issue until you finish. Then switch roles. Do this until the hat is empty, you're out of time, or you're laughed out. (By the way, I have encountered all of these issues in my clinical work.)

Client Issues for Exercise 7.6

Cut out along the lines.

Bed wetting	Body odor
Sexually suggestive comments	Lack of humor
Excessive nose hair	Multiple tattoos
Multiple body piercings	Wearing headphones
Very out-of-date clothes	Very revealing clothes
Late arriving	Long-windedness
Bad breath	False teeth shaped like vampire fangs
Smells of alcohol	Appears high
Wearing flip-flops (sandals) on a snowy day	Wearing multiple layers of clothes (during the hot summer)
Severe eczema or acne	Client is falling asleep during your meeting

Chapter 8

Working with Ambivalence

Opening

"Sorry, but next Tuesday doesn't work for me." The supervisor didn't offer an alternative time.

The Department of Health Services practice coach had been trying to reach this supervisor for a week. The coach, charged with assisting supervisors to learn and implement a new intervention model, had been worried about this supervisor. Carrie was very quiet during the initial training session and seemed slow to embrace the new model in practice exercises. Like most supervisors, she is harried by multiple job demands and also a veteran of many prior initiatives—some of which were short-lived. Yet, the coach knew from conversations with Carrie during the initial training that she remains very committed to the welfare of the children and families the department serves. The coach observed a tape of Carrie in practice last week and noted very little use of the intervention model.

"Well, what will work for you?"

"I don't know. I am pretty jammed right now. How about if we push it back another couple of weeks?"

"I can imagine it feels like there are not enough hours in the workday, given everything the department asks of you, and yet you know that the department requires this training as a priority. They also said that this first meeting must happen within 6 weeks of the training. Unfortunately, we are right at the end of that period, so we can't postpone any longer. Given that, how can we get this accomplished?"

"Well, I can't do Tuesday. I think I can spare about 30 minutes on Wednesday morning."

Carrie, like all participants at the initial training, received information (written and oral) about the timing and length (45 minutes) of the first follow-up meeting. They also received a follow-up e-mail and phone call with the same information. She knew that 45 minutes was the expectation.

"Actually, Carrie, we will need the full 45 minutes."

"OK. I know we need to get this done. Can you start early then, say 7:45 A.M. on Wednesday?"

"You bet."

While it might be easy to view this supervisor as simply resistant, we also know that she is committed to providing good quality care to her charges. At the same time she is skeptical of initiatives because in the past these have not necessarily lasted. Thus, it is probably more helpful to think of her as ambivalent. The question is, *If you were the coach in this situation, how would you engage this individual when you met next Wednesday?*

A Deeper Look

We first brought up ambivalence in Chapter 2, and it has cropped up throughout the text. Recall the definition of MI: *"a client-centered, directive method for enhancing intrinsic motivation to change by **exploring and resolving ambivalence**"* (Miller & Rollnick, 2002, p. 25; italics in original, bold emphasis added). Merriam-Webster's Online Dictionary (*www. merriam-webster.com/dictionary*; accessed February 9, 2008) defines ambivalence as: "**1:** simultaneous and contradictory attitudes or feelings (as attraction and repulsion) toward an object, person, or action; **2 a:** continual fluctuation (as between one thing and its opposite) **b:** uncertainty as to which approach to follow." These definitions seem apt descriptions of Carrie's situation and mindset.

Ambivalence is a complex concept. Engle and Arkowitz (2006) devote an entire book to understanding the dimensions of ambivalence. Despite this complexity and its centrality in the definition and conceptualization of MI, there is surprisingly little direct guidance in MI-1 or MI-2 on strategies that specifically target ambivalence.

Perhaps as a result, some MI practitioners focus on decisional balance activities (i.e., weighing the pros and cons of the status quo, change, or both) to resolve ambivalence. Miller and Rollnick (2009), as indicated in Chapter 5, have noted this approach may be problematic. Data suggest that change talk, in relation to sustain talk, may be an important predictor of when change does and does not occur. Given this finding, Miller and Rollnick (2009) have begun moving away from techniques like the decisional balance activities that elicit sustain or status quo talk. Although they do not prohibit the use of decisional balance activities, they note that they are probably most useful in a very targeted situation for people; that is, when clients are early in their readiness and reluctant to discuss change.

So then, how does the practitioner explore and resolve ambivalence beyond that early stage? The answer, which flows from the previous chapters and has been present since the earliest writing on MI (Miller, 1983), is to be directive and selectively elicit and reinforce change talk. Exploration of sustain talk is limited, happens early, and is done in the context of moving toward change talk. Stated more plainly, within MI, people resolve ambivalence by talking themselves into changing.

In this chapter we focus on four approaches to resolving ambivalence: using evocative questions, picking the flowers (i.e., finding and reinforcing the change talk), collecting bouquets (i.e., using summaries), and contrasting values and behaviors (i.e., value sorting). In addition to these four approaches, all of the other activities noted in Chapter 5 for eliciting change talk are appropriate.

Evocative Questions

These queries ask clients to directly identify reasons why they might change. Early in the change process this method can be particularly helpful, though it is not limited to that time frame. The practitioner uses the questions to steer the conversation toward change elements and away from sustain factors. If we were to return to Carrie and think about the coach's upcoming meeting with her, some examples of evocative questions might be the following:

"What concerns you now about your current work?"

"What worries you about how your supervisees are working with people?"

"What would you like to see more of in your work with supervisees?"

"In what ways does this new model fit for you?"

"Besides more time, how would you like things to be different in your work with people?"

"How would things be better if you changed?"

Picking the Flowers

Although we may ask for change talk, this does not mean the client will speak only of these elements. Indeed, because the client is ambivalent, we would expect to hear both change and sustain talk, as well as more neutral language. However, we listen for and selectively reinforce the elements that focus on change.

MI practitioners do not give equal weight to all elements; this is what clients are already doing and has allowed them to remain stuck. Instead, we pay attention to the things clients tell us about possible change. Miller likens this aspect of MI to walking with a client through a garden, listening to the client's description of the flowers and then picking only those that have the greatest salience for them. The picking, in this instance, is the use of targeted reflective listening. In this way, we may hear descriptions of flowers of lesser value, as well as those clients don't like; we provide only limited attention to those elements.

Returning to Carrie, we might note her heavy workload, but we don't remain focused on it. Instead, we focus on the required change—embracing the new practice model. A double-sided reflection may work well and require that we refer back to information conveyed previously.

"I can imagine it feels like there are not enough hours in the workday, given everything the department asks of you, and yet you know that the department requires this training as a priority."

Although the second part of this statement is not change talk, per se, it is the element that focuses on change. As such, it is an initial step toward change.

Providing Bouquets

People who are ambivalent are typically well aware of being stuck. They don't need our help to know that they've been unable to make a change. What they need help with is moving forward.

As a result, our job may not be complete by just picking flowers. Clients may need our help organizing this material. Thus, after selectively choosing the flowers, we also collect these together in bouquets. These arrangements help clients see the types of flowers, the relations between the flowers, and the elements still needed. Summaries are the way we accomplish this task of providing bouquets.

All three summary types can be used. A *collecting summary* gathers together what clients have said, keeps the momentum moving forward, and shows clients their most important thoughts on change. It may do this by placing elements in contrast or in relation to each other. The *linking summary* adds the element of contrasting current ideas with those offered in the past or from other sources. This linking can be used to highlight particular relationships or areas of conflict. Finally, the *transitional summary* helps clients not only see the relationships but also to consider additional options or directions.

If we return to the interaction between the coach and Carrie, the coach offers this linking summary that contrasts present information with other information that has already been conveyed. Although not a traditional transitional summary, the question is both joining and focused on the first step in change (i.e., meeting).

> "I can imagine it feels like there are not enough hours in the workday, given everything the department asks of you, and yet you know that the department requires this training as a priority. They also said that this first meeting must happen within 6 weeks of the training. Unfortunately, we are right at the end of that period, so we can't postpone any longer. Given that, how can we get this accomplished?"

Exploring Values

Another approach is to ask more directly about values. Values questions might include queries about what things are most important to clients. For example, "When you have to make a major decision in your life, what things factor in?" This inquiry can also be done through an activity such as a values card sort (VCS).

The VCS involves using a deck of cards that can be sorted into different piles. The cards can be obtained through the MINT website (*www.motivationalinterview.org*). Allan Zuckoff provides a description of how he uses the VCS.[1] It is based on his observation of Bill Miller demonstrating the technique, with some modifications.

---

[1] Adapted by permission.

Begin by asking clients to sort the cards into "Not Important" and "Important" piles. When many cards inevitably end up in the "Important" pile, take a moment to affirm that many things are important to the client. Then note that most of us, in fact, have many values that sometimes come into conflict with each other, and that this is sometimes what makes it hard for us to make important life decisions. This helps detoxify the client's likely feelings of frustration, anger, and/or disgust with self for being stuck for so long.

Then ask clients to sort the "Important" cards into "Important" and "Most Important" piles, with no more than five in the "Most Important" pile. Then have the clients tell, in any order, what the word on each of the Most Important values cards means to them. Listen empathically, working to understand the unique meanings each value holds for the client and listening for underlying themes, connections, or tensions among them.

The next step is to ask clients in what ways they are currently succeeding in living out each of these values; listen empathically and ask for elaboration and examples. This elicits self-affirming statements and gives the therapist opportunities to offer affirmations as well. This is followed by asking clients in what ways they are not currently living out these values as fully as they would like. Developing discrepancy this way is intended to prime clients in favor of change, broadly speaking. This requires a high level of trust on the part of clients, and has the potential to, at least temporarily, leave clients feeling worse.

Finally, ask clients how the target behavior fits with these values or what effects the target behavior has on their ability to live out these values. If clients don't spontaneously describe any conflicts between the values and the target behavior, ask about such conflicts or tensions. Ask clients what they would need to do or to change in order to live out these values more fully.

This activity permits clients to explore how current behaviors fit in with important values. As always, practitioners hold themselves in a nonjudgmental position as clients explore the meaning and implication of a behavior. At times, this exercise can bring in clear relief that a "problem" behavior is very low on the person's list of important values and therefore change is unlikely. It's simply not as important as other values. At other times, the exercise can illuminate a stark contrast and, as Zuckoff wisely notes, the possibility of shame is real. Allowing this shame to become the focus may immobilize the person from changing the behaviors. Again, the target is change, so this is where the practitioner will focus.

Although practitioners sometimes feel this activity is highly technical and complex, it is something that can be done by people learning the MI method. Using instructions and cues will help, but the essential elements are these:

1. Identify the most important values.

2. Ask the client what each value means.

3. Inquire about how the client is living out this value.

4. Inquire about how the client is not living out this value.

5. Note links (or lack thereof) between the problem behavior and values.

As always, use OARS liberally!

Concept Quiz—Test Yourself!

True or false:

1.   T F   Ambivalence is common as people consider changing a behavior.

2.   T F   Ambivalence and resistance are the same concept.

3.   T F   Sometimes using OARS alone is enough to sort through contradictory feelings and arrive at a decision point.

4.   T F   A decisional balance activity is necessary to do MI.

5.   T F   Within MI, ambivalence is resolved by being directive and focusing on change talk.

6.   T F   Evocative questions are those that evoke emotion.

7.   T F   *Picking the flowers* refers to listening and selectively reinforcing the elements in the conversation that focus on change.

8.   T F   Selectively reinforcing change talk is sometimes not enough. Clients may need help organizing the information in a way that is useful to them.

9.   T F   The VCS is a highly technical activity that requires significant skill in MI.

10.   T F   The VCS exercise can be both affirming and shaming for clients.

Answers

1.   T   OK. I've probably asked this question one too many times, but it's only to build a rhythmic chant that feels like breathing. *Breathe in*: Ambivalence is normal. *Breathe out*: Reflect.

2.   F   Engle and Arkowitz (2006) make a clear differentiation between the uncertainty of making a change and the active pushing back in which clients sometimes engage. This assertion is similar to the comments made in Chapter 6 about sustain talk and resistance.

3.   T   OARS alone can be enough, though sometimes a more formal approach can yield a fuller picture of the situation and assist the person in moving forward toward readiness.

4.   F   Decisional balance is not MI (Miller & Rollnick, 2009). Although it may be useful in some specific situations, it is not necessary and may even be problematic because it elicits status quo talk.

5.   T   Although the definition of MI refers to an exploration of ambivalence, this focus is not meant to involve a lengthy elicitation of all the reasons for the status quo. Instead, it is a targeted approach that selectively elicits and reinforces change talk.[2]

---

[2]There are differing perspectives about how best to explore ambivalence. One end of the continuum tends to favor the full exploration of ambivalence, a propensity that may be more in line with humanistic traditions in psychotherapy. Conversely, the other end, which may come from a more cognitive-behavioral bent, notes the importance of self-perception theory to the understanding of what occurs in MI and worries that elicitation of the pros of the present behavior or situation may reinforce the status quo. There are some data to support this concern. However, it is important to note that there is not one cohesive view about this matter. The good news is that this is a testable proposition that will (hopefully) be answered by research in the coming years.   (*cont.*)

6. F   Although evocative questions may indeed evoke emotion, that is not the intent behind these types of questions. These queries are meant to draw attention to elements focused on change and ask the client to speak directly to these elements.

7. T   Most of the time picking the flowers involves change talk. However, there may be times when preliminary steps—like in the conversation with Carrie—focus on the change element but don't meet the standard for change talk (i.e., noting the department's requirement that she must engage in this activity). This is not the same as change talk, yet it puts us on the path where change talk may happen. We may need to attend to these elements until change talk emerges. Once it does, change talk is the primary focus.

8. T   As noted a few times in this text, clients may need our assistance in organizing their experience. This may be especially the case when clients are ambivalent: They know they are stuck and have been unable to resolve this dilemma on their own. In this case pointing out the relation between ideas, behaviors, or values may assist them in moving forward.

9. F   The VCS technique is not highly technical, though some practice and experience with it is clearly important to use it effectively. Like many of the areas we've discussed, it will be the small nuances and skilled reflections and questions that ultimately determine the effectiveness of the technique. However, this does not prevent people who are learning MI from using this technique effectively. You should bear in mind the information in the next answer when using this technique.

10. T   This exercise can elicit both of these emotions, and both can serve as motivators, though the latter is a much more complicated situation. In general, MI does not seek to elicit shame because this response does not create a safe environment for change. On the other hand, in the course of careful review and discussion, people might become quite aware that their behavior has not matched their expectations for themselves (or that others held). The aim is not to elicit feelings of shame, but, if they are brought forth, then the goal is to move to a situation where behavior feels more congruent with values. This process requires skill. It is the art of doing MI well and for which there is nothing like practice, feedback, and coaching.

In Practice

We return to the Department of Health Services practice coach and the supervisor, Carrie. This is the start of the Wednesday meeting negotiated between the coach and Carrie. The change goal for the coach in this situation is for Carrie to embrace the model. He begins by establishing rapport and finding a mutual agenda in this process. Again, the coach observed a tape of the supervisor in practice last week and noted that she used very little of the

---

For now, my position is toward the middle of the continuum: to explore the pros but to elaborate more fully the cons of the status quo as a stepping-off point for eliciting change talk. My experience in the addiction setting is that people have rarely been asked what they like about their use, and so there is disarming quality to this inquiry and a sense from clients that there is value in the practitioner's genuine interest and curiosity in their situation. This inquiry also helps me understand what clients will have to replace if they make this change, and this understanding will aid in the development of a change plan, when that time arrives. However, this is not a purposeful excavation of every bit of sustain talk. Rather, the point is to develop some understanding of what maintains the behavior, *while focusing on the change elements.*

intervention model. In the following dialogue, the C represents the coach and the S is the supervisor (Carrie).

Statement	*Commentary*
C: I'm here to chat about the intervention model, but I'd like to find out a little more about how things are going for you first. I know there are lots of demands on your time.	Starts with opening statement that is broad and elicits information about the supervisor's context.
S: It's true. Between families, paperwork, and personnel issues, it's nonstop. But, I've good a good staff here—for the most part—and that makes it easier.	Talks about struggles and assets. She also drops a hint.
C: You feel like your staff functions pretty well.	Picking the flowers. A complex reflection targets the change elements and might allow further exploration.
S: For the most part …	Reinforces the hint.
C: But not entirely …	Picking the flowers again. This complex reflection addresses the hint.
S: Yeah. Well, I have this issue with Don. I spend what seems like a half hour each morning dealing with the fallout of his interactions with clients. He just doesn't seem to get along with folks. I've talked with him multiple times, and it just doesn't change. I think I'm at the point where I just need to write him up [make a personnel report], but if I do that, then I have union trouble. Who needs it?	Describes the agenda item that is important to her—and it's not the intervention model.
C: It's just one more headache on top of all the others.	Links this back to the other demands with a reflection. Builds rapport, but focuses on sustain element.
S: And then with all these new policy initiatives, it's like one after the other. I've got no time, and families are supposed to come first.	Describes ambivalence about the initiative.

Statement	*Commentary*
C: It's like tasks stacked on top of tasks. Then there is Don. Then somebody comes and adds this huge new task—doing this intervention—on top of that. I can imagine it feels like there is no way this can all be balanced. I can also imagine your feeling a little frustrated and maybe even a little resentful that this intervention model gets thrown on top.	With a summary and metaphor, the coach acknowledges the burden the initiative creates, then adds a feeling element. Again, the focus is on building rapport, which involves some limited focus on the sustain talk.
S: Yeah. You got it.	Feels understood, but ambivalence is not resolved.
C: And throughout all of this, you're trying to keep your eye on the target—families. You sound like someone who really cares, even when it might've been easier to just do your job and build some walls around your heart.	Providing bouquets. This brief linking summary affirms supervisor's strength while attending to potential source of motivation (change elements) to engage with intervention.
S: I do care. It's why I've stayed in the business. But it just feels harder and harder, especially when you're asked to do more and more, but without any extra help.	Endorses this motivation and reiterates the challenge.
C: And that's what this feels like—"more bricks, less straw."	Metaphor.
S: No offense, but yeah.	Supervisor feels understood and engaged with coach, though not the program.
C: I wonder if I could offer a little bit of information. [S: Yes.] Well, our aim is not to make your life harder. So, I'm wondering if there are any ways you could see our presence being of assistance rather than a hindrance to you.	Provides targeted information and then asks an evocative question that attempts to see if the client can observe any benefits from engagement.
S: If you could make my problem with Don go away, that would be a start!	Supervisor is very clear.
C: So, helping with Don would be a good start.	Picking the flowers.

Statement	*Commentary*
S: Can you talk with him?	The supervisor likely knows this is not how the system works. Still, ambivalence about engagement is present.
C: That's not exactly how the model works. What we are trying to do is help folks deal effectively with the Don-types themselves—along with other things—so when these things come up, they feel able to address them. The hope would be that you could have more of the outcomes you'd like.	Coach provides information directed to the ambivalence and attempts to engage the part that might benefit the supervisor. Starts to be close to persuasion.
S: So, you're not going to talk with him?	Feels the persuasion and presses the point.
C: No, but there might be other possibilities.	Responds directly, but offers another option.
S: Well, maybe I could meet with him and you could watch and see how hard he is to deal with.	Provides the option herself.
C: That would be helpful for you.	Coach picks the flower and reinforces this engagement.
S: You might have some ideas, but you'd also see what I am up against.	Engagement is present though still tentative. This is the beginning of moving from ambivalence into change.
C: You're hopeful, but realistic. And you want me to be realistic as well. That's a value for both of us. It's unlikely that we'll come up with something that fixes this situation in one meeting. But, if we could reduce the time spent with Don-related problems each morning—say from 30 minutes to 15 minutes—how would that fit?	Providing the bouquet. The coach offers some additional information about realistic expectations and follows this up with an evocative question.
S: It would cut my headache in half.	Buy in.
C: It would be a start. So, what would be helpful for me to watch for in this meeting?	Reinforces change talk. Moves to target the intervention to supervisor's needs and to reinforce engagement.

Try This!

Ambivalence is a tough area to practice without talking with others. However, we'll start with some imagination exercises, as well as self-focused work, and then move toward conversations with others.

Exercise 8.1. Tipping the Balance?

This is an exercise in imagination and ambivalence. You will find a worksheet of common problem areas encountered by practitioners using MI. For each area, you will be asked to imagine what things might sustain this behavior or the status quo and what might be problematic. Then you will write an evocative question designed to elicit from the change side of this ambivalence.

Exercise 8.2. Finding and Picking the Flowers

In this exercise you'll practice identifying and reinforcing the areas that might have change talk inherent in a client statement. You'll practice finding this "flower" and reinforcing it through reflection. Sometimes the flower will be difficult to see, so look carefully.

Exercise 8.3. Arranging the Bouquet

Using the information you generated in Exercise 8.1, write a summary that helps to organize the information and present it in a manner that focuses on the change elements. The questions are listed on the worksheet, along with space for your summary. However, you will need your completed forms for Exercise 8.1 to do this exercise. An example is included on the worksheet for your reference.

Exercise 8.4. Sorting Your Values

In this exercise you will be working on sorting through your own values and thinking about these in relation to a behavior you would like to change. Begin by obtaining the VCS from the MI website (*www.motivationalinterview.org/library/valuescardsort.pdf*). Once you've done this, cut the cards up and sort them into unimportant and important categories. From the important category, choose the five most important values, then complete the questions on the worksheet for Exercise 8.4.

Exercise 8.5. Everyday Ambivalence

This is an opportunity to practice asking about ambivalence in everyday encounters. You might start with friends, family, or coworkers and then work your way up to strangers. Listen for opportunities or inquire about subjects that typically contain ambivalence. If it is political season in your area, new candidates can be a ripe subject, but you can also ask about current leaders. There are sample questions provided to help you start this process.

Partner Work

All of the activities in this section could be done with your partner. For Exercise 8.1, Tipping the Balance?, make this into a game. Take turns adding items onto the list. The last person adding an item scores a point. Every evocative question scores 2 points. The person with the most points wins. Make a friendly wager for the loser to buy the winner a cup of coffee. You can also use the prompts in Exercise 8.5 to practice having conversations with your partner, and you can practice the VCS with your partner. Use the instructions in the chapter in relation to a behavior change your partner is considering. Make sure to use the prompts.

Exercise 8.6. My Client Isn't Changing

Think about a client who has all the observable reasons for changing and yet does not. Then play this client and have your partner do the VCS. Don't caricature your client. Instead, try to guess at what things might be happening below the surface. Remember, people tend to do things for reasons. See if you come to any new understandings.

Other Thoughts . . .

When asking for more information in an area, the "What else?" query is very useful. A subtle shift to a closed question (e.g., "Anything else?") can also be helpful in demarcating the discussion. The beauty of this query is that clients typically recognize the shift, and if there is more to say, they will typically offer it. So, although it can close down an area of inquiry, it does not shut down the client or feel disrespectful.

Tipping the Balance?

This is an exercise in imagination and ambivalence. Listed on this worksheet you will find problem areas that are frequently encountered by practitioners using MI. However, most of these will not match your work area. Try, for each area, to imagine what things might sustain this behavior or the status quo. Then try to identify what might be more problematic about this situation. Some categories will obviously overlap, but some will be unique. Try to identify as many items as you can for each category. Then write an evocative question that might elicit some of the change side of this ambivalence and begin tipping the balance.

Why does a diabetic continue to eat foods with high sugar content?

Sustains status quo	Problems with status quo
1.	1.
2.	2.
3.	3.
4.	4.
5.	5.

Evocative question:

Why does a parolee continue to hang out with problematic friends from the old neighborhood?

Sustains status quo	Problems with status quo
1.	1.
2.	2.
3.	3.
4.	4.
5.	5.

Evocative question:

(*cont.*)

Why does a young man (woman) continue to have unprotected sex with multiple partners?

Sustains status quo	Problems with status quo
1.	1.
2.	2.
3.	3.
4.	4.
5.	5.

Evocative question:

Why does a recent cardiac patient continue to smoke?

Sustains status quo	Problems with status quo
1.	1.
2.	2.
3.	3.
4.	4.
5.	5.

Evocative question:

Why does a young mother with two children stay with her physically abusive husband?

Sustains status quo	Problems with status quo
1.	1.
2.	2.
3.	3.
4.	4.
5.	5.

Evocative question:

Why does the shopper continue to buy unnecessary items that are on sale despite his or her partner's concerns about finances?

Sustains status quo   Problems with status quo

1.   1.

2.   2.

3.   3.

4.   4.

5.   5.

Evocative question:

Why does the recent addictions treatment program graduate continue to throw darts in his old bar?

Sustains status quo   Problems with status quo

1.   1.

2.   2.

3.   3.

4.   4.

5.   5.

Evocative question:

Why does the high school freshman continue to play video games despite falling grades and parental anger?

Sustains status quo   Problems with status quo

1.   1.

2.   2.

3.   3.

4.   4.

5.   5.

Evocative question:

Sample Responses for Exercise 8.1

Why does a diabetic continue to eat foods with high sugar content?

> Evocative question: *In what ways do your eating patterns concern you?*

Why does a parolee continue to hang out with problematic friends from the old neighborhood?

> Evocative question: *So, there are obviously good things about hanging out with old friends, and some risks associated with that. What are some of the risks you see?*

Why does a young man (woman) continue to have unprotected sex with multiple partners?

> Evocative question: *What would be better for you if you decided to be safer in the sex you're having?*

Why does a recent cardiac patient continue to smoke?

> Evocative question: *What benefits do you think might accrue if you stopped smoking?*

Why does a young mother with two children stay with her physically abusive husband?

> Evocative question: *What do you hope for either you or your children if you could start fresh in a relationship?*

Why does the shopper continue to buy unnecessary items that are on sale despite his or her partner's concerns about finances?

> Evocative question: *If you made changes in your shopping patterns, how would things be better with your partner?*

Why does the recent addictions treatment program graduate continue to throw darts in his old bar?

> Evocative question: *What might others say are the risky spots for you in throwing darts?*

Why does the high school freshman continue to play video games despite falling grades and parental anger?

> Evocative question: *How would life be better for you if your parents weren't always on your case?*

Finding and Picking the Flowers

In this exercise you'll practice identifying and reinforcing the areas that might have change talk inherent in a client statement. You'll practice finding this flower and then picking it. You'll pick the flower by using a reflection. Sometimes this will require you to take a guess at what is implied in the client's statements.

"I wish people would just back off about my smoking. I'm not an idiot. The more people tell me I have to stop, the more annoyed I get."

"I thought drinking wine was supposed to be good for my heart. Now you say I have to give that up, as well as all of my favorite foods. This makes absolutely no sense to me. Is this a life worth living?"

"It doesn't work. The kids continue to misbehave and fight with each other. They only stop when I yell."

"I'm happy with things as they are. Really, I am. This is everybody else's issue, not mine. If they'd back off, I'd be fine. I'm just trying to lose some weight and be healthy."

"Hemp is a naturally occurring plant that has been used for hundreds, maybe thousands, of years. It is not physically addicting. I think I'm more focused and can get things done when I have smoked a little."

"You don't know me. You don't know what I've had to put up with or how hard it has been. If you did, you wouldn't make these stupid suggestions."

Sample Responses for Exercise 8.2

"I wish people would just back off about my smoking. I'm not an idiot. The more people tell me I have to stop, the more annoyed I get."

You're aware that you are in some danger. You're just not ready to do something yet.

"I thought drinking wine was supposed to be good for my heart. Now you say I have to give that up, as well as all of my favorite foods. This makes absolutely no sense to me. Is this a life worth living?"

It's hard to imagine that your lifestyle had become so hard on your health.

"It doesn't work. The kids continue to misbehave and fight with each other. They only stop when I yell."

You've been willing to try because you see some advantages to it.

"I'm happy with how I am eating. Really, I am. This is everybody else's issue, not mine. If they'd back off, I'd be fine. I'm just trying to lose some weight and be healthy."

There are potential elements in virtually every line. Here are a couple of examples.

You're perfectly satisfied with how you're controlling your weight.
You want to be healthy, and it's confusing to you that others view your behavior as unhealthy.

"Hemp is a naturally occurring plant that has been used for hundreds, maybe thousands, of years. It is not physically addicting. I think I'm more focused and can get things done when I have smoked a little."

You're someone who's willing to look at the evidence and weigh it out for yourself.

"You don't know me. You don't know what I've had to put up with or how hard it has been. If you did, you wouldn't make these stupid suggestions."

If I knew you, then I might make some suggestions that are helpful; that has not been the case so far.

Arranging the Bouquet

Using the information you generated in Exercise 8.1, write a summary that helps to organize the information and present it in a manner that focuses on the change elements. The questions are listed below, along with space for your summary. Choose any three of the questions to do this exercise. You do not have to do each item. However, you will need your completed forms for Exercise 8.1 to do this exercise. A sample is included below, using a different scenario than those presented before.

Sample:

Why does the person continue to drink, despite clear evidence of health consequences and warnings from doctor and family?

Sustains status quo

1. *Doesn't feel he can change.*
2. *Thinks he only hurts himself.*
3. *Provides relief from the troubles of his life.*
4. *Doesn't want to be told what to do.*
5. *Believes he likes it.*

Problems with status quo

1. *His health is suffering.*
2. *His behavior is affecting others.*
3. *Others are worried.*
4. *He may be afraid.*
5. *Life may not have much of the other things he wants.*

Bouquet/Summary:

> "*Some issues with your health have cropped up, and that is a source of concern for others and perhaps you. Drinking is something you've done for a long time, and you may feel as though it provides you with a little respite from the world and all of your troubles. While you don't like being told what to do, it may also be clear to you that these folks have a point, and you may be a little afraid of what might happen if you don't make some changes. You might like to have some other things in your life and not have folks on your back all the time.*"

Why does a diabetic continue to eat foods with high sugar content?

Bouquet/Summary:

Why does a parolee continue to hang out with problematic friends from the old neighborhood?

Bouquet/Summary:

(cont.)

Why does a young man (woman) continue to have unprotected sex with multiple partners?

Bouquet/Summary:

Why does a recent cardiac patient continue to smoke?

Bouquet/Summary:

Why does a young mother with two children stay with her physically abusive husband?

Bouquet/Summary:

Why does the shopper continue to buy unnecessary items that are on sale despite his or her partner's concerns about finances?

Bouquet/Summary:

Why does the recent addictions treatment program graduate continue to throw darts in his old bar?

Bouquet/Summary:

Why does the high school freshman continue to play video games despite falling grades and parental anger?

Bouquet/Summary:

Sorting Your Values

In this exercise you will be working on sorting through your own values and thinking about these in relation to a behavior you would like to change. Choose a behavior that you have struggled to change or that someone else has suggested you need to change. Begin by obtaining the VCS from the MI website (*www.motivationalinterview.org*), cutting up the cards, and then sorting them into unimportant and important categories. From the important category, choose the five most important values, then complete the following questions.

In the spaces below, record your five most important values and what each means to you.

1. Value: _____ This value means to me:

_____

_____

_____

2. Value: _____ This value means to me:

_____

_____

_____

3. Value: _____ This value means to me:

_____

_____

_____

4. Value: _____ This value means to me:

_____

_____

_____

5. Value: _____ This value means to me:

_____

_____

_____

(*cont.*)

Now choose one of these values that seems particularly important to you. Then answer the following questions. You can copy the following page and repeat for each value, if you like.

Value: _____

In what ways are you succeeding in living out this value?

_____

_____

_____

_____

_____

In what ways are you not living out this value as fully as you would like?

_____

_____

_____

_____

_____

How does your target behavior (i.e., the behavior you would like to change) fit with this value? How does the target behavior affect your ability to live out this value? Are there any conflicts or tensions?

_____

_____

_____

_____

_____

What would you need to do or change to more fully live out this value?

_____

_____

_____

_____

Everyday Ambivalence

This is an opportunity to practice asking about ambivalence in everyday encounters. You might start with friends, family, or coworkers and then work your way up to strangers. Listen for opportunities or inquire about subjects that typically contain ambivalence. If it is political season in your area, new candidates can be a ripe subject, but you can also ask about current leaders.

Here are some examples of questions you might ask:

- "So, what do you think about the prime minister [president/governor/mayor]? What do you like about the job she [or he] is doing? What aren't you happy about? [Don't forget to ask for examples.] What was a decision that you had a reaction to?"
- "What are your thoughts about the upcoming election? Whom do you like? What worries you?"

Other areas or topics you might explore are global warming, tourism, movies, kids and TV or video games, testing to standards in schools, subsidized health care, "big box" stores versus mom-and-pop stores, the impact of cell phones on society, etc. Here are two questions you might use.

- "What do you think about what the researchers and politicians are saying about global warming? What makes you feel that way? Anything that makes you pause?"
- "People seem to have these love–hate feelings about tourism. What do you think about tourists here? Why do you think some people are so in favor of (or against) the tourism industry? What gains do they see? How about the folks who don't like it?"

Asking the questions could feel a bit odd, so try to work them into your conversations in a manner that fits your style. Remember to ask about both sides and try to elicit examples. Also, remember that you aren't trying to convince people of a particular position, but instead to understand their views and explore areas where ambivalence may arise. This is not the same as what you will do in MI; rather, it provides practice in eliciting this information.

Think about a client who has all the observable reasons for changing and yet does not. Then play this client and have your partner do the VCS. Don't caricature your client. Instead, try to guess at what things might be happening below the surface. Remember, people tend to do things for reasons. See if you come to any new understandings. The instructions written by Allan Zuckoff for the VCS are included below.[3]

- Ask clients to sort the cards into "Not Important" and "Important" piles. When many cards inevitably end up in the "Important" pile, take a moment to affirm that many things are important to the client. Then note that most of us, in fact, have many values that sometimes come into conflict with each other, and that this is sometimes what makes it hard for us to make important life decisions. (This helps detoxify the client's likely feelings of frustration, anger and/or disgust with self for being stuck for so long.)

- Ask clients to sort the "Important" cards into "Important" and "Most Important" piles, with no more than five in the "Most Important" pile.

- Ask clients to tell, in any order, what the word on each of the Most Important values cards means to them. Listen empathically, working to understand the unique meanings each value holds for the client and listening for underlying themes, connections, or tensions among them.

- Ask clients in what ways they are currently succeeding in living out each of these values; listen empathically and ask for elaboration and examples. (This elicits self-affirming statements and gives the therapist opportunities to offer affirmations as well.)

- Ask clients in what ways they are not currently living out these values as fully as they would like. (Developing discrepancy this way is intended to prime clients in favor of change, broadly speaking. This requires a high level of trust on the part of clients, and has the potential to, at least temporarily, leave clients feeling worse.)

- Ask clients how the target behavior fits with these values (or what effects the target behavior has on their ability to live out these values).

- If clients don't spontaneously describe any conflicts between the values and the target behavior, ask about such conflicts or tensions.

- Ask clients what they would need to do or to change in order to live out these values more fully.

---

[3] Adapted by permission.

Chapter 9

Information Sharing, Offering a Concern, and Giving Advice

Opening

"My doc thought I should come here and talk about my diabetes, but I think he's making too big of a deal about it."

Walt sprawled on the couch as he talked. A 29-year-old carrying 50 extra pounds of weight and a similarly proportioned chip on his shoulder, he wore his flat-billed baseball cap at a jaunty angle. His physician, in making the referral, indicated that Walt had twice made trips to the ER in the last 4 months because of blood sugars so high these wouldn't register on his glucometer (above 600, 80–120 is normal). His last A1c was 14, whereas his target goal was 7 or below. His doctor diagnosed the diabetes when Walt was 6. His single mother had tried her best to encourage good self-care habits, but Walt had become increasingly truculent over the years. School had always been a struggle, and he'd received special education services prior to dropping out his senior year. Drifting in and out of work for a decade, he was now taking a welding program at a local vocational-technical school. This is the first meeting, picked up midconversation, with the practitioner responding to Walt's statement.

"Too big a deal ... "

"Yeah. He wants me to check my blood sugar more often, and he's always bugging me to exercise and watch my diet."

"It feels like he's nagging you."

"Like my mom."

"Your mom does the same thing."

"She's always in my face about something. She says I'm a slob, and if I don't take care of my diabetes I'm going to go blind, or my kidneys will quit working, or they'll amputate my feet. She's full of sh—crap. Sorry."

"I don't care if you swear, just as long as you can spell it right."

Walt laughs. "There's nothing wrong with my eyesight or those other things. I take pretty good care of my diabetes. She's just trying to scare me."

"And that's what your doctor does too."

"Well, not like her. But he does keep saying we need to get this under control or something bad will happen."

"And that's a little hard to believe, since nothing bad has happened yet."

"Well, nothing really bad."

"But a few things have worried you a little."

"Did my doc tell you why he sent me here?"

"He filled me in a bit. Told me that you'd struggled to get your A1c where he wanted it to be and that you'd had a couple of trips to the ER over the last few months."

"Yeah, this last time I was feeling pretty crappy. I thought I had the flu. I was throwing up and feeling out of it. I tried checking my blood, but nothing happened."

"Nothing happened ... "

"The glucometer told me that my blood sugar was too high to register. I'd already injected a sh—, uh, boat load of insulin, so I knew I was in trouble. I called my mom and she called 911."

"It scared you."

"I wasn't scared ... I just needed some help."

" ... which was hard, because you don't want to be treated like a kid. You want to make your own decisions."

"What do you mean?"

"Maybe I misunderstood. It seemed you were saying that you're a guy who doesn't like it when folks nag you and tell you what to do. You like to make up your own mind."

"That's true. I do."

"And this was a situation where you couldn't quite do it on your own."

"Yeah, and so now everyone is bugging me, making this big deal out of this situation and making me come to see you."

"You resent that and at the same time you came. I wonder why."

"I guess it does worry me a little, but I'm not going blind, am I?"

The practitioner worked hard to build rapport with Walt. Through this process (with the interviewer mostly listening), Walt has begun to provide small openings and to offer some tentative change talk, and now he's asked for the practitioner's opinion. What would you say? If you don't work in diabetes or health care settings, you might feel that you wouldn't have any information to offer. I challenge you to think beyond your setting and consider the information the doctor told this practitioner: (1) The client has made two trips to the ER because of very high blood sugars; (2) he has an A1c (a lab test that provides an "average" blood glucose level over the past 90 days) that is very high (14 vs. the 7); and (3) his doctor is concerned enough to send him for a treatment consult. Knowing just these things, what would you say? How would you say it?

A Deeper Look

In their most recent book, *Motivational Interviewing in Health Care*, Rollnick et al. (2008) describe three communication styles (directing, following, and guiding) and three primary communication tools within those styles (asking, listening, and informing). Each of the communication styles is well suited to some situations and a mismatch with others. The goal is not for practitioners to use only one style but rather to move flexibly and skillfully among them as the situation dictates.

A directing style involves the practitioner providing expertise, often in the form of advice or a plan of action. There is a problem-solving quality to this process. The person directing is typically in charge. Before surgeons insert a pacemaker/defibrillator, they communicate to patients the problem, the solution, and how they will accomplish this task. The technical expertise that the practitioner brings to the encounter may be quite helpful to the client, but there is also an implication of an uneven relationship as a result. The client depends on the practitioner for decisions, advice, and action. This approach may save lives. For example, a child runs into a street, and the parent responds quickly with a command to stop to prevent harm. The implicit message in this style is, "I have ideas about how to solve this situation."

In contrast, in a following style the practitioner, not surprisingly, follows the client's lead as the client explores an area. Following is an approach wherein the client is primarily in charge. The goal is to listen well and understand the situation. The practitioner sets aside concerns and focuses on how the client sees the problem. For example, a man considers either staying in a stable job, where he is valued but not entirely fulfilled, or leaving for self-employment that might be more fulfilling but also has significant financial risk. There is no correct choice generally, so the practitioner helps the client understand his situation more clearly, primarily through listening and avoiding the temptation to give advice. This style may be particularly helpful in situations in which the client has received some powerful news or is overwhelmed by emotion. The conversation moves at the client's pace and direction. The practitioner's implicit message is, "I accept and trust your wisdom about what is needed."

A guiding style involves an approach in which a client and practitioner work as a team. The practitioner and client "walk" together, but this time the practitioner points out routes and options, serving as a resource about what is possible, what others have done, and what the risks and benefits might be of each approach. As the practitioner points out possible paths, the client receives assistance in choosing the direction that fits best for him or her. However, it is the client who must ultimately choose the way. In this style the implicit message is, according to Rollnick et al. (2008), "I'll help you solve this yourself." MI is a refined form of this guiding style.

Within each of these styles, practitioners might listen, ask questions, or advise/provide information, though some skills may predominate within a particular style. Each of these styles can be enacted in a manner that is either consistent or inconsistent with MI principles. Finally, although the distinction of the styles make intuitive sense, it may be difficult to draw clear boundaries between them as one moves from following to guiding to directing. In practice, this boundary question is of only minor importance, as the goal is not to do one style only, as mentioned, but rather to move fluidly between all three and decide at which point a particular style is likely to be most effective.

This chapter focuses on how to provide information, offer a concern, and give advice, using both guiding and directing styles of communication. Let's begin by reviewing some basic concepts about providing information, offering a concern, and giving advice.

Basic Concepts

Here are some ideas to keep in mind when you are communicating new or discrepant information to a client. Many of these ideas can and should be combined together.

• *Offer information, don't impose it.* You may think that clients are entirely inaccurate in their perception of the information, but to argue the correctness of your data (or error of their conclusions) is likely to engender resistance. Remember, we are not trying to pin an opponent in a wrestling match.

• *Find out if clients want the information before you give it.* If clients ask for your opinion, check before you offer it. Many times people ask what we think as a lead-in for telling us what they think. Returning to our example of Walt, you might say, "I'm happy to answer that, but first I'm wondering what you think?"

• *Ask permission, especially if clients haven't asked for the information.* Sometimes we have information that we think would be really helpful to clients in sorting through their situation. However, it's only helpful if the client wants to hear it. Responding to Walt, you could say, "I have some information that might be helpful. Would you be interested in hearing it?" Most clients will answer in the affirmative, but if they say "no," you should respect their wishes. To do otherwise is to fail to respect autonomy and likely to engage resistance. Having said all this, there will be situations when you do not ask permission to provide information—for example, when there is a risk of harm to others. Also, once clients grant their consent, permission does not need to be requested every time. Indeed clients will likely become annoyed if this is done repeatedly. Still, permission should be reaffirmed occasionally: "Is it OK if I share a little more?"

• *Provide information in the context of other clients.* As practitioners, we often bring a wealth of experience to the interaction. Use this information in providing ideas or solutions. You might say, "In my work with clients like yourself, Walt, they have found. … " Clients tend to respond well to what others like themselves have done. This approach also prevents a dynamic wherein clients resist you if they don't view any of your suggestions as fitting for them.

• *Give clients implicit or explicit permission to disagree with you.* In so doing, you actually increase the chance that clients will be able to hear your concern. This can be done through simple prefacing with phrases such as the following:

"This may or may not be of concern to you … "

"I don't know if this will make sense to you, but … "

"You may not agree with me on this … "

• *Use a menu of options.* Typically, there is more than one correct way to solve a problem. Again, our experience can serve us well. Provide more than one way to solve the problem and ask which way seems to fit best for a particular client. You can combine this approach with a prior concept and use your clients' methods to demonstrate multiple paths to success. Using Walt as an example, you might say: "There is more than one way to develop better control. Some clients have chosen to keep logs of their blood sugars. Others try to focus on eating a consistent diet—the same times, types of foods, and amounts each day. Still others have tried to increase their exercise while checking their blood sugars more often. Which of these makes the most sense to you?" This approach avoids the situation where we offer suggestions one at a time, and clients shoot them down one at a time, like a skeet shooter targeting clay pigeons.

• *Use client statements.* In MI, the practitioner acts as a mirror for clients so that they can observe what they've said and organize the different elements and make sense of these. By returning to their statements, we provide a powerful reminder of how they've looked at the situation. Remember Bem's self-perception theory and the importance of change talk. Given Walt's statements, you might say, "Although others are making too big a deal, you also know that your glucose control is related to feeling crappy recently and needing some help you'd prefer not to receive."

• *Give information that is factually or normatively based, rather than just opinion.* Present data as information for clients to consider. Since general information is often less helpful, provide information that speaks to each person's situation or behavior. Using diabetes as an example, here is a statement made at a global level: "There are risks for poor blood glucose control. The Diabetes Control and Complications Trial (DCCT Research Group, 1993), a study completed in the early 90s, showed that poor or fluctuating blood glucose control led to serious side effects in 80% of participants, including blindness, amputation, kidney failure, and death." Instead, you might use specific findings from an examination: "Compared to a year ago, your visual field examination is showing decreased sensitivity in two quadrants." Or "Last year, your A1c was 7.0, whereas now it is 14.0"

• *Invite clients to decide what the information means for them.* There is a tendency to draw the conclusion as to what the data imply, but, remember, it is much more powerful (and less likely to engage resistance) if clients decide the implications. You might say: "In a typical year, the average diabetic has zero ER visits. You've had two in the past 4 months. I wonder what you make of that information."

• *Remember, your client is a person, not an information receptacle.* Rollnick et al. (2008) provide this very helpful reminder. At times it is easy to feel that there is significant information that clients *must* know, and we feel pressured to provide it all at once. In this situation our expertise can be an impediment; our training indicates that clients need to know all of this information, so we bury them under a barrage of data. This issue becomes particularly salient when information provision is part of our job description. It's taken you many years to acquire this knowledge, and it's probably not realistic to expect that clients can process it all in a matter of minutes.

With these principles in mind, here are some techniques that you might consider for engaging in what Rollnick et al. (2008) describe as "information exchange."

Information Sharing

Rollnick et al. (2008) note a richness of context that often occurs when we share ideas about issues with clients. When done well, information provision is mutually interactive. We provide information, and clients offer information back to us. This process is a dialogue, not a monologue. The interactive nature of this process is lost if we label it as information provision, so instead we use the more user-friendly term *information sharing*.

There are many ways to accomplish information sharing. In addition to using approaches suggested by the above principles (e.g., asking permission), you might use one of the methods described below.

Elicit–Provide–Elicit (E-P-E)

This method, described by Rollnick and colleagues in *Health Behavior Change* (Rollnick et al., 1999), starts by asking clients what they know already (or want to know) about an area of interest (*elicit*). Once clients describe what they know, then the practitioner can add to it (*provide*). This method avoids telling clients what they already know, respects their skills and knowledge, and allows the practitioner to provide only the information that clients need. It also permits the practitioner to ask the clients view on what is offered (*elicit*). Here is an example of a student with test anxiety:

"What do you know about reducing text anxiety?"

"I know it would be good if I could."

"Yeah, I bet. And my guess is that you've probably tried some things already."

" … like telling myself not to worry so much."

"And that didn't work so well."

"Nope."

"I wonder if you'd be interested in some ideas that others like yourself have used."

"That's why I'm here."

"One approach people have tried is some simple breathing exercises. Others have tried our biofeedback machine, which helps them learn to relax their body when they want to. Still others have tried different studying regimens. Finally, some do an evaluation to receive more formal accommodations, such as additional time or taking tests in quiet environments, away from other people. What do you think of those ideas?"

Chunk–Check–Chunk

This approach is a variation on the E-P-E model (Rollnick et al., 2008). It is useful when the practitioner must convey a large volume of information, but wants to do so in a manner that still engages clients. The practitioner begins by providing a "chunk" of information. A chunk is a unit of information that is cohesive and can be delivered in a self-contained manner. Consider the following chunk about driving violations given to a driver who had four speeding tickets in a year:

> "The average driver in the State of Washington has zero moving violations, including speeding tickets. In fact, they make up about 85% of the licensed drivers in the state. If we add in the numbers for one violation, we account for 95% of the drivers. In fact, fewer than 1 in a 100 has four or more violations in a year or five in 2 years. What do you make of that information?"

After delivering the chunk, the practitioner stops to talk with the client about the information. This exchange is followed by another chunk of information. Here is a lengthier exchange, typical of my evaluation practice:

"Let me fill you in a little bit about what is we are doing here today. The Division of Vocational Rehabilitation [DVR] asked me to do this evaluation for a couple of reasons. First, they need to have a diagnosis under which they can provide services. These can be things like depression or anxiety, substance use or learning disabilities. Now I understand you've had some struggles with depression, as well as some challenges in learning. We'll spend some time getting specific information in areas like that. How's this fitting so far?"

"It makes sense. I know they talked about disabilities in the orientation meeting."

"This is no surprise."

"Not really."

"In addition to those specific areas, I'll also spend some time finding out a little bit about your history and your interests. I want to understand how these things fit into the big picture of your life. I'll ask you some questions about your family, schooling, medical history, and things like that. This information gives me a better perspective on those other things. What do you think about that?"

"It seems to me you'd need to know that stuff."

"It might help me understand you."

"Right."

"Then the last thing DVR wants is some information about what areas make sense for you in terms of your skills, ability, and if training is needed, what situation would work best for you. To accomplish that, I'll have you do some tests that look at how you think and solve problems. Some will make sense to you, and some may seem a bit goofy, but these all help me understand how your brain works. Then I'll also have you do some academic-style tasks to see where your reading, writing, and math skills are at. This is not the kind of thing you could've studied for—you just do your best. How does that sound?"

"I hate math, but I guess that's what you need to do."

"You'd prefer not to do it, and you also see why we would do this to understand your learning challenges."

"Let's do it."

A lot of information is conveyed, along with periodic check-ins. Client responses are brief, but reflected. At the end of this exchange, the client is moving with me and also ready to begin. As is evident, other MI skills should be at play in these methods.

Offering a Concern

As noted throughout this book, practitioners create safe situations by accepting client statements about their view of situations, but this is not the same as agreeing with this view. Practitioners *should* offer concerns about clients' harmful or detrimental decisions or positions, but it is the manner used that is critical. Practitioners avoid arguing with clients or telling clients that they are wrong. Instead, MI practitioners offer an alternative for clients' to consider or additional information that may shift their viewpoint. It is tempting at this juncture to offer the "overwhelming" evidence to persuade clients. Yet persuasion is likely to lead to resistance—either passively or openly. Once again, clients are left to make the final decision about the accuracy and meaning of the practitioner's statement.

For example, in the opening with Walt, the practitioner has information about Walt's difficulty managing his diabetes based on his A1c and his two trips to the ER, despite his statements about "taking good care of my diabetes." So, without being a specialist in diabetes, a practitioner could offer a concern in this manner:

> "So, as you look at the situation, it feels like you're taking good care of your diabetes. At the same time, I can also see there are some things you're less happy about. As I look at the situation, I have a couple of concerns I'd like to talk about with you. Is it OK if I share those with you [asking permission]?
>
> "Your A1c indicates that even though you've been working to stay in control of your diabetes, you're having trouble hitting the targets that your doc thinks are important. Also, you've had to make a couple of trips to the ER lately, and that probably doesn't feel real good to you, especially since it has other people making decisions on your behalf. We've talked about your liking to be the guy who calls the shots. So, it concerns me that your efforts at control might not be giving you the things you would like [offering multiple concerns].
>
> "That's what I think. What do you think about these things [asking client's view]?"

As noted in Chapter 7, offering a concern is helpful in situations where we need to raise a topic but there is no path immediately available. Consider this example with a person who is obviously suffering health problems but is not discussing these in the course of a probation officer meeting.

> "So, Janine, we've talked about a number of things. There is one more thing I'd like to raise, if I might? I've noticed over the last few meetings that you seem much more tired that you did before. I saw you coming up the stairs, and you looked really winded when you got to the top step. In addition, your skin looks yellow. These things suggest it's more than just a cold or the flu, but I'm not a doctor. So I am concerned about your health. What's happening?"

As noted before, even when well done, this approach may lead to "dissonance" in the relationship. If that happens, we work to bring the relationship back in tune. There will also be times when we directly disagree with a client's decisions or behaviors. Here is an example of an interaction with an 18-year-old freshman girl.

> "I'm concerned about your decision to hang out at the frat with the senior guys. You've told me that you tend to use alcohol, pot, and 'X' when you're in that situation, and that those drugs have led to you making risky sexual decisions. Although you may enjoy the attention and sex at the time, afterward you've told me that you've been embarrassed and uncomfortable. You've also told me that you don't want to end up in that situation

again. Of course, you will have to decide what is right for you. What do you think about those concerns?"

As was noted in Chapter 7, there are three elements in this statement. First, there is a direct report of the practitioner's concerns. The statement is made without judgment and uses prior client statements when possible. Then there is a statement of the client's responsibility for choice and change. Finally, the client's view is solicited.

Giving Advice

In many ways this topic of giving advice has already been covered in the previous sections. Yet, for many people, it feels like this is a primary component of their jobs, so we will review how the preceding components (basic concepts, information sharing, and expressing a concern) might fit into the context of giving advice. To accomplish this, let's consider a few types of sessions where advice feels not only important but essential.

Some practitioners work in settings where clients engage in harmful behavior to self or others. For example, an individual working in an eating disorder treatment unit routinely sees individuals engaged in self-destructive behavior. At times, this behavior threatens clients' lives. For this practitioner, there is a strong pull to warn that a failure to change could result in death. The question is not should this warning be given but how to maximize its effectiveness.

Practitioners feel even more strongly when the behavior not only endangers the client's life, but also others—especially children. So, when an abused woman expresses a desire to leave a domestic violence shelter and return to the home of a violent partner, towing her children back into this volatile situation, practitioners sometimes find it very hard to stay within a client-centered approach. It feels too dangerous to do anything less than confront the mother in the strongest terms possible to try to protect the children.

So, how do we "confront" these clients? First, if the goal is to change the behavior, and we don't have the capacity to control all aspects of this client's life, our power to enforce change is limited. Therefore, we will need the client's participation for this change to occur. In some situations a sober assessment of a dire situation may be enough. In others—like when a child runs into the street—we deliver the message in very strong terms. Second, we need to be aware that if we make dire predictions, the client may brush these off if others have delivered similar messages. Finally, we must consider client context. The option the client is choosing may feel like the only one available. Conversely, the option offered by the practitioner is so low on the client's priority list that other options take much greater precedence. In the case of the woman returning to her violent partner, ponder these contextual factors and then consider these two approaches: one MI consistent, the other not. We'll start with the second.

"You can't do this! If you do this, not only are your putting your life in danger, but also your children's lives. This guy beat you so badly that when the children saw your face, they didn't know it was you. He choked you until you blacked out. I know he says he's sorry now, but this is just part of a cycle. He broke his promise! This has happened before and will happen again. Given how much worse the violence has gotten, it seems pretty clear to me that he will kill you. Or maybe it will be the kids. You've told me you love your children, and you want them to be safe. Do you? If you do, how can you do this to them?"

This is strong medicine. In some situations such an approach may jolt a woman into a more accurate assessment of her situation. At other times, it might draw a more resistant response—either active or passive. As an alternative, here is a more MI-consistent confrontation.

> "I need to say something here. I am terrified of the decision you are making to return to your partner. I see all kinds of danger signs that the violence is getting worse. You've described how it's escalated over time. The last time he choked you until you passed out. Your face was so badly bruised that your children didn't recognize you. I know there all sorts of reasons why you might want to return to him, including his promises to never do this again—something you'd really like to believe. And I know you balance that against your past experience. I also know you love your children, and it must be hard to think about how this must affect them, as well as the risk you feel for them. So, I cannot control your decision. This must be your choice to make—and I must say, in the strongest terms, I hope you will reconsider and make a different choice."

Both statements present strong warnings. Both press the client to consider a different choice. The first tells the client that she cannot do this, whereas the second acknowledges that the client will choose. Both provide information, though the first presents it in the form of support for the argument that the mother must change, whereas the second supports the practitioner statement that she is terrified. Both address her experience with the abusive cycle and concern for her children. Again, the manner this information is presented differs, with the second version placing it in the context of the client's experience and view, whereas the first buttresses the argument already made. Finally, they both end with a plea to reconsider, but the second provides both choice and an avenue for the client to rethink the decision, whereas the first requires a capitulation. Finally, the literature consistently suggests that women in domestic violence situations will often return to the abuse perpetrators. The second approach might make it easier for her to return to the *practitioner*, if she returns home and then must leave again; it leaves the door open, perhaps making it easier for the client to walk back in, if that time should come.

As noted, for some clients, the first approach might work. It might also work for certain practitioners. If it works consistently well for you, I encourage you to continue doing it. There is no sense changing something that is consistently effective. However, if it works only occasionally, then you might consider the second approach as an alternative.

In discussing this area, we have considered many ideas. Here are some clear guidelines that might be helpful as you think about advice giving. These guidelines form the acronym FOCUS, which also expresses an important idea about advice generally.

- **F**irst ask permission. Make sure the client is interested in what you are about to offer.
- **O**ffer ideas. Don't try to persuade.

- Concise. Don't ramble. Be direct and succinct. If you offer too many concerns, you do not help clients organize and respond effectively to their situations.
- Use a menu. That is, provide different ways or ideas the client might use to address the situation; do this in the context of a menu from which they select one or multiple ways to succeed.
- Solicit what the client thinks. Always begin and end with the client.

Concept Quiz—Test Yourself!

True or false:

1.   T F   An MI practitioner should not use directing as a communication style.

2.   T F   MI is most like guiding.

3.   T F   Practitioners should strive to move flexibly between the communication styles of directing, following, and guiding.

4.   T F   The implicit message in guiding is, "I'll help you solve this for yourself."

5.   T F   If clients are inaccurate in their perceptions, it is acceptable in MI to correct their misperceptions.

6.   T F   You must always ask permission before giving information in MI.

7.   T F   Clients typically find personal information more helpful in feedback, then general information about a behavior.

8.   T F   Clients are typically uninterested in what others have done to either address similar challenges or solve comparable problems.

9.   T F   It is often useful to integrate prior client statements when providing information.

10. T F   Because clients don't have the technical expertise to understand certain kinds of the information, it is our job to provide the conclusions of what it means for them.

Answers

1. F   In fact, MI practitioners use directing when needed. The issue is how to use it effectively. All three of the communication styles can be used in an MI-consistent manner, as well as in an MI-inconsistent way.

2. T   MI is a refined form of guiding, according to Rollnick et al. (2008). Practitioners provide expertise and guidance about directions, but also provide options and allow clients to choose directions that make sense to them.

3. T   As suggested by the two previous answers, there may be a preference for guiding as a style in MI, but the practitioner will need to be flexible and facile in all three to be successful. Different situations call for different skills, just as different household problems require different tools. A pencil, hammer, and plunger are all the right tools in some situations and very wrong in another.

4.   T   Throughout this workbook, we have focused on empowering clients to use their own resources to solve problems. Guiding is in step with this approach. We might have opinions about options that will be harder and easier, but ultimately the client will choose and then must enact the decision. Our job is to support that effort.

5.   T   We should correct misperceptions, though it is important to be thoughtful in how we do it. There are times when providing contrary information will simply heighten resistance in an argumentative client. In this situation, delaying might make sense or choosing not to address that issue, if it is a minor point. However, even in situations where it might temporarily increase disagreement (and hence resistance), it may be important to present alternative information. When an adolescent says "Pot can't hurt you because it's a natural substance," you might say: "It's interesting how people hold to that idea. It's clearly a popular one, and probably because there was so much misinformation spread about pot by folks in authority, people started tuning out other messages. Actually, there is research showing that weed can impact teens negatively. I wonder if you'd be interested in hearing about that."

6.   F   Although it is often very helpful to ask permission, there will be times when you will provide information without doing so first. As noted earlier, in situations where there is an imminent threat to the safety of a client or others, our ethics indicate that we must act. In other situations, for example, when providing significant amounts of information, it would annoy the client to continually ask permission. In that situation, occasionally checking in with the client to see if it is OK to continue would be more helpful then repeatedly asking permission.

7.   T   Although normative information can be very helpful, it is the application of these data to clients' personal situations that they seem to find most useful. People want to know what is significant for *them*. It's not that people who smoke are at greater risk of lung cancer, but it's the finding of abnormal cells that, in combination with a history of smoking and cancer in the family, is more likely to prompt a client's consideration of change.

8.   F   Clients often find it very helpful to hear about how others have addressed similar challenges. In addition to providing options for consideration, these statements also give a message of hope and an explicit communication that there are many paths to success. Providing this kind of information might also have the salutary effect of reminding you that change is possible even in difficult situations and bolster your expectancies of a client. As noted in Chapter 2, our expectations are strong determinants of clients' ultimate success.

9.   T   "Holding up a mirror" by repeating client statements can serve as both a powerful reminder of what they've already said about the situation and as a tool for helping to organize their experience. It's important, however, not to "use their words against them," as this will likely elicit resistance. Instead, it's part of the mosaic they've presented, which at times may be contradictory.

10.   F   This is a challenging question. It is true that we bring technical expertise, and we may provide information that helps clients to interpret information. However, it is not our role to tell clients what that information means to them; that is their job. Our job is to provide context and then allow them to decide how this information fits and affects them. Thus, we might indicate that behavioral effects from alcohol intake begin to show up at even .06 and that serious reaction time changes happen at .08, but they will ultimately decide if the DUI at .085 was significant or "just barely over the legal limit."

In Practice

Here is a common experience for many of us—talking with our dental hygienist about flossing (or lack thereof). It is an example of information sharing in practice. While it demonstrates techniques, it is also less than a perfect example; this is intentional.

"You know that we think flossing is really important, but I wonder what you know about why."

"Well, I know it can lead to cavities if you don't."

"That's true. It can lead to cavities and also to gum disease."

"Is that a big deal? I mean, really?"

"Well, there are a couple of things that can happen. First, you get little pockets of bacteria that can cause decay, and you know what happens then. It can also cause your gums to recede, which can put you at risk for exposing nerve roots. This can lead to things like root canals and tooth loss eventually."

"But none of my teeth hurt now!"

"And I'm really glad of that. There are some things we can do once your gums recede, but it becomes much harder. So we encourage people to prevent that from happening. Of course, you've got to decide what makes sense for you."

"Well, I do floss sometimes. It just gets easy to drop when I'm late in the morning or it gets busy. Then I think I'll do it later, and sometimes later ends up being a few days and then it hurts."

"So, flossing is important. It's just hard to do it consistently. My guess is you've probably had times when you were more consistent and times when you were less. When you were doing it more consistently, how were you doing that?"

"It usually happens after I see you folks. Then I think I need to do better."

"So having someone or something outside reminding you helps to keep your eye on the target."

"Then I try to make sure I have floss in a couple of places—like, I keep some in the downstairs bathroom and some at my office—that helps."

"How about when you're feeling pressed for time, since that sounds like a hard one for you?"

"That's a tough one."

"Would you be interested in hearing what other folks have done about that time issue in managing flossing?

"Sure."

"People have told me a bunch of different things. Some people set their alarm for 3 minutes earlier in the morning. Given that it's only 3 minutes, it doesn't feel like that big a deal to them, and they use that 3 minutes for flossing. Others have switched flossing times to after dinner or before bed, since they don't feel quite as pressed for time then. Others have put floss containers in a bowl in their family room so that they can floss while they're watching the news—and then it becomes a habit. Other people don't like floss, so they've switched to picks or those kinds of things and keep those handy—like where they watch TV or read. There is no one right way to do this. Which of those makes the most sense to you?"

"Part of the issue with me is dealing with the string and all of that stuff. I wonder if the picks on the coffee table wouldn't work better."

"And that would replace your flossing in the morning."

"No. I don't think that's such a good idea. But I think I could make it a backup plan."

" … just in case you missed in the morning."

"Exactly."

"What do you know about using picks?"

"Truthfully? Not much."

"Would it be helpful if I spent a few minutes just showing you how to use a pick and then having you do a little practice? Sometimes it helps if people just get a feel for when they're doing it right. Of course, that's up to you."

"How long will it take?"

"Less than 5 minutes."

"I can do that, but then I need to get back."

"OK, I'll grab the picks. But first, I just want to check—it sounds like you're feeling pretty committed to working on the flossing."

"Yeah, I guess I am. I really do think it's important. I just need a jump start on it sometimes."

"And you feel like you got that today."

"Yeah."

"Great."

Here the dental hygienist tackles a common problem and begins by asking the client what he knows. She provides targeted information, and then she recognizes and reinforces the client's prior efforts. Other client efforts are used to develop ideas about how to be more effective. Once the client has decided on a plan, she also seeks to cement his commitment.

Try This!

Exercise 9.1. Monday Morning Quarterbacking

As any sports fan will tell you, part of the joy of watching sports is the rehashing of what happened and the offering of what you would've done instead. This is a version of that activity. You will find an exchange between a practitioner and a client. You will decide what type of response the practitioner employed and then will offer alternatives. As with Monday morning quarterbacking, the fact that you may not have any expertise in the matter should not stop you from offering your thoughts!

Exercise 9.2. Advice Columnists

In this exercise, you'll read letters to an imaginary advice columnist and then write responses. If you find this exercise helpful, you can get additional practice by looking at advice columns in your local newspaper, on the Internet (e.g., "Aunt Sally," in the *London Times*, or "Ask Amy" in the *Chicago Tribune*), or from specific individuals (e.g., "Dear

Abby"). Remember your goal is to provide MI-consistent advice to someone that has asked for help.

Exercise 9.3. "I Can Fix That!"

Here are some sample bits of advice that need a little rehabbing. Most are confrontational. Write down how you might spruce each up.

Exercise 9.4. "I Can Build That!"

This time you will read some scenarios and construct your own bit of advice. Try to come up with MI-consistent advice using the FOCUS guidelines to create your answers.

Exercise 9.5. Practice in Life

This exercise is more opportunistic. In our everyday encounters we experience people talking about the struggles in their life. Listen for opportunities and then try out offering the advice you would have typically given, but doing it in a manner that is consistent with the skills discussed. You might also try this with your clients.

Partner Work

The first four exercises in this chapter can all be done with your practice partner. Take turns coming up with alternative responses. If you want some real-time practice, have your partner pretend he or she is in one of the situations described in Exercise 9.4. Have him or her describe the situation to you and then ask for your input. In addition to these situations, consider doing Exercise 9.6.

Exercise 9.6. "My Dilemma Is … "

In this exercise your partner will offer an issue or a concern that is a struggle for him or her currently.

This does not have to be his or her deepest, darkest secret—in fact, it shouldn't be-but it should be something that he or she can talk about for a few minutes, so it should have some substance. When you feel you have enough information, provide some additional information, offer a concern, or give some advice. Continue with your MI skills, however your partner responds. Switch roles and repeat.

While you should try to do this exercise seriously, there may be situations that leave you completely flummoxed (e.g., your partner wants to become a deep sea diver). In those situations, call a time out and ask your partner for opinions about advice to give. Then restart the session. Alternatively, give each other permission to make things up beforehand. If you do this, the exercise has the potential to be fun. Try to stay within the MI methodology, however.

Repeat this exercise for as many dilemmas as you can identify or have time to cover. Examples of topics might include international politics, the local sports team, an upcoming election, a change in habit, or a relationship quandary.

Other Thoughts ...

Keep the context in mind. The bit of information or advice you are offering in a particular session may feel like the most important thing that the client must keep in mind, but remember that your client must navigate many spheres. A behavior that appears very maladaptive in one area may serve a very important purpose in another. Likewise, there may be other issues that are much larger and more important than your concern.

Consider Walt: Whereas getting his blood sugar under control might be the most important consideration in our view, he may be worrying about his finances and how expensive it would be to eat "better" or what the diabetes supplies might cost him. As a young man about to turn 30, he may be struggling with identity and life direction issues, and being diabetic might be low on his priority list. He may worry that his teachers, seeing him as less capable if they know he has a chronic health condition, won't give the strong recommendations he needs to get a good job. All or none of these might be true and might influence how he receives advice. The only way of learning about this kind of information is for Walt to tell us. This is part of why asking for clients' perspectives on the information given is so important; in their answers some of these other contextual factors may emerge.

Monday Morning Quarterbacking

As any sports fan will tell you, part of the joy of watching sports is the rehashing of what happened and the offering of what you would've done instead. This is a version of that activity. Below you will find the exchange with the dental hygienist; her statements are shaded. Now most of you are not dental hygienists, but it's likely that you will have gone to see one and been told about flossing. Use that experience both to discern what response (e.g., reflection, asking permission, E-P-E) was used and to offer an alternative way you might have handled that exchange. It is not a perfect interaction; this does not assume that responses in this interchange were "bad" or "problematic," just that there are always alternative paths. Although you'll need to read the client statements as well, it is the dental hygienist's statements to which you should provide responses. Like with Monday morning quarterbacking, the fact that we have no expertise in the matter never stops us from offering our opinions! And if you are a dental hygienist, it's all the better. So, go ahead and be the expert!

Statement	Response type and alternative response
"You know that we think flossing is really important, but I wonder what you know about why."	
"Well, I know it can lead to cavities if you don't."	
"That's true. It can lead to cavities and also to gum disease."	
"Is that a big deal? I mean, really?"	
"Well, there are a couple of things that can happen. First, you get little pockets of bacteria that can cause decay, and you know what happens then. It can also cause your gums to recede, which can put you at risk for exposing nerve roots. This can lead to things like root canals and tooth loss eventually."	
"But none of my teeth hurt now!"	
"And I'm really glad of that. There are some things we can do once that happens, but it becomes much harder. So we work with people to prevent that from happening. Of course, you've got to decide what makes sense for you."	
"Well, I do floss sometimes. It just gets easy to drop when I'm late in the morning or it gets busy. Then I think I'll do it later, and sometimes later ends up being a few days and then it hurts."	

(cont.)

"So, flossing is important. It's just hard to do it consistently. My guess is you've probably had times when you were more consistent and times when you were less. When you were doing it more consistently, how were you doing that?"	
"It usually happens after I see you folks. Then I think I need to do better."	
"So having someone or something outside reminding you helps to keep your eye on the target."	
"Then I try to make sure I have floss in a couple of places—like, I keep some in the downstairs bathroom and some at my office—that helps."	
"How about when you're feeling pressed for time, since that sounds like a hard one for you?"	
"That's a tough one."	
"Would you be interested in hearing what other folks have done about that time issue in managing flossing?	
"Sure."	
"People have told me a bunch of different things. Some people set their alarm for 3 minutes earlier in the morning. Given that it's only 3 minutes, it doesn't feel like that big a deal to them, and they use that 3 minutes for flossing. Others have switched times to after dinner or before bed, since they don't feel quite as pressed for time then. Others have put floss containers in a bowl in their family room so that they can floss while they're watching the news—and then it becomes a habit. Other people don't like floss, so they've switched to picks or those kinds of things and keep those handy—like where they watch TV or read. There is no one right way to do this. Which of those makes the most sense to you?"	
"Part of the issue with me is dealing with the string and all of that stuff. I wonder if the picks on the coffee table wouldn't work better."	

"And that would replace your flossing in the morning."	
"No. I don't think that's such a good idea. But I think I could make it like a backup plan."	
" ... just in case you missed in the morning."	
"Exactly."	
"What do you know about using picks?"	
"Truthfully? Not much."	
"Would it be helpful if I spent a few minutes just showing you and then having you do a little practice? Sometimes it helps if people just get a feel for when they're doing it right. Of course, that's up to you."	
"How long will it take?"	
"Less than 5 minutes."	
"I can do that, but then I need to get back."	
"OK, I'll grab the picks. But first, I just want to check—it sounds like you're feeling pretty committed to working on the flossing."	
"Yeah, I guess I am. I really do think it's important. I just need a jumpstart on it sometimes."	
"And you feel like you got that today."	
"Yeah."	
"Great."	

Advice Columnists

Advice columns in some ways are a peculiarly American phenomenon, though a quick search of the Internet reveals that these are now offered around the world. People write with problems and the columnist offers advice. In this exercise, you'll respond to a couple of fictional letters to our imaginary columnist, "Uncle Todd." If you find this useful and want more practice, you could search out letters to advice columnists in your local newspaper. If you don't have any locally, then you might use the Internet to find them in newspapers from around the world (e.g., "Aunt Sally" in the *London Times*, or "Ask Amy" in the *Chicago Tribune*) or from specific individuals (e.g., "Dear Abby"). Regardless of the source, the goal is to provide your "advice" in an MI-consistent manner, though like any good newspaper columnist, you want to add a little humor for readers.

Dear Uncle Todd—

I have a friend, "Hannah." We're living in a dorm in college. We have this tight group of four friends, but we also want to expand our social sphere since we are all freshmen. Unfortunately, Hannah focuses all of her energy only on us. She's always hanging around my room and asking what I'm going to do. She does the same with the others in the group. Lately, I often feel guilty because I want to do things without her. I've found myself telling her that I'm going out to the library when I was really going to meet some other friends. It feels as if she invades my personal space, and I have taken to shutting my door, which I don't want to do. Help, Uncle Todd.

From, Tangled in Cling Wrap

Dear Tangled—

Uncle Todd

(cont.)

Dear Uncle Todd—

Once again the holidays are here. Don't get me wrong, I love my family. But it always feels like there is tension. We have out-of-town guests, and that changes the household routine. People don't sleep as well and get a little grouchy. My uncle drinks too much sometimes and gets opinionated when he does. We spend hours in preparation for the big day and then it all happens so fast and it always feels a bit disappointing. Part of me wants to just skip the whole thing, but I know I wouldn't like that either. And there are moments that are precious to me—just not enough. How can I make it less tense?

From, Holiday Blues

Dear Holiday Blues—

Uncle Todd

Sample Responses for Exercise 9.2

Dear Tangled—

You sound like you're wrapped air tight. You don't want to hurt this person's feelings, and yet the decisions you're now making put you at risk for really doing that. It also seems like she's starting to make you angry. I have a couple of ideas.

One thing some freshmen have done is be real explicit about what their goals are—they want to meet new people—but that doesn't mean they're replacing the friends they already have. A second thing some young women have done is have a direct talk about how the behavior of the clingy friend is making them feel and then see if there are ways that they can help that person to make other friends. A third thing is to involve the Resident Assistant by discussing your concerns and seeing if there are some suggestions that she has. Finally, some people have set "date nights," so that clingy friends can count on a fixed time for socializing with the sought-after friends. Then other nights are free for other activities without the clingy friends.

So, Tangled, which of these seems to sit best with you?

Uncle Todd

Dear Holiday Blues—

You do sound stuck between a rock and a suitcase. Leaving might feel like a good option, but probably not one you are ready to exercise, so you are left to manage the situation—and yourself—as best you can. I have a few thoughts; you'll have to decide which, if any, make sense to you.

One thing that some families have done is try to structure their holidays a bit. Without overdoing, they try to have a game plan laid out for how they'll spend their time. This seems to keep them from having too much time on their hands. Some people use big outings. Others put out puzzles. Others do some baking or cooking. This gives people a focus.

Another option people sometimes use is splitting up the responsibility. Everybody has a day they're in charge of, including meals. People sometimes pair up if it's too much for one person. This approach seems to lessen any single individual or small group of individuals being overburdened.

Alcohol use at holiday time is often a concern. People tell me different approaches work for them. Some provide snacks when alcohol is served so that no one drinks on an empty stomach. Some limit the amount of alcohol or the type of alcohol available. Others have tried approaching the individual that struggles (apart from others) and talking about their concerns. Still others decide to offer no or low alcohol options only.

My last thought is that you might work on your own reactions to the situation. Some people have told me that their expectations get them into trouble, so changing those help. Others say it is their reactions that escalate the situation and so they have to be sensitive to those. Finally, still others say it is their focus that trips them up. If they focus on the things they like or want, they are much happier—even when things go wrong—than if they focus on the negatives or the problems that come up. And let's face it, when there is a house full of family, problems are likely to come up.

So, that is a long answer, Blues. Any of those ideas fitting for you?

Uncle Todd

Here are some sample bits of advice that need rehabbing. Most are confrontational. See if you can tone down the confrontation using some of the techniques discussed in the chapter. Some existing elements may be fine, so, like any repair job, decide what can stay and what needs to be replaced or reworked. Be aware that in some situations you may need to start over entirely. Write down how you might spruce up or rebuild each statement. You don't need to stay true to the words, but try to express the ideas being conveyed in each example.

1. "You really do need to start eating more fruits and laying off the fried food. If you don't, you are risking another heart attack. And the fact of the matter is, a second heart attack is more likely to be deadly, so you've got a real stake in making these changes."

2. "I know your meds have some side effects, but you can't just take them when you think that you need them. Antidepressants don't work that way. They need to be at a therapeutic level, and when you only take them every few days, you're at nontherapeutic levels. You're getting all the side effects and none of the benefit."

3. "I think it is a really bad idea for you to return to drinking, especially now. Although your troubles weren't with alcohol before, you're somebody who has a history of dependence and are likely to substitute addictions. In addition, you've been feeling depressed, and the alcohol is likely to make you feel more depressed. Finally, you didn't consult your sponsor because you know that he would've said, 'No!'—and so you've got no support while you're trying this risky experiment. You're playing with fire!"

(cont.)

4. "It's your life, but I don't think you want to spend it having sex with guys who aren't interested in relationships. Hooking up may feel like it's giving you sexual power, but who's getting and who's receiving? Are they returning the favors? Most of the time it's the girl who's giving, and let's face it—guys' reputations don't get wrecked because they've hooked up. But yours can."

5. "Here's my dilemma. I don't want to take your kids away. I think you do care about your kids. But, if you continue to engage in this behavior, I will be forced to do that. Now you don't want to put me in a position where that is what I have to do. This means that you have to go to these parenting classes, and you have to participate. Otherwise I will take the kids away, and it'll be your fault, not mine."

6. "If you don't start taking better care of your diabetes, these consequences are going to get worse—even deadly. Your A1c was at 14; that's twice where it should be. You already have some reduced sensation in your feet—which means that the diabetes is damaging your circulation and your nerves. You could lose a foot or a kidney. You have a family history of stroke, and that's without the problems that diabetes causes in circulation. Your father died of a heart attack. It just keeps getting worse. This is not a joke. If you don't get this under control—and I mean soon—you're going to be in big trouble!"

Sample Responses for Exercise 9.3

1. "You really do need to start eating more fruits and laying off the fried food."

   Concerns: *The advice is solid, and the context is problematic. It does not ask permission, and it warns of dire consequences. The rehab for this response could occur by asking permission and providing information or using E-P-E.*

   Response: *"What do you already know about diet and its role in preventing another heart attack?"*
   "You're right—eating more fruits and vegetables is important to the health of your heart, as is laying off the fried foods."
   "What do you know about the severity of a second heart attack?"
   "It does seem that when the heart has been damaged once, the risk for an even worse outcome—like death—goes up. What are your reactions to that information?"

   Techniques: *E-P-E*

2. "I know your meds have some side effects, but you can't just take them when you think that you need them."

   Concerns: *As with the last example, this advice is trying to persuade the client. Again, it's likely to be more effective to ask permission, provide information, and get the client's take. Alternatively, you could use a chunk–check–chunk approach.*

   Response: *"May I share a little information about how antidepressant medications work? Please stop me if you already know this stuff."*
   "With this kind of medication, it takes a little while to build up to a therapeutic dose, and then you need to keep it at that level, which means taking it every day. How does this fit with what you know?"
   "If the medications aren't taken every day, then you don't reach those levels where the medication is helping. Instead you just get side effects. Taking them every once in a while doesn't really help."
   "Although I think the meds could help you, it is your decision about whether you will or won't take them. What do you think about all that?"

   Techniques: *Asks permissions, chunk–check–chunk*

3. "I think it is a really bad idea for you to return to drinking, especially now."

   Concerns: *In this situation, the practitioner has lots of good information, but slips into chastising to bring home the importance of the point. It's better to stay neutral when offering the concern to avoid building resistance.*

   Response: *"I'm worried about your decision. May I share why?"*
   "There are a few reasons. You've been feeling depressed, and alcohol can make you feel more depressed, even though it may make you feel a little better initially. Also, your sponsor doesn't know, so you've lost that support and feedback system, during a time when it might be really helpful to have another set of eyes watching your back. Although your history of dependence doesn't preclude you from making this choice, the data show that you are at higher risk for other substance problems. So that is what has me concerned. What are your thoughts?"

   Techniques: *Statement of concern, asks permission, provides information, and checks client's view*

(cont.)

4. "It's your life, but I don't think you want to spend it having sex with guys who aren't interested in relationships."

Concerns: *This is a sensitive topic. The practitioner's tone needs to be less harsh and more concerned. Many of the elements can be retained, but there are elements of warning, and the practitioner may be better served by placing the information sharing in the context of other women.*

Response: *"Is it OK if I share a little information that I've learned from other young women like you? These women have taught me that it feels very powerful to have this sort of sexual agency. They like it—generally. There are a few things they are less crazy about. One of the things they like less is that it's often a one-way street—they're doing the giving and not receiving in kind. What do you think?*

  "A second thing they don't like—and perhaps is even more frustrating for these women—is that men and women's reputations are perceived differently as a result of hooking up. Men's reputations still tend to be polished by this behavior, whereas women's aren't. It makes them angry. What's your take on that?"

Techniques: *Asks permission, chunk–check–chunk*

5. "Here's my dilemma. I don't want to take your kids away."

Concerns: *Again, there are many useful elements here. Beware of the <u>but</u>, though, because it wipes away the concern the practitioner noted for the client. Also, the responsibility element at the end has a quality of blaming, which is likely to draw the client's ire.*

Response: *"Here's my dilemma. The court says that certain things must be done if the kids are to stay with you, including attending and participating in the parenting classes. The court requires that I report to it about whether those things have or have not happened. I need to be truthful not only for the court, but also for you and the children. I think you do care about your kids, and we have this requirement that must be met. I can't decide for you, though I hope you will go—for your and the children's sake. But, this is your call. What do you think?"*

Techniques: *Chunk–check–chunk*

6. "If you don't start taking better care of your diabetes, these consequences are going to get worse—even deadly."

Concerns: *Legitimate concerns about real problems. It's also unidirectional. A more collaborative strategy will help.*

Response: *"What do you know about the risks you have currently because of your diabetes?"* (*Client answers.*)

  "There are a few other things you might know about as well. The reduced feeling in your feet is kind of like the canary in the coal mine tunnel. It lets us know that there might be some other risks happening. Typically, it means that your body is having some trouble with circulation. This is not uncommon for diabetics who are having some struggles with control. Unfortunately, the risks get much greater as these things begin to happen. What do you know about these more serious risks?"

Techniques: *E-P-E*

"I Can Build That!"

This time you will read scenarios and construct your own bit of advice. These are situations you may either encounter or hear about others encountering in daily life. Try to come up with MI-consistent advice using the FOCUS guidelines to create your answers. These are repeated below for your convenience. Also be aware that this exercise can be a tough one. Try to really imagine, if you were asked to provide advice in this situation, what options/thoughts you might offer. You may feel that you need more specifics, and I've chosen not to provide those elements. This approach was taken so that you can respond with ideas that make sense to you.

- **F**irst ask permission.
- **O**ffer ideas.
- **C**oncise.
- **U**se a menu.
- **S**olicit what the client thinks.

Choosing a College

Your 18-year-old son tells you about his struggle to choose between several good college options. Some are nearby and some are not; some are public and some are private. Nearby options will cost less but also have fewer offerings in terms of majors and opportunities. There is merit scholarship money available from the private schools, though such a college would still cost more than you can afford, and so your son, by agreement, would need to take out some large loans. Individual contact and attention from professors is more likely at the private colleges. And forget the "follow your heart" speech—he did that in choosing the colleges to which he applied, and now he is thoroughly ambivalent.

Advice:

(*cont.*)

A Change in Careers

Your friend is considering a change in careers. For as long as you've known her, she has worked multiple jobs to make ends meet. This practice began out of economic necessity as she went from a two-income family to single parenthood. It has continued for nearly 15 years. During this time, a new relationship blossomed and became established, but her partner makes considerably less money and works fewer hours than she. Now she has an opportunity to become an independent consultant with a large contract from a single provider. This contract will provide a year of very good income and allow her time to build up other parts of her consultant business. But it will also necessitate that she leave the part-time job that has provided financial stability. She is excited about the consulting possibility, but also worried about an economy that is tumbling into recession and the uncertainty beyond the first year. She asks what you think she should do.

Advice:

An Aging Parent

Your coworker confides that he is struggling with a big decision. His elderly mother and father were living in a distant city until very recently. His father, whose health had been declining, finally died during the last year. Your mother didn't want to rush into decisions after his death, but it has become clear that she is struggling to live independently. She has used a home health aide, but her funds are running out, and so the choice is now to move her into a retirement facility or into his home. While his spouse is supportive, he also admits that she and his mother have always done best in small doses—and this would be a long-term commitment. They also have an active household with several children, and taking in his mother would require reconfiguring bedrooms and routines. The children would like to have their grandmother live there, but they are already complaining about having to share bedrooms and a bathroom. The retirement facilities your coworker has toured have ranged from dismal to passable. None seems great, and he feels guilty for even thinking about putting his mother into this type of assisted-care facility. He promised his father that he would care for her after he died. He wants your advice on what to do.

Advice:

Your Best Friend Is Getting Married

You've known this friend since childhood. You were a member of her wedding party, and you consoled her though the breakup of that marriage. You talked to her throughout her father's descent into Alzheimer's disease and offered support through her mother's battle and ultimate defeat by cancer. As long as you've known her, she has wanted two things: a partner to love and a child of her own. She found the former, but he doesn't want the latter. This conundrum has led to an on-again/off-again relationship as she tries to decide if she can be OK without a child. During some of her "off periods" with her partner, she has gone so far as to explore adoption, since she cannot become pregnant for medical reasons. Now as the two of you dine, she announces that a wedding date has been set. With her bravest face, she tells you that she has decided that she would be an auntie to others' children and that would have to be enough. You know your friend, and it seems that she has finally acted to end this interminable uncertainty plaguing her. You also know that she will be unhappy if she follows through with this decision. She asks what you think.

Advice:

Sample Responses for Exercise 9.4

Choosing a College

Your 18-year-old son tells you about his struggle to choose between several good college options (etc.).

"I have some ideas, but I want to make sure it's OK that I share them. But first, my guess is that you've tried some strategies to sort this though and I don't want to repeat what you've already done. What have you tried?" (The young man answers.)

"Here are some ideas you might consider, based on what other parents have told me. One is to spend some time on each campus, including a schoolday. Sleep in the dorm, attend classes, and eat in the school cafeteria. Another approach is to talk to older siblings of some of your friends about their choices and what made the decision for them. Sometimes it helps to hear what their critical factors were and how these played out for them, once they arrived on campus. Others call and talk to a few students and get their view of their school. They usually have a list of questions, and that helps them make sure that they get similar information across students. Asking their reasons for going to the school can also be helpful. What do you think about those ideas?"

A Change in Careers

Your friend is considering a change in careers (etc.).

"You're sure? Sometimes people ask when what they really want to do is say more about how they're thinking, and that's OK. Well, I know you really worry about the money and the insurance, so I can see why you're spending this time making sure. I'm also really struck by how excited and happy this opportunity seems to make you. It seems almost like you can dream about your life in a whole new way. Maybe part of you distrusts that possibility of happiness, and yet you seem to have lined everything up. I wonder if you probably already know what you want to do, and it's just a matter of allowing yourself to really have it or to hear from people who care about you that it's OK. I think it's a great choice, but it's not my call to make. What do you think?"

An Aging Parent

Your coworker confides that he is struggling with a big decision (etc.).

"That is a tough situation. There are so many different pulls. You know your mom needs more than she's getting now, and you want to honor that commitment you made to your dad, buts it's not quite clear what will serve everyone best. It seems to me that no matter what you decide, it is not going to feel good, and at the same time, you're hoping it will. I have a couple of thoughts or reactions about what might be important to consider. May I share these?

"You didn't mention your mom's view on all of this. That seems pretty important. What does she think?

"I am also curious about what taking care of your mom means to you. It seems like you feel that this means having her live with you, but I could also imagine it meaning other things as well. It seems like if you broadened that horizon a little, it might help you. What do you think?

"Finally, I wonder if part of making the decision is coming to terms with being unable to make everyone happy—perhaps, even more, that you are responsible for everyone's happiness. I wonder if this might be an easier choice if you let go of those things. What are your thoughts about that?"

Sample Responses for Exercise 9.4 (*cont.*)

Your Best Friend Is Getting Married

You've known this friend since childhood (etc.).

"Are you sure? I'm concerned about this decision—not because I think he's a bad guy. He's a good guy and I know you love him; that's part of what has made this so hard for you. What I know is how badly you've wanted a child and how difficult it is to be stuck in this limbo. I'm concerned you've made this choice to end the uncertainty, and you will regret it and then resent him for 'forcing' you to make a choice. So, those are my worries. What's your reaction to all of that?"

This is a more opportunistic activity. In our everyday encounters we experience people talking about the struggles in their life. Friends, to whom we may have already provided our opinions liberally, might be open to suggestions. Listen for opportunities and then try offering the advice you would typically have given, but it in a manner that is consistent with the skills discussed.

Similarly, if you tend to give advice to your clients, then pay attention when this situation arises. When it does, consciously decide to try out one of the MI consistent forms for sharing information, offering a concern, or giving advice. Make sure to pay attention to how your client responds.

If you don't normally give advice, you might watch for situations where some additional guidance would be helpful to your client and then offer some information.

As always, use your OARS liberally!

In this exercise, your partner will offer an issue or a concern that he or she is currently struggling with. It does not have to be a deep, dark secret—in fact, it shouldn't be—but it should be something of substance that he or she can speak about for a few minutes. Begin this conversation with the prompt, "So what's your dilemma?" Then use all of your other MI skills as the person describes the dilemma. When you feel you have enough information, provide some information, offer a concern, or give some advice. Then continue with your MI skills, however your partner responds.

Then switch roles and repeat. While you should try to do this seriously, there may be situations that leave you completely flummoxed. In those situations, call time out and ask your partner for opinions about advice to give. Then restart the session. Or alternatively, give each other permission to make things up beforehand. If you do this, the exercise has the potential to be fun. Try to stay within the MI methodology, however.

Do this for as many dilemmas as you can identify or have time for. Examples of topics might include international politics, the local sports team, an upcoming election, a change in habit, or a relationship quandary.

Chapter 10

The Key Question

Opening

Tanya left this message on the answering service:

> "I've been doing my best, but I'm at the end of my rope. It's been the year from hell, and things just aren't getting any better. Normally, I don't believe in this kind of thing, but I gotta do something. I've left messages for several different people, and I hope that I can see someone soon. Please call me as soon as you can."

Making multiple calls to practitioners suggests that Tanya is ready for a change. There is urgency to her efforts, even though we don't know yet what the problem is or what she has tried. Clearly, though, she is ready to have something be different. Our questions, predicated on this assessment, would inquire about what had been happening, how she'd like her situation to be different, and what she'd thought about or tried already. The following conversation skips over the introductions and begins with the practitioner.

"Your message started with 'I've been doing my best, but I am at the end of my rope.' What's been happening?"

"It started when I injured my back at work. I fell off a shelf when I was picking parts for this company. I wasn't supposed to be climbing, but it's what everybody does to meet their quotas. You're supposed to get a ladder, but if I did that for every item, it would be impossible to keep up. The company knows it and just ignores it, until something happens. Then they say it's your fault. Anyway, I fell, hurt my back, and haven't been able to work because I'm in constant pain. Normally, I'm really active. I played on a soccer team every week, went to all my kids' sports events, and did things like backpacking and hiking. Now I can't even sleep because I can't get comfortable. I can't lift anything. It's hard to walk more than a block. I'm miserable, and it's impacting my mood, my kids, and my husband. Oh, yeah, in the middle of all of this, we—my husband and I—we're remodeling the kitchen. The house is torn apart. We were doing it together. In fact, don't tell him I said this, but

I'm a better carpenter then he is. Now he has to do it all himself. He has to get the kids ready for school, get them to places, and make meals—all the stuff I used to do. You get the picture?"

Our guesses about readiness seem on target. Tanya appears highly motivated to feel better. But now we need to help her translate this desire into specific behaviors or situations to target and secure commitment to plans for changing those things. How best to do that? Where would you go next? What question(s) might you ask to get there?

A Deeper Look

As we noted in Chapter 1, Chapters 3–9 all deal with Phase I, wherein practitioner goals are to raise the importance of a change, enhance confidence, and resolve ambivalence. During Phase II the practitioner seeks to solidify commitment to change and to negotiate a change plan. The transition between these phases is a time (or window) of opportunity. The client stands at the brink of a change, but has not yet made the decision to undertake it. This is the swimmer perched at the edge of the dock, deciding whether or not to jump in.

This point in the therapeutic process hinges on good timing. The practitioner must respond when the client is ready or risk having the client return to an earlier state of readiness. It is simply too uncomfortable psychologically to remain aware of a motivating discrepancy and fail to act on it. An individual who is in this situation for too long will engage in strategies to reduce the perception of risk. The swimmer will decide it's too cold, too deep, or not the right time and head back to the shore. Thus the therapist must be attuned to when the person is ready and respond by assisting with a commitment and moving forward on a plan.

Signs of Readiness

Writers and researchers have offered both data and models about what factors influence and indicate readiness to change. DiClemente (2003) refers to these as *markers of change* and notes the importance of decisional balance (Janis & Mann, 1977; Prochaska, DiClemente, & Norcross, 1992; Prochaska, Velicer, et al., 2004) and self-efficacy (Bandura, 1997; Carbonari & DiClemente, 2000). DiClemente (2003, p. 36) also notes other factors such as "intrinsic and extrinsic motivation (Curry, Wagner, & Grothaus, 1990; DiClemente, 1999), rationalization and harm minimization (Daniels, 1998), and beliefs and barriers to change (Werch & DiClemente, 1994)." Miller and Rollnick (2002) offer a list of potential markers of readiness, while encouraging further research in this area (see Figure 10.1).

The seven signs in Figure 10.1 are cues that a client may be ready to shift from considering a change to actually making it. The practitioner, on recognizing these signs, also shifts strategies and communication styles. There is less following and more directing and guiding, though behavior remains MI consistent. The Other Thoughts section at the end of this chapter discusses the pitfalls to watch for during this time, but for now, the focus is

Signs of Readiness for Change

Decreased resistance. The wind seems to have gone out of the sails of resistance. Dissonance in the counseling relationship diminishes, and resistance decreases.

Decreased discussion about the problem. The client seems to have talked enough about the area of concern. If the client has been asking questions about the problem area, these stop. There is a feeling of at least partial completion or waiting for the next step.

Resolve. The client appears to have reached some resolution and may seem more peaceful, relaxed, calm, unburdened, or settled. This can also have a tone of loss, tearfulness, or resignation.

Change talk. Whereas resistance diminishes, change talk increases. Clients make direct statements about a desire to change, the ability to change, the reasons or benefits of change, and the need to change (the disadvantages of the status quo). They may also make statements about intention to change.

Questions about change. Clients may begin to ask what they could do about the problem, how people change once they decide to, and the like.

Envisioning. The client talks about how life might be after a change. This can be mistaken for resistance; that is, looking ahead to change often causes a person to anticipate difficulties if a change were made. Of course, the client may also envision positive outcomes of change.

Experimenting. The client may have begun experimenting with possible change actions since the last session.

Figure 10.1. Signs of readiness for change. Adapted from Miller and Rollnick (2002). Copyright 2002 by The Guilford Press. Adapted by permission.

on the first two components of Phase II: recapitulations and key questions. We discuss the third component, negotiating change plans, in Chapter 11.

Recapitulation

This component typically begins with a transitional summary that bridges the ending of Phase I and leads into the key question. Remembering that summaries help organize clients' experiences, the aim is to include the elements necessary without overwhelming clients with information. Brevity remains important, though transitional summaries tend to be slightly longer. Miller and Rollnick (2002, p. 130) suggest that certain elements be included in a transitional summary:

- A statement indicating that you are pulling together what the client has said.
- A summary of the client's perceptions of the issue, including any reasons or need for change noted by the client.
- A summary of the client's ambivalence, including the benefits of the status quo.

- Objective evidence relevant to the importance of change.
- A restatement of desire, ability, and commitment to change.
- Your assessment of the client's situation, especially when it matches the client's concern.

It is often hard for practitioners to keep all of these elements in mind, especially as they are learning MI. My suggestion to beginning MI practitioners is to simplify the elements and use an acronym (I CAN) to remember them:

- **I**ndicate that this is a summary and include
- **C**hange talk,
- **A**mbivalence, and then ask about the
- **N**ext step.

As clinicians become more comfortable with this transition, they add in the other elements suggested by Miller and Rollnick (2002). The goal with both approaches is for clients to arrive at that last element (i.e., next step) cognizant of their ambivalence and fully aware of their motivations for change.

Key Question

Miller and Rollnick (1991, 2002) introduced the concept of the key question as a way to solidify commitment to change. It is not made key by the exact content included, indeed there are many ways to ask a key question. Rather, it is the timing of when it is asked and the intent of the question. The key question is posed when the client stands at the precipice of change; the answer indicates whether the client is ready to jump. Miller and Rollnick (2002) use the analogy of Phase I being like the tough slogging of snowshoeing up to the summit of a mountain, and Phase II as skiing down the other side. The key question asks if the client is ready to go down the hill (or mountain). In essence, a key question asks "What next?" and thereby evokes the client's own thoughts about change rather than imposing the practitioner's. Examples of key questions include:

"Given what you've told me, what do you think you will do next?"

"Where do you think you would like to go from here?"

"What's your next step?"

Sometimes there is a clear summing up and a central key question, but sometimes—as with Tanya—there are multiple behaviors that might be addressed and multiple key questions as a result. These queries would happen at several points during Phase II and be targeted to specific areas.

This is often a time when clients ask for advice. Using the skills described in Chapter 10, offering specific ideas can be very helpful to clients. As before, these activities continue to be done in an MI-consistent manner. Chapter 11 discusses these issues further.

Concept Quiz—Test Yourself!

True or false:

1.   T   F   The goals of Phase II are to solidify commitment to change and negotiate a change plan.

2.   T   F   If a practitioner is too slow in moving into Phase II, the client may slip into defensive responding.

3.   T   F   When clients begin to ask questions about how they might change, this may signal a readiness to move toward Phase II.

4.   T   F   If clients begin talking about difficulties that may occur with a change, they are indicating that they are not yet ready to change.

5.   T   F   A key question typically starts the transition from Phase I to Phase II.

6.   T   F   A key question is made key not by the content but by its timing and intent.

7.   T   F   Only one key question is needed to secure commitment and begin the planning process.

8.   T   F   The clinician communication styles in Phase II remain the same as Phase I.

9.   T   F   Clients may appear more settled and less resistant when ready to move into Phase II.

10.   T   F   Ambivalence is no longer present in Phase II.

Answers

1.   T   Whereas Phase I builds motivation for change, Phase II solidifies commitment for a specific change and assists the client in developing a plan by which to achieve this aim.

2.   T   This is an area where the practitioner should avoid getting too far ahead or behind. Indeed, when there is research in which MI does not work as well (Project MATCH Research Group, 1997b, 1998b), it seems to be with clients who were already primed for a change. In that situation, continuing to either explore ambivalence or build motivation can get in the way of change. Miller and Rollnick (2002) indicate that clients may slip into defensive responding in this situation.

3.   T   Clients' questions about mechanisms for change often signal increased readiness for change. This situation is especially true when these queries occur in combination with other signals such as reduced resistance and increased change talk.

4.   F   Envisioning is a process that clients use to anticipate what the future might look like after a change occurs. This process may include some of the difficulties that change creates. Remember back in Chapter 2 when the concept of ambivalence was first raised? Difficult changes almost always include ambivalence, and it is not surprising to hear it at this critical juncture. However, if this occurs in combination with tepid commitment to change, then the practitioner may need to return to further exploration of ambivalence and motivation, before strengthening of commitment.

5.   F   While a key question is usually part of the transition, the process typically begins with a transitional summary that assists clients with organizing their thoughts about the change. The acronym of "I CAN" was offered as a simplified form of this summary.

6. T   Key questions do not contain particular wording, but they are typically open-ended questions that ask for the client's thoughts about change. The "key" part is the intention of the question in combination with when it is asked.

7. F   Oh, if it only were true! Although the process of answering a key question may help solidify commitment, there are often multiple issues, behaviors, and plans that require attention. Key questions may be needed for all. So, although one key question may shift the session into treatment planning, this is not always the case and may not be the usual case. However, it is an important marker.

8. F   While the clinician will continue to use the same guiding style and microskills as used in Phase I, there is often a shift into a more directing style as well. The amount of time in each style may shift.

9. T   To paraphrase Miller and Rollnick, it may feel as though the wind has gone out of their resistance/sustain talk sails. There may be a quieting that occurs, as well as a new sense of resolve.

10. F   Back to our mantra: Ambivalence is normal, even as people move actively into the planning and change process, though its intensity will typically have diminished. Strong sustain talk may indicate that more work is needed on resolving the ambivalence, rather than on just reaffirming commitment.

In Practice

Let's pick up the interchange with Tanya. She had just described the range of difficulties in her life. We'll start with the practitioner's last statement. As noted before, this is an instance in which general motivation may be high, but she will likely need to define a target behavior and then make specific commitments to a plan. Thus, there will be an interplay between transitional summaries, key questions, and determining the planning agenda.

Statement	*Commentary*
P: It sounds like the year from hell. You're hurt, you can't do the things you like and enjoy, let alone the things you must do. It's affected almost every aspect of your life. It just feels overwhelming.	Start of transitional summary.
C: Exactly. I'm tired of being in pain. I did physical therapy—was religious about doing my exercises—and it helped a little but not much. My doctor sent me to a consultant for back surgery; I'd just as soon not go there if I don't have to—but I may have to. I take Oxycontin for the pain, and it helps, but it also makes me spacey. I don't like the way I feel on it. I've been pushing for some cortisone injections, but my doctor hasn't been too enthusiastic. He	Client provides more information.

Statement	*Commentary*
doesn't think it will help. I'm desperate and getting depressed, so I figured I would see what you folks could do to help.	
P: You sound like you are ready to do something, though you aren't quite sure what would be helpful here.	Continues summary and reinforces commitment to action. Practitioner also acknowledges her uncertainty, but doesn't leave her mired in it.
C: Exactly. What do you suggest?	Client asks for information.
P: I have some ideas, based on what other people like yourself have done, but I also want to find out what area feels most important to you. Where would you like to begin?	Practitioner will respond to request, but first wants to check for the client's priorities; this leads to a key question.
C: Well, if we could begin with the pain, that would be great.	Client responds directly.
P: The pain feels like it is driving this bus.	Simile/metaphor.
C: Yeah. I think if I could just feel a little bit better physically, then everything else would be easier to do. You know what I mean?	Client begins articulating a path for change.
P: Yeah. Like if you could just turn down the volume, then you could deal with all this other noise.	Another complex reflection.
C: Exactly.	
P: You seem pretty clear about how this works for you. Tell me a little more about what you know about how emotions—and especially depression—and pain work together.	Affirmation, then moves to the beginning of E-P-E.
C: I know that when I'm in pain, I don't do things, and I don't feel well. I don't see my friends. I get angry more easily. I snap at my kids and my husband. Then I feel crappy and get depressed.	Client draws clear connections.
P: So you see how being down starts with the pain and the things that happen around the pain. The other part—and you may already know this—is that the feeling down can then intensify the pain. What do you think about that?	Provides information, then elicits client's view.

Statement	Commentary
C: It makes sense. When I'm depressed, everything feels worse.	Client agrees.
P: So, one of the things that other people have found is that, if they can start to get a handle on the depression side, then other things—including the pain—can feel a little easier. It won't cure the pain, but it may help it feel more manageable. How does that seem to you?	Provides an additional bit of information, based on the client's response. Again elicits client reaction.
C: It seems like a good place to start.	Client agrees. There is now the start of a mutual agenda.
P: You have probably tried some things to manage your feeling down. Tell me about what you've been doing already or about what has worked in the past.	Elicits information on current or prior efforts at change in this area. It might be better to simplify this query into one question.
C: Well … I talked with my doc about it, and he suggested some antidepressants, but I've been reluctant to use those. It feels like it would be a crutch.	Client provides important data.
P: You've thought about antidepressants. What else?	Acknowledges, but doesn't jump into discussion about medication. Probes for more.
C: Before I hurt my back, I used to exercise, and that really helped when I felt down.	Additional information.
P: Getting out and being active helped.	Complex reflection reorients the meaning slightly.
C: But I can't do that now.	Slight up-tick in resistance?
P: Not in the way you did before. What else?	Reorients again, followed by a probe.
C: I tried counseling once before—when I hit a rough patch—and that seemed to help, to have a place where I could talk about things.	Additional information.
P: A place where you could sort through some of the struggles. Anything else?	Reflection and a probe that signals a possible closing of the discussion.
C: That's about it.	Client agrees.

Statement	*Commentary*
P: You know some things that have helped or may help, but you've also got some concerns about how things might work now. Would it be OK if I shared some information about a couple of those things?	A summary and permission requested to share information directly.
C: Absolutely. That's why I'm here.	Agreement.
P: It's not uncommon for people to have mixed feelings about antidepressants. There is great concern about these medicines being overprescribed, especially for people who may not need them. Given what you've told me so far, though, I think these may be appropriate for you, but you would need to talk with a physician to be sure. I can say there is reason to be hopeful. First, medication often helps with depression. Second, certain kinds of counseling can help with depression. Third, the two together seem to have the best success rate. What do you think about that?	Addresses possible concerns underlying the use of medication. Places in the context of others. Also gives clear information that this avenue might be helpful for the client. Finally, provides some factual data about medication use. Then asks for clients perceptions.
C: I guess it makes sense. I just don't want to get addicted to those things and feel like I would have to take them. I want to be myself.	Client articulates her concerns.
P: And that's your worry … that somehow you would lose your ability to control that decision making.	A couple of reflections add depth to the discussion.
C: Yeah. That's right—I know that's not really true, but that's what I'm afraid of.	Client is able to take some perspective.
P: There's a part of you that has this fear, but another part knows that this is not likely to be the case and that it could be helpful.	Double-sided reflection that acknowledges ambivalence and reinforces hope.
C: I think it would be helpful. I guess I just needed to say that out loud. Now that I did that—I'm not so worried about it. I won't get addicted, right?	Client reinforces hope, but still wants some reassurance.
P: That's not how these medicines work. It's not the same as when people become dependent on alcohol or heroin—where they crave the medications and feel as though they cannot live without them.	Offers (after the client provides permission by the question) factual information that addresses the addiction fear.
C: I knew that. Some of my friends have used them at times, and they said they really helped.	Client presents more balanced and hopeful view.

Statement	*Commentary*
P: There are a couple of reasons to think that it might be helpful for you, though it will ultimately be up to you decide whether or not medication makes sense in your situation. What some docs have told me is that antidepressants not only help alleviate the depression, but because of their action in the brain, they may also have some direct impact on the experience of pain. So, I do think in your situation there is some reason to consider using an antidepressant medication. What do you think?	Practitioner reinforces this reasoning and adds additional information. Again, checks for client's view.
C: Yeah. I think I should.	Change talk, but notice that it's desire and not clear commitment.
P: It sounds like you are thinking pretty strongly about it. Now, I do have a bias in this area. I think it's important for people to talk with a psychiatrist, not just a family physician, about these types of medications. My reason for this bias is that these people are the specialists in these medications. These medications are not like antibiotics. There is a certain amount of fussing that goes into finding the right medications at the right dose. So I want people talking to the experts in these medications. What do you think?	Reinforces the change talk and adds a bit of emphasis. Practitioner, now in the directing style, adds an opinion and labels it as such, along with the reasoning behind it. This builds toward a plan the practitioner feels will be most helpful. Again, asks client's view.
C: It makes sense to me.	Client concurs.
P: Where do you stand on this medication idea?	Key question asks for commitment.
C: I am going to do it.	Commitment!
P: You're committed.	Reinforces.

This is an example of an extended discussion in the transition to a plan. Tanya indicates a readiness to change but does not include any specific target behaviors. As a result, commitment to change remains defuse. This discussion and the key question lead to a commitment to a specific action. The style is a combination of directing and guiding. This excerpt also illustrates how information exchange is woven into this process, as well as how agenda setting can remain an ongoing activity. It is also a natural segue into a negotiated plan, which we discuss in Chapter 11.

Try This!

Here are some exercises to hone your skills in identifying commitment language, practicing transitional summaries, and asking key questions. Working with a partner will allow some practice in the interactive aspects. However, as in the last few chapters, it is important to begin inserting these skills into your clinical encounters. If you are finding that this is still difficult, then it's time to seek out additional training and/or supervision and coaching. Even if practicing in your setting is not difficult for you, the research data about the importance of supervision and coaching to skill acquisition and maintenance are clear, as we discuss in Chapter 12.

Exercise 10.1. Are They Ready?

In this exercise you read client statements and then decide—using the seven signs of readiness described in Figure 10.1—if the client is ready to move into Phase II. Describe your reasoning.

Exercise 10.2. Stuck in the Middle with You . . .

Having worked at identifying readiness for the transition, this next exercise asks you to practice developing transitional summaries. We begin with using the "I CAN" strategy for the first three summaries and then switch to the more nuanced Miller and Rollnick strategy for the last three. (P.S. In practice, these may not look terribly different.)

Exercise 10.3. So, What's Next?

Adept at identifying readiness for Phase II and constructing transitional summaries, now you have an opportunity to practice asking key questions. There is a prompt for each of several different times that key questions might be asked (e.g., commitment, goals and options). Practice developing your questions for each form.

Partner Work

Exercises 10.1–10.3 will all work well as shared exercises. Here are some modified instructions for each.

Exercise 10.1. Are They Ready?

Read the client statements and then decide independently—using the seven signs of readiness described in Figure 10.1—if the client is ready to move into Phase II. Describe your reasoning. If you have a discrepancy, then talk it through until you reach an agreement (or agree to disagree).

Exercise 10.2. Stuck in the Middle with You . . .

This exercise asks you to practice developing transitional summaries. Try to generate two different summaries to each statement. If you are feeling ambitious, you might alternate the "I CAN" and Miller and Rollnick strategies on each item. Talk about which approach seems to fit your style best or helps you organize the materials most effectively.

Exercise 10.3. So, What's Next?

Take turns asking key questions, using the prompt provided. Make a game of it. Alternate and see who runs out of "original" questions first.

Other Thoughts . . .

There are challenges in the transition to, and working in, Phase II. Miller and Rollnick (2002) refer to three specific hazards: underestimating ambivalence, overprescription, and insufficient direction. We'll focus on underestimating ambivalence in this chapter and return to the last two in Chapter 11.

It can be a long, hard struggle getting to the summit of motivation. Once at that point with clients, we may find it dismaying to suddenly encounter a resurgence of ambivalence within the client. Although we've talked about change as a process and not typically a transformative event (cf. Miller & C'de Baca, 2001), where suddenly the client knows and must act upon change intentions, still the reappearance of ambivalence can lead the best of us to want to nudge that client over the edge and into change. It is as if we have abandoned our MI spirit and given in to what we "know" will be "good" for them. Unfortunately, this shift seems to engender the same sort of reactive pattern from clients discussed in Chapter 6. Indeed, Miller has described data (Amrhein et al., 2003; Miller et al., 2003) indicating that motivation diminished among drug-addicted clients during the last moments of an MI session, when therapists were required to complete a change plan. It is important to normalize this ambivalence, address it, and, if the client is ready, to move forward. However, if the client is still contemplating change and not ready to act, then it is time to shift back into strategies better suited to individuals who need assistance in resolving ambivalence. Listening is your ally at this moment.

In considering this information, we may find ourselves recalling exceptions to it. Indeed, we may have experience where a nudge at the summit either helped us or our clients to go forward with a change. This does indeed happen but, on balance, most people respond with resistance when this occurs. So, my counsel is to try to avoid this tendency, unless you have a clear sense that a nudge is needed. To return to hesitant swimmers, they are typically much better served if we clasp their hand and offer to jump in together than if we give them a shove.

Read the client statements and then decide—using the seven signs of readiness—if the client is ready to move into Phase II. Describe your reasoning.

Signs of Readiness for Change[1]

- *Decreased resistance.* The wind seems to have gone out of the sails of resistance. Dissonance in the counseling relationship diminishes, and resistance decreases.

- *Decreased discussion about the problem.* The client seems to have talked enough about the area of concern. If the client has been asking questions about the problem area, these stop. There is a feeling of at least partial completion, of waiting for the next step.

- *Resolve.* The client appears to have reached some resolution and may seem more peaceful, relaxed, calm, unburdened, or settled. This can also have a tone of loss, tearfulness, or resignation.

- *Change talk.* Whereas resistance diminishes, change talk increases. Clients make direct statements about a desire to change, the ability to change, the reasons or benefits of change, and the need to change (the disadvantages of the status quo). They may also make statements of intention to change.

- *Questions about change.* Clients may begin to ask what they could do about the problem, how people change once they decide to, and the like.

- *Envisioning.* The client talks about how life might be after a change. This can be mistaken for resistance; that is, looking ahead to change often causes a person to anticipate difficulties if a change were made. Of course, the client may also envision positive outcomes of change.

- *Experimenting.* The client may have begun experimenting with possible change actions since the last session.

Sample

This is not what I expected. I thought you would be more in my face about the DUI. It's been more like a workshop than a jail term. It's made me really think about some things, and I wasn't expecting to do that.

Do these statements signal a possible readiness to shift phases?   No _____   Yes __*X*__

If yes, what kind?

X	Decreased resistance		Questions about change
	Decreased discussion about problem		Envisioning
	Resolve		Experimenting
	Change talk		

Reasoning for your choice?

The client is clearly talking about how expectations were not met and how this caused a shift. Whether or not he is ready to shift is not clear, but the response indicates it is possible.

---

[1]Adapted from Miller and Rollnick (2002). Copyright 2002 by The Guilford Press. Adapted by permission.

(*cont.*)

Statement 1

So, what do your other clients say about this?

Does this signal a possible readiness to shift phases?   No _____ Yes _____

If yes, what kind?

	Decreased resistance		Questions about change
	Decreased discussion about problem		Envisioning
	Resolve		Experimenting
	Change talk		

Reasoning for your choice?

Statement 2

I agree it would be good to make some low-risk choices, but I also like to have fun with my friends. I have too much fun with them.

Do these statements signal a possible readiness to shift phases?   No _____ Yes _____

If yes, what kind?

	Decreased resistance		Questions about change
	Decreased discussion about problem		Envisioning
	Resolve		Experimenting
	Change talk		

Reasoning for your choice?

Statement 3

You don't understand. These guys aren't going to take "No, thanks" for an answer. They're going to hound me. I've got to come back with something stronger.

Do these statements signal a possible readiness to shift phases?   No _____ Yes _____

If yes, what kind?

	Decreased resistance		Questions about change
	Decreased discussion about problem		Envisioning
	Resolve		Experimenting
	Change talk		

Reasoning for your choice?

Statement 4

I won't be in this situation again. It sucks. I'm so embarrassed.

Do these statements signal a possible readiness to shift phases?   No _____   Yes _____

If yes, what kind?

	Decreased resistance		Questions about change
	Decreased discussion about problem		Envisioning
	Resolve		Experimenting
	Change talk		

Reasoning for your choice?

Statement 5

You know I am not very social, but I have been trying to speak up here.

Does this signal a possible readiness to shift phases?   No _____   Yes _____

If yes, what kind?

	Decreased resistance		Questions about change
	Decreased discussion about problem		Envisioning
	Resolve		Experimenting
	Change talk		

Reasoning for your choice?

Statement 6

I don't see any point in talking about it.

Does this signal a possible readiness to shift phases?   No _____ Yes _____

If yes, what kind?

Decreased resistance		Questions about change	
Decreased discussion about problem		Envisioning	
Resolve		Experimenting	
Change talk			

Reasoning for your choice?

Statement 7

I feel like we're going over it and over it. I get it. I just need to figure out how.

Do these statements signal a possible readiness to shift phases?   No _____ Yes _____

If yes, what kind?

Decreased resistance		Questions about change	
Decreased discussion about problem		Envisioning	
Resolve		Experimenting	
Change talk			

Reasoning for your choice?

Key for Exercise 10.1

Statement 1

So, what do your other clients say about this?

> Yes, question about change.
>
> Although we don't know the entire context, the question implies a curiosity about the issue and an interest in hearing about others' views.

Statement 2

I agree it would be good to make some low-risk choices, but I also like to have fun with my friends. I have too much fun with them.

> No.
>
> This statement has some change talk in the first part; the *but* then negates it. The "yes, but … " suggests that ambivalence remains strong.

Statement 3

You don't understand. These guys aren't going to take "No, thanks" for an answer. They're going to hound me. I've got to come back with something stronger.

> Yes, envisioning.
>
> This man seems to be thinking about what it would be like to make a change, especially about the challenges he might encounter. He is thinking about what he must "come back with" if he's to be successful.

Statement 4

I won't be in this situation again. It sucks. I'm so embarrassed.

> Yes, change talk and apparent resolve.
>
> The client is very clear in her statement and provides the rationale for why.

Statement 5

You know I am not very social, but I have been trying to speak up here.

> Yes, experimenting.
>
> The client is trying out new behaviors. Of course, we don't know the target behavior, and this statement may be unrelated to the issue for which the client has sought help. However, there is an effort at change embedded in this statement.

Sample Responses for Exercise 10.1 (*cont.*)

Statement 6

I don't see any point in talking about it.

> No.
> Although this client may be indicating a decreased need to talk about the situation, there is not enough information to know. As it stands, it appears to be a resistance or status quo statement.

Statement 7

I feel like we're going over it and over it. I get it. I just need to figure out how.

> Yes. Decreased need to talk.
> There is also an element of resistance, though it seems to be a function of the therapist failing to keep pace. The client is not arguing with the need. The client wants some help imagining how to do it.

Stuck in the Middle with You . . .

Having worked at identifying readiness for the transition, this next exercise asks you to practice developing transitional summaries. We begin with using the "I CAN" strategy for the first three summaries and then switch to the more nuanced Miller and Rollnick strategy for the last three. (P.S. In practice, these may not look terribly different.)
Here is the "I CAN" strategy:

- **I**ndicate this is a summary, and include
- **C**hange talk,
- **A**mbivalence, and then ask about the
- **N**ext step.

Here are the elements Miller and Rollnick (2002) suggest.

- A statement indicating that you are pulling together what the client has said.
- A summary of the client's perceptions of the issue, including any reasons or need for change noted by the client.
- A summary of the client's ambivalence, including the benefits of the status quo.
- Objective evidence relevant to the importance of change.
- A restatement of desire, ability, and commitment to change.
- Your assessment of the client's situation, especially when it matches the client's concern.

Client Statement 1

Target behavior: Studying for school

"I don't want my mother brought into this. I don't see why she would need to be. I know some things need to change, and I have been talking about this with my dad. I live with him and he pays the bills, so I think it makes sense to talk with him. I know I need to get some things going, if I'm going to graduate. I've been talking with my teachers—more or less—and I think I know what I need to do. I am a little worried about all the things that I have to do between now and the end of the year."

(cont.)

From *Building Motivational Interviewing Skills: A Practitioner Workbook* by David B. Rosengren. Copyright 2009 by The Guilford Press. Permission to photocopy this exercise is granted to purchasers of this book for personal use only (see copyright page for details).

Client Statement 2

Target behavior: Writing

"I wasted another evening last night. I sat down to write and then I started fiddling with transferring files from my old computer to my new one. Then I checked my e-mail because I realized that I'd forgotten to send an e-mail I promised to take care of. I also checked my personal account and responded to a few things there. Then my computer froze. Next thing I knew, it was 9 o'clock and I was still on the first page. The last few weeks just haven't been productive because 'things' come up, but I am running out of time to get this done. I have to do it or I'm toast!"

Client Statement 3

Target behavior: Improving intimate relationship

"I am willing to apologize, but he has to admit that he wronged me as well. I admit that what I did was wrong. I shouldn't have said it. But he also said some things that were pretty mean and won't acknowledge it. There was a context, and now all of our friends have turned against me. Still, I know it's not doing me any good staying angry. I just feel worse and more depressed. So, I know that I should let go, but it's hard."

Client Statement 4

Target behavior: Consideration of medications

"I didn't like the way I felt on the medications. There were just too many side effects. So, I stopped. I haven't taken anything since I was 18. But I think I need to do something. Nothing feels good. I'm always anxious. I can never get comfortable. Sometimes I just sit at home because it just feels like too much of an effort to go out. But then I start get-ting depressed and nothing feels good. That's where I'm at now. This is my first time out of the house in 3 weeks."

Client Statement 5

Target behavior: Eating healthier

"I have made a decision to eat healthier. I just think it would be better for my health if I did that. My follow-through isn't always as good as my intentions, and I do have a sweet tooth. But I've tried to be more judicious in my eating of those things generally. I would like to eat more salads. I really do like salad for lunch. Breakfast and lunch, and even dinner, for that matter, are generally OK. I have one problem area currently—snacking at night. I like ice cream, and that is a problem. I'm not crazy about fruit as a substitute, even though I know it would be better for me. I can manage those other areas, but that nighttime stuff needs some work."

Client Statement 6

Target behavior: Drinking

"Here is the deal. I came in here thinking it was just bad luck I got caught. I mean my BAC was only 1.0 when the cop pulled me over. I really hadn't drunk that much, but I was tired, and you've taught me about how that can interact with the alcohol. I guess now I feel lucky that nobody got hurt. I'm not ready to stop drinking entirely, but I am thinking hard about making more low-risk drinking choices. It's just not worth it. I don't want to be here doing this again."

Sample Responses for Exercise 10.2

Client Statement 1. Target behavior: Studying for school

"I don't want my mother brought into this (etc.)."

(I CAN Transitional Summary)

Let me see if I understand all of this. You've filled your dad in on the situation, but you're not so sure you want to bring your mom into the discussion. You want to graduate and are worried about getting everything done. You know things need to change. What do you think you'll do?

Client Statement 2. Target behavior: Writing

"I wasted another evening last night (etc.)."

(I CAN Transitional Summary)

Let me see if I've got it. You're feeling the heat. There's a deadline approaching, and you have tasks to do. You try to do these things, but other tasks seem to jump ahead in priority when you have time to do the work. The lack of productivity is a real concern. You're ready to do something and not quite clear what. What happens now?

Client Statement 3. Target behavior: Improving intimate relationship

"I am willing to apologize, but he has to admit that he was wrong as well (etc.)."

(I CAN Transitional Summary)

I think I've got it, but let me check. You're feeling stuck because you can't put your anger down. From your vantage, it feels like his unwillingness to admit his part keeps you stuck, though there is also some recognition that hanging onto this view may be costing you. Where do you think you want to go from here with waiting for his apology?

Client Statement 4. Target behavior: Consideration of medications

"I didn't like the way I felt on the medications (etc.)."

(Miller and Rollnick's format for a transition summary)

Let me see if I've understood what you've told me. Nothing feels good to you right now. You're uncomfortable at home and when you go out. And while you want to feel better, you're also worried about medications. Still, you've been so immobilized that this is your first time out in 3 weeks. You think you need to do something. Given what you've told me, it does seem like at least talking about medications makes sense. Where do you stand on that discussion?

Sample Responses for Exercise 10.2 (*cont.*)

Client Statement 5. Target behavior: Eating healthier

"I have made a decision to eat healthier (etc.)."

(Miller and Rollnick's format for a transition summary)

There are a couple of different pieces here. You've made a decision to eat better and be healthier, and then followed this up with changes to your meals. A sweet tooth and the evenings are your trouble spots. Fruit is a good idea in theory, but just doesn't work for you. Still, you're committed. You want to be healthier and have experienced some success toward that goal. What do you think your next step will be?

Client Statement 6. Target behavior: Drinking

"Here is the deal. I came in here thinking it was just bad luck I got caught (etc.)."

(Miller and Rollnick's format for a transition summary)

That's a lot of change in a short period of time. You came in with one idea about what happened, and your thinking has really shifted. You feel lucky now instead of unlucky. You're not sure that stopping entirely is what you want to do, but you're pretty clear that this low-risk drinking has some merit. And, of course, another DUI would likely be even more problematic for you, and you're clear that's not what you want. This is a big shift, and it seems like quite a powerful one for you. What happens next?

So, What's Next?

Here is an opportunity to practice asking key questions. There is a prompt indicating the various times that key questions might be asked (i.e., when seeking commitment, goals, or options). Practice developing your questions for each form.

When you are asking for ... commitment to change ...

Sample response: *Where does this leave you now?*

1.

2.

3.

When you are asking for ... setting specific goals ...

Sample response: *What would you like to be different?*

1.

2.

3.

When you are asking for ... development of a plan ...

Sample response: *How might you go about doing this?*

1.

2.

3.

(cont.)

When you are asking for ... commitment to the plan ...

Sample response: *Now that you have a plan, where do you stand with doing it?*

1.

2.

3.

When you are asking for ... setting the alarm ...

Sample response: *Since now might not be the right time, what will need to happen for it to be the right time?*

1.

2.

3.

When you are asking for ... a follow-up discussion, after the client did not commit.

Sample response: *When last we talked, you weren't quite ready to jump in. I'm wondering where that is sitting for you now.*

1.

2.

3.

Sample Responses for Exercise 10.3

When you are asking for ... commitment to change ...

1. *What happens now?*

2. *What do you think you'll do?*

3. *Where do you go from here?*

When you are asking for ... setting specific goals ...

1. *How would you like things to be better?*

2. *What specifically are you hoping will change?*

3. *What do you see as the first change?*

When you are asking for ... development of a plan ...

1. *What have you considered doing?*

2. *What's the first step?*

3. *What's worked for you before?*

When you are asking for ... commitment to the plan ...

1. *When do you start doing this?*

2. *What do you think about doing this plan?*

3. *What worries you about the plan?* (This is a tricky one, because it could elicit ambivalence—though it may also elicit a consolidating response.)

When you are asking for ... setting the alarm ...

1. *When could you see this changing?*

2. *What would need to change for this to feel like now is the time?*

3. *What things will you watch for to know when that time has come?*

When you are asking for ... a follow-up discussion, after the client did not commit ...

1. *What are your thoughts now about it?*

2. *Since we last met, what came up for you as you thought about this?*

3. *So, what's been going on in your head about this decision?*

Chapter 11

Negotiating a Treatment Plan

Opening

"I've been doing my best, but I'm at the end of my rope. It's been the year from hell, and things just aren't getting any better. Normally, I don't believe in this kind of thing, but I gotta do something. I've left messages for several different people, and I hope that I can see someone soon. Please call me as soon as you can."

This was Tanya leaving a message on the answering service in Chapter 10, where we observed a practitioner guiding and directing her to the point of a key question. Let's return to the end of that process. Recall that Tanya had decided to focus on her depression as one way to begin managing her pain, and the discussion had turned to the use of medications. Here is the end of that interchange, repeated from Chapter 10. We'll begin with the practitioner offering some information about antidepressants.

"It's not uncommon for people to have mixed feelings about antidepressants. There is great concern about these medicines being overprescribed, especially for people who may not need them. Given what you've told me so far, though, I think these may be appropriate for you, but you would need to talk with a physician to be sure. I can say there is reason to be hopeful. First, medication often helps with depression. Second, certain kinds of counseling can help with depression. Third, the two together seem to have the best success rate. What do you think about that?"

"I guess it makes sense. I just don't want to get addicted to those things and feel like I would have to take them. I want to be myself."

"And that's your worry ... that somehow you would lose your ability to control that decision making."

"Yeah. That's right—I know that's not really true, but that's what I'm afraid of."

"There's a part of you that has this fear, but another part knows that this is not likely to be the case and that it could be helpful."

"I think it would be helpful. I guess I just needed to say that out loud. Now that I did that—I'm not so worried about it. I won't get addicted, right?"

"That's not how these medicines work. It's not the same as when people become dependent on alcohol or heroin—where they crave the medications and feel as though they cannot live without them."

"I knew that. Some of my friends have used them at times, and they said they really helped."

"There are a couple of reasons to think that it might be helpful for you, though it will ultimately be up to you decide whether or not medication makes sense in your situation. What some docs have told me is that antidepressants not only help alleviate the depression, but because of their action in the brain, they may also have some direct impact on the experience of pain. So, I do think in your situation there is some reason to consider using an antidepressant medication. What do you think?"

"Yeah. I think I should."

"It sounds like you are thinking pretty strongly about it. Now, I do have a bias in this area. I think it's important for people to talk with a psychiatrist, not just a family physician, about these types of medications. My reason for this bias is that these people are the specialists in these medications. These medications are not like antibiotics. There is a certain amount of fussing that goes into finding the right medications at the right dose. So I want people talking to the experts in these medications. What do you think?"

"It makes sense to me."

"Where do you stand on this medication idea?"

"I am going to do it."

"You're committed."

Through this dialogue, Tanya has resolved her ambivalence. She is ready to seek out medication. But there is no plan for how to proceed. Now we need to help her translate this commitment into specific behaviors for change. Where would you go next? What question(s) might you ask to get there?

A Deeper Look

In Chapter 10 we noted that Phase II has two primary parts: solidifying commitment and negotiating a change plan. Although we've separated these two parts for ease of understanding, there is an ongoing and dynamic interplay between them. Although the client has now moved further into Phase II, we will return to issues of commitment even as we negotiate plans.

Returning to the skiing analogy we used in Chapter 10, Miller and Rollnick (2002) note that this planning process can become much easier—like swooshing down the slopes—though practitioners remain active guides. They don't just shout "Good luck!" as novice skiers position their skis downhill. Miller and Rollnick (2002) suggest four elements in putting together an effective change plan. I have relabeled these four to form the acronym SOAR: set goals, sort options, arrive at a plan, and then reaffirm commitment.

Set Goals

We remain consistent with MI principles as we help clients decide which goals are important to them. Again, our desires for clients may not match their needs or situations, and so we must be sure that we inquire about their hopes and expectations and then narrow these to specific goals. Questions are a good way to access this information.

"How would you like your life to be different?"

"What would you like to see change?"

"If things were better, what would be different?"

"What would you like to have more of? Less of?"

You would follow up these queries with the other OARS skills, especially reflections and summaries. Miller and Rollnick (2002) remind practitioners to keep a broad focus initially, as it is easy to become so problem directed that other important aspects of the client's life are missed. However, once goals are identified, it is helpful to prune these down to achievable aims and then to consider options for making changes.

Sort Options

This is an area in which practitioner expertise can be particularly beneficial to clients. Still, caution is needed to avoid becoming overly directive. The elicit–provide–elicit (E-P-E) model can be very helpful throughout this task. Find out what the client has considered doing and then add ideas to it.

As with many problem-solving approaches, it is helpful to have the client brainstorm a range of ideas, including some that may seem unreasonable. This approach may provide a broader palate for clients' consideration as they develop a plan. If clients are unable to come up with ideas on their own, provide a menu of options with some more extreme elements added. As always, clients will choose the alternatives that fit best for them.

Arrive at a Plan

Planning is a negotiated process in MI. That is, practitioners do not sit idly by as clients develop overly elaborate or underdeveloped plans. Instead like any good guide, they assist clients in thinking through the steps of an option, difficulties they might encounter, how they might address these, what resources they might bring to this process, and how they will evaluate the plan. This process is typically begun with an open-ended question.

"What will you do first?"

"What specific steps will need to be done?"

"What's your plan?"

In Project MATCH (Miller et al., 1992), therapists in the MET condition used a change plan that included writing out the specific steps. Miller and Rollnick (2002) include a similar plan in their book. For some clients, a written document can be very helpful. For others, it will feel artificial, intimidating, or unnecessary. The client should take the lead in whether the writing aspect is included, but the practitioner can provide information about why some clients find this helpful (e.g., adds clarity, serves as a memory aid, reinforces commitment to oneself). Practitioners might also provide a form that matches their work environments and clients' needs. A sample change plan worksheet, based on the MATCH (Miller et al., 1992) and Miller and Rollnick (2002) forms, is included in Exercise 11.2. Your introduction to this form might go like this:

"We've been talking about what you might do. Some clients find it very helpful to write down possible options, so they can have a tangible reference. Posting it in a public place can also aid in maintaining commitment. There are data indicating that people who state their intentions and make them known to others are more successful in making the change they want. The written document also serves as a visual reminder of their decision. Still, this is your decision, and some people choose not to do it. What makes sense to you?"

It is important that the practitioner express concern if there is something about the plan that appears unworkable. This feedback should be given in the manner described in Chapter 9. Here is an example of practitioner feedback regarding an overly elaborate plan:

"It's clear that you would very much like to get this change moving, and there are many pieces you've chosen to work on all at once. I do have a concern about that. May I share my concern with you?

"My clients' experiences have been that if they spread themselves thin on too many tasks, then they begin to have trouble meeting all their goals. As a result, they start to see themselves as slipping, which can undermine their commitment. What they've often found helpful is to narrow their focus and start to experience success in one area and then begin to expand that outward to other areas. How does that sound to you?"

Alternatively, if a client has an underdeveloped plan, the practitioner might offer something like this:

"You've told me that you are someone who doesn't like to spend lots of time *thinking* about things but rather *doing* them. Once you've made the decision to go, you want to go now. That eagerness to act can work in your favor, and I also want to make sure we are helping you put enough structure into your action so that it can succeed. My concern at this moment is that you might not have given yourself the best chance at success. May I share with you why?"

Presuming the client agrees, the practitioner would note his or her concerns and end with an invitation to hear the client's view. Given that it will be the client's job to implement and monitor the plan, he or she might choose to ignore the practitioner's advice. In this situation it can be helpful to offer an alternative to a client's flat "No." The practitioner might say something like this:

> "You're not so worried about those things. You feel like you can improvise as needed, and it often seems to you, when the plan is left more open, it frees you to make the choices that best fit the particular situation. I wonder if it would be OK if we just checked back on that decision the next time you come in. We would see how it's working, as well as talk about the other parts of your plan. How does that sound?"

Reaffirm Commitment

The final task that Miller and Rollnick (2002) describe is that of securing the client's commitment to the plan. In some cases, this commitment is already evident, and it would be redundant and perhaps patronizing to ask for specific commitment. In others, though, especially after significant negotiation, it may be useful to review the plan and then ask a simple closed question, *"Is that what you plan to do?"*

This is also a time for the practitioner to be alert to hesitation on the part of the client. It is a natural point for ambivalence to arise. Note that it may appear in the use of less active verbs such as *hope, try,* or *consider.* This is not necessarily a problem, but it does require that the practitioner respond. If the client is uncertain, then the practitioner either helps reaffirm commitment or explores the root of the ambivalence and helps the client address this situation. Sometimes this exploration can be accomplished by simply using a double-sided reflection. For example:

> "It worries you to think about what you would have to give up to start this plan. At the same time, you are clear that continuing with how things are at present is no longer an option."

If the client is not ready to choose commitment, then avoid the trap of pressing for it. This can be an especially trying moment for you as a practitioner, because you've worked hard to help get the client to the top of the mountain, only to see him or her turning back in the direction just traveled. Your tendency will be to press harder to "close the deal," yet doing so is likely to undermine the client's commitment and lead to either active or passive resistance. As tough as it may be, this is a time to switch back to OARS and make sure that the door is left open for the client to revisit this issue. One technique is "setting the alarm." That is, you are merely setting the clock to awaken yourself in the morning, not setting the burglar alarm or sounding the warning. In this approach you simply acknowledge the client's position:

> "It sounds like you aren't quite ready to take this on now. As you look down the road, when can you see this happening? What would need to happen for that to occur?"

This approach avoids building resistance and encourages clients to take an active rather than a passive role in looking toward the future, toward events that might need to transpire to increase their readiness. It also encourages them to think about a time in the future when this change could occur. As with setting the alarm for a morning wake-up, the setting of it doesn't ensure that we will rise, but it does increase the likelihood. Thus, we set the alarm for possible future change.

Finally, it is useful to check back with clients about a decision to forego change—at least for now. Language is important when returning to this earlier choice. Rather than asking, *"Have you made a decision?"*, it is more productive to ask, *"Where's your thinking now about this decision?"* This wording sidesteps a closed question and opens the possibility of a discussion about this area.

Concept Quiz—Test Yourself!

True or false:

1.   T F   During Phase II active guidance is less important to clients.

2.   T F   SOAR refers to the four elements in negotiating a change plan.

3.   T F   Once the client commits to a change, you should begin brainstorming ideas with clients for how to change.

4.   T F   It is helpful to funnel broad goals down to achievable aims.

5.   T F   We should encourage clients to consider options broadly, sometimes including extremes to help them do so.

6.   T F   Since clients will enact the change, the plan must ultimately be theirs, and this means that they may choose to ignore our advice.

7.   T F   Since these are clients plans, we should not interfere if they choose problematic goals.

8.   T F   Clients should write down their change plans.

9.   T F   *Reaffirming commitment* refers to securing the client's commitment to the change plan.

10. T F   If clients balk at commitment to action in Phase II, then "setting the alarm" can help them return to a more active process in contemplating change.

Answers

1.   F   During Phase II active guidance becomes an even more salient strategy. Practitioners work actively with clients to develop change plans that are workable for them. Receiving information about possible choices, along with attendant risks and benefits, can be quite helpful for clients.

2.   T   Miller and Rollnick (2002) suggest that four elements be included when negotiating a change plan. These four have been renamed to form the acronym SOAR: **s**et goals, sort **o**ptions, **a**rrive at a plan, and **r**eaffirm commitment.

3.   F   Brainstorming is an important strategy, though it typically follows assessment of clients' goals for change. The first step than after hearing a commitment statement is to find out what the client would like to change, then developing strategies that target these areas. It is at this point that brainstorming is usually done.

4. T We start broadly when eliciting goals. This breadth allows attention to other client needs and contexts that may be more important. However, once these broad goals have been developed, honing them into more focused, achievable aims helps clients develop appropriate strategies, measure progress, and determine if alterations are needed.

5. T While we don't want clients to act recklessly, we do want them to think broadly and creatively about what will work for them. As with many problem-solving approaches, including extremes can assist people with identifying novel, or at least unconsidered paths, to success.

6. T Clients are responsible for the change and therefore they must be invested in the plan. They must feel that the plan is theirs and not ours. Without this sense of ownership, sustainable change will be less likely to occur.

7. F As good guides, we don't let clients choose problematic goals without offering our concerns. Although clients must choose their own goals, this does not mean that we stand by quietly. Again, learning how to express our feedback in an MI-consistent way is the essence of good MI practice.

8. F Although there are many reasons why writing down a plan may be helpful, this is not the only way to construct a plan, and for some people it simply does not fit. In some situations it might even be dangerous. For example, victims of interpersonal violence are usually strongly encouraged to create a safety plan, if they return to their partner, as a step in changing their circumstance, but not typically encouraged to write down this information.

9. T Although the client has already indicated global commitment to a change, this step secures specific commitment to the plan that has just been negotiated. However, this step may feel redundant or patronizing in some instances. The practitioner should decide whether a reaffirmation is needed, based on the negotiation process. If there seems to be uncertainty, than asking for a commitment can be helpful.

10. T Hesitation and ambivalence are normal. Some clients will realize they are not yet ready to take action. Helping them to "set the alarm" puts them into a more active mode where they are identifying and looking for signs that indicate their readiness.

In Practice

Let's return to the interchange with Tanya. She has just decided that she will pursue antidepressant medications, but there is no plan in place. Here we see a brief, but active planning process.

Statement	*Commentary*
P: Where do you stand on this medication idea?	Key question asks for commitment.
C: I am going to do it.	Commitment!
P: You're committed.	Reinforces.

Statement	*Commentary*
C: Yeah. I am. I think I know someone I could talk to about them. When I talked with my friend before, she gave me her psychiatrist's name, and I still have it at home. She liked her.	Agreement and then offers thoughts about how to do it. This is both goal setting and considering options.
P: That feels like a good option. And if she isn't available?	Reinforces and checks for how obstacles might be handled. This is a form of sorting through options.
C: I guess I'll ask for some other names from their office.	Client provides an option.
P: I could also provide some names.	Offers resources, but may be pressing practitioner's agenda.
C: Let me start with this person and then if that doesn't work, I'll call.	Client asserts her autonomy and chooses a form that makes sense to her.
P: It sounds like you have a plan. When do you think you'll do this?	Reinforces plan. Asks another key question about timing.
C: Probably as soon as I get home today.	Tentative statement.
P: Probably . . .	Picks up on the weak modifier and asks her to reaffirm her commitment.
C: (*Laughs.*) OK. As soon as I get home.	Client is moving with provider and handles this press without problems.
P: (*Laughs.*) Other clients have taught me that it's good to have a firm idea about when.	Reinforces and uses other clients as an aid in this process.
C: I can see that. Today. I'll do it today.	Firm commitment to plan.

This is an example of plan that is not written, but it includes specific elements and has a timeline in it. The practitioner checks to see that the client has the resources needed to succeed and follows the client's lead, but also addresses when ambivalence arises or less than clear commitment is communicated. The style is a combination of directing and guiding. Previously, we observed how information exchange is woven into this process, though it was also evident in small doses here. This plan is also negotiated. Finally, although Tanya may add other elements to this planning process later, on this topic there is a clear agreement on what will be done, when it will be done, and what will happen if problems arise. It is also manageable, and she feels capable of handling it. Notice how her mood and attitude have shifted during the course of this encounter.

Try This!

Here are a few exercises to hone your skills in negotiating a change plan. Working with a partner will allow some practice in the interactive aspects, though it is also important to begin inserting these skills into your clinical encounters. Again, if this is still feeling difficult, it's probably time to seek out additional training and/or supervision and coaching.

Exercise 11.1. Negotiating a Change Plan

In this activity we return to the interaction with Tanya and practice developing change plans for the areas that were mentioned but not addressed in the interchange.

Exercise 11.2. Developing a Change Plan Form

Here is an opportunity to develop your personal form for use with clients. Begin with the form provided in the exercise at the end of the chapter, and then modify it to a format that fits your style, work context and clients. Once you've designed it, try it out with a client. Don't forget to write a brief preamble that you might use with your clients. Remember, this preamble is not to be read to your clients, but just an aid in organizing your thoughts. Once you've designed it, try the form out with a client. After this pilot test, revise it and then try it with another client. Continue this process until you feel comfortable with the introduction and use of the form.

Partner Work

Exercise 11.1 can be done as a shared exercise. Work as a team to complete this interaction with Tanya, developing change plans for these other areas.

Exercise 11.3. Back to the Future

If more practice is desired, partners could return to their completed worksheets for Exercise 10.2 and use these as launching pads for negotiating change plans. One partner plays the client suggested by the scenario. You'll work to a conclusion and a confirmation of commitment (if appropriate). Then choose another scenario and switch roles. You can also play a client becoming tentative and deciding not to change. Practice setting the alarm in this scenario.

Other Thoughts ...

Challenges remain in Phase II. We addressed one of the three specific challenges Miller and Rollnick (2002) identified, underestimating ambivalence, in Chapter 10. Now we tackle overprescription and insufficient direction.

Overprescription is a variation on underestimating ambivalence. In this situation we fail to attend to client resources and needs in the planning process. Our expertise and experience can be significant resources to clients, but only if these fit with clients' views of how change can occur for them. That is, they must embrace these ideas as suitable and appropriate to *their* situation. Otherwise we risk developing an elegant but ultimately flawed blueprint for change because we failed to attend to the most important element—the person who must enact the change. A "yes, but … " response should be viewed as a cue that clients feel that the solutions are ours, not theirs.

The final challenge is the opposite of overprescription. In this situation we have left clients entirely to their own devices. It would be as though we moved into a following style when the client needed us to continue guiding or even directing. Reflections are still intermixed into this process, especially when ambivalence appears, but information should also be provided about options, as well as benefits and risks attendant to those. If the client develops a plan that has serious flaws, good guides would not be content to simply shrug their shoulders and say, "It's his plan." Instead, good guides would express their concerns directly, especially when the client is making a dangerous choice. However, this is the difference between offering a concern and stating a warning. A warning is, "If you continue to drink, given the fragile health of your liver, you are likely to die." A concern is expressed in this way: "I'm a very worried about your decision to drink, given the compromised state of your liver. My fear is your liver will fail and you could die. It's still your choice—not mine—but I am very concerned. What are your thoughts?"

Negotiating a Change Plan

In this activity we will return to the interaction with Tanya and practice developing additional change plans for areas that weren't addressed initially. The dialogue, originally encountered in Chapter 10, has been reprinted, along with commentary, below.

Following this interchange are directions to focus your attention on a particular point in the dialogue where the interaction could have gone productively in another direction. After this instruction, the dialogue takes you on this new branch. The form asks you to respond to specific prompts and then imagine the client's response. You complete the dialogue for both practitioner and client. Continue this process through the end of the form. Then you will have another opportunity to practice.

Original Dialogue	*Commentary*
P: *You sound like you are ready to do something, though you aren't quite sure what would be helpful here.*	Reinforces commitment to action. Practitioner also acknowledges her uncertainty, but doesn't leave her mired in it.
C: *Exactly. What do you suggest?*	Client asks for information.
P: *I have some ideas, based on what other people like yourself have done, but I also want to find out what area feels most important to you.*	Practitioner will respond to request, but first checks for the client's priorities.
C: *Well, if we could begin with the pain, that would be great.*	Client responds directly.
P: *The pain feels like it is driving this bus.*	Simile/metaphor.
C: *Yeah. I think if I could just feel a little bit better physically, then everything else would be easier to do. You know what I mean?*	Client begins articulating a path for change.
P: *Yeah. Like if you could just turn down the volume, then you could deal with all this other noise.*	Another complex reflection.
C: *Exactly.*	
P: *You seem pretty clear about how this works for you. Tell me a little more about what you know about how emotions—and especially depression—and pain work together.*	Affirmation, then moves to the beginning of E-P-E.
C: *I know that when I'm in pain, I don't do things, and I don't feel well. I don't see my friends. I get angry more easily. I snap at my kids and my husband. Then I feel crappy and get depressed.*	Client draws clear connections.

A New Branch

Focus on this client statement, "*I don't do things, and I don't feel well. I don't see my friends.*" Read the new dialogue and then fill in the boxes according to the prompts provided. Don't worry if you don't know the specifics in this area

(cont.)

as a practitioner. Use your good sense about what might work for a person in pain. As for the client responses, try to imagine what it would be like if you were in chronic pain. Again, the goal is to negotiate a change plan.

P:	*You don't do things.*	Simple reflection targets an area.
C:	*Yeah. I ended up sitting home, doing nothing. Then I just focus on how bad I feel.*	Client provides additional information.
P:	*One thing just piles on top of another, like bricks on top of bricks.*	A little deeper reflection—the metaphor may add emotional resonance.
C:	*And I end up buried beneath it all.*	Client agrees. There is now the start of a mutual agenda.
P:		Elicit information on current or prior efforts at change in this area.
C:		Client provides important data.
P:		Acknowledges but doesn't jump into problem solving. Probe for more.
C:		Client provides additional information.
P:		Reframe the response slightly.
C:		Client provides additional information.
P:		Reflection and a probe that signals a possible closing of the discussion.
C:		Client agrees.
P:		A summary and a key question.
C:		Client commits to making a change, but does not specify how.
P:		Reflection and then ask a key question about client goals.

C:		Client articulates things she would like to have, or conversely, would like to avoid or not have.
P:		A reflection or two.
C:		Client adds an additional goal or two.
P:		Summary and key question about how she might accomplish these goals.
C:		Client is unsure how to proceed.
P:		Provide some ideas in the form of a menu. Don't forget to ask permission.
C:		Client chooses all the suggestions.
P:		Help Tanya narrow this down. Provide an explanation as to why a more focused plan might bear more fruit.
C:		Client agreement and articulation of how she might accomplish this plan.
P:		Add an idea to her plan and ask her view.
C:		Client concurs with plan.
P:		Key question asks for commitment to plan.
C:		Commitment!
P:		Reinforce commitment.

Now use the same strategy for these statements. Note the prompts have changed slightly.

"I get angry more easily."

"I snap at my kids and my husband."

P:	*You get angry more easily, and you're responding in a way you don't like with your family.*	Simple reflection, followed by a reframe.
C:	*Yeah. I never used to be this way. Now little things just set me off. It's like, who is this person?*	Client provides additional information.
P:	*Like someone else entirely and not someone you particularly care for . . .*	A little deeper reflection.
C:	*Sometimes they deserve it. It's like they don't get how uncomfortable I am.*	Some resistance to this deeper reflection.
P:		Respond to the resistance and return to her concern.
C:		Client provides important data.
P:		Acknowledges but doesn't jump into problem solving. Probe for more.
C:		Client provides additional information.
P:		Reframe the response slightly.
C:		Client provides additional information, but also shows ambivalence.
P:		Summarize, taking care to acknowledge the ambivalence. Ask a key question.
C:		Client commits to making a change, but does not specify how.
P:		Provide reflection, then ask a key question about client goals.
C:		Client articulates things she would like to have, or conversely, she would like to avoid or not have.
P:		A reflection or two.

C:	Client agrees but again notes ambivalence.
P:	Summary, with attention to ambivalence. Ask a key question about how she might accomplish these goals.
C:	Client is unsure how to proceed.
P:	Provide some ideas in the form of a menu. Don't forget to ask permission.
C:	Client is unsure if she likes these options.
P:	Find out more about what concerns her.
C:	Client describes concerns and articulates how she might accomplish this goal.
P:	Suggest an alteration to her plan and ask her view.
C:	Client concurs with plan.
P:	Key question asks for commitment to plan.
C:	Commitment language is weak.
P:	Explore her uncertainty.
C:	Client isn't ready to commit.
P:	Set the alarm for when she might be ready.
C:	Client articulates when she might be ready.
P:	Provide a summary.

Developing a Change Plan Form

Here is an opportunity to develop your personal form for use with clients. Begin with the form on the next page, and then modify it to a format that fits your style, work context and clients. Don't forget to write a brief preamble that you might use with your clients. Once you've designed it, try out the form with a client. After this pilot test, revise it and then try it with another client. Continue this process until you feel comfortable with the introduction and use of the form.

Sample preamble from the chapter:

> *"We've been talking about what you might do. Some clients find it very helpful to write down possible options, so they can have a tangible reference. Posting it in a public place can also aid in maintaining commitment. There are data indicating that people who state their intentions and make them known to others are more successful in making the change they want. The written document also serves as a visual reminder of their decision. Still, this is your decision and some people choose not to do it. What makes sense to you?"*

Your preamble:

Change Plan Worksheet[1]

The most important reasons why I want to make this change are:

My main goals for myself in making this change are:

I plan to do these specific things in order to accomplish my goals:

Specific action   *When?*

Other people could help me with change in these ways:

Person   *Possible ways to help*

These are some possible obstacles to change, and how I might handle them:

Possible obstacle to change   *How to respond*

I will know my plan is working when I see these results:

[1]From Miller and Rollnick (2002). Copyright 2002 by The Guilford Press. Reprinted by permission.

From *Building Motivational Interviewing Skills: A Practitioner Workbook* by David B. Rosengren. Copyright 2009 by The Guilford Press. Permission to photocopy this worksheet is granted to purchasers of this book for personal use only (see copyright page for details).

Back to the Future

In this exercise you will need the completed worksheets for Exercise 10.2. Use these scenarios as launching pads for negotiating change plans. One partner plays the client suggested by the scenario.

Here is the process:

- Partner-practitioner provides the transitional summary and then asks a key question. You should read this over and then say it in your own words, rather than reading it, to build authenticity.

- "Client" responds affirmatively to the key question and then creates the remainder of the story as the exercise unfolds

- Practitioner works through negotiating a change plan. Remember to use the four elements of SOAR. Work to a conclusion and a confirmation of commitment.

- Then choose another scenario and switch roles.

- Also play a client becoming tentative and deciding not to change. Practice setting the alarm in this scenario.

Chapter 12

Learning MI

The purpose of this book is to review basic MI concepts and to provide an opportunity and a means to develop greater comfort and facility with MI skills. However, it is not meant to supplant participation in a MI training experience. Indeed, as is made clear in the following pages, there is little research support for learning MI skills through reading alone. What is less clear is the degree to which natural skills and abilities may be enhanced by completion of this type of workbook.

My work as a trainer has convinced me that slowing down the training process often aids people in learning. MI skills often look deceptively simple at first viewing. Many people have made the comment that "simple is not easy," and that seems to be especially true of these types of skills. Indeed, Simpson (2002), in evaluating the complexity of substance abuse interventions, has placed MI at the complex end of the intervention continuum. As a result of this complexity, my training often uses a five-step format:

1. Tell—brief didactic or exercise designed to elicit information.
2. See—observe or recognize the skill in action.
3. Do in slow motion—often a writing task or a skill in isolation, many times done in a group situation.
4. Perform—isolate skills and do them in real time.
5. Build—work from easier to more complex and chain more complicated skills together.

The reasons for this process are fourfold:

1. Using multiple modalities engages different learning styles.
2. Slowing the learning down enough to see the nuances allows people to experience the complexity of the skills.
3. Stepping people through the skill, before asking them to produce it in "real time," builds confidence in their ability to do so.
4. Participants feel readier to take on complex skills as well as learn the nuance of technique.

This workbook is an extension of that thinking. The exercises have attempted to work from the less complex to the more complex, as well as from recognition to production in isolation to performance in real time. Although this approach has a reasoned intent, the evidence to support it is still anecdotal. That is, the format of my teaching approach and this book is based on belief, not on research. There are, however, data available about learning MI. This chapter provides a more thorough review of the available data on what works when learning MI.

The learning of MI can be divided into four basic questions:

1. Can the skills of MI be learned?
2. What are the best methods for teaching MI?
3. Does MI skill matter in terms of client outcomes?
4. Based on these findings, how should MI learning occur?

Can the Skills of MI Be Learned?

The simple answer is yes. There is evidence that aspects of MI can be learned. Yet, the full answer is really more complex that a simple yes. Questions about "What instruments were used to evaluate the learning?", "What is the focus of the researcher?", and "Who is the learner?" all influence our understanding of the learning process. A study of these factors is beyond the scope of this workbook, but I do offer them as points to consider as you read through this overview.

Knowledge of MI basic principles appears to be relatively easily transmitted through a variety of methods. For example, Voss and Wolf (2004) describe transmission of MI principles and skill concepts to medical residents through a 3.5-hour combination of lecture and video-based demonstrations. Handmaker, Hester, and Delaney (1999) taught basic principles and microskills for obstetricians using a 20-minute video; they also noted skill gain in expressing empathy, minimizing patient defensiveness, and supporting women's beliefs in their ability to change.

Evidence is also accumulating for *skill acquisition post MI training*. Miller and Mount (2005) describe an increase in MI-consistent skills following a 2-day workshop and suppression of MI-inconsistent skills in probation officers. These authors also note that maintenance of skill gain was an issue.

Baer et al. (2004) also report skill gains with addictions and mental health professionals. This study showed a significant increase in knowledge on questionnaires, as well as measures of observed skills, and also noted less need to suppress problematic behaviors in this sample of highly educated treatment professionals.

Miller et al. (2004) implemented a larger-scale training effort that investigated the learning of MI via self-directed methods (reading and watching videotapes) versus receiving workshop training followed by one of four conditions: no additional services, coaching, feedback, or coaching plus feedback. All four workshop conditions demonstrated skill acquisition posttraining. However, increased skill proficiency was greatest in the condition that received coaching plus feedback posttraining, whereas workshop-only participants retreated toward baseline levels.

Schoener, Madeja, Henderson, Ondersma, and Janisse (2006) report skill increase using a representative sample of mental health therapists that included gains in six of seven studied areas. Of particular importance, these researchers noted an increase in client change talk in session following the training. The increase in this form of in-session client utterances is noteworthy because prior research has linked it to prediction of clients' subsequent behavior change. However, Schoener et al. (2006) did not collect data about subsequent client behavior (i.e., behavior change) in this study. Still, the results are significant because they occurred in a population with co-occurring mental health and substance abuse disorders—a particularly difficult treatment population.

Tober and colleagues (Tober, Godfrey, Parrott, Copello, Farrin, et al., 2005) report that therapists in the UK Alcohol Treatment Trial (UKATT) were trained to research criterion (i.e., predetermined levels of proficiency in MI skills); this is significant because therapists were not hired for this study, but were already working in agencies and were randomly assigned to an intervention condition. This methodology stands in contrasts to those in studies such as Project MATCH (Carroll, Kadden, Donovan, Zweben, & Rounsaville, 1994), wherein research therapists were hired based on their skills and then trained to criterion. Tober et al. (2005) did find that supervision was critical in reaching competence and that training to criterion in MI took longer than for an alternative therapy (Social Behavior and Network Therapy), originally hypothesized to require more time to train. This finding reflects the complexity of the skill requirements in MI.

Martino, Ball, Nich, Frankforter, and Carroll (2008) also found that community therapists could be trained to deliver MI or MET services in a competent and adherent manner after participating in an initial 2-day workshop with follow-up supervision. Again, these findings are important because the therapists, although volunteers, were not preselected according to MI knowledge, skill, or potential.

Others have found similar findings. Moyers and colleagues (Moyers et al., 2008) demonstrated that substance abuse counselors in the U.S. military could make significant skill gains following a 2-day workshop. Baer and colleagues (Baer et al., 2009) also demonstrated skill gain with community addictions therapists. Others have found improvements with medical providers, including dietitians (Brug et al., 2007), specialist nurses (Lane, Johnson, Rollnick, Edwards, & Lyons, 2003), medical students (Martino, Haeseler, Belitsky, Pantalon, & Fortin, 2007; Poirier et al., 2004), residents (Chossis et al., 2007), and general practitioners (Rubak et al., 2006; Saitz, Sullivan, & Samet, 2000; Thijs, 2007).

It's unclear if prior knowledge may influence subsequent training. Moyers et al. (2008) describe a study in which a waiting-list control group seemed to benefit more from training once it was provided, then did two training conditions in which training was provided immediately. Although Moyers and colleagues (Moyers et al., 2008) attributed this finding to the possible benefits of positive anticipation of training, it might also represent the priming effect of prior review of reading and videos. However, it should also be noted that Miller et al. (2004) found no such result for their waiting-list control group. Nor has our research shown that report of prior MI training correlates with baseline skill levels (Baer et al., 2004, 2009).

Taken as a whole, these findings suggest that the knowledge and skills necessary to implement MI can be taught and learned. Also, these skills can be acquired by a range of individuals and professional types, not just substance abuse counselors predisposed to learning MI skills.

What Are the Best Teaching Methods for Learning MI?

Miller, Sorensen, Selzer, and Brigham (2006), in a recent review article about diffusion and dissemination practices in substance abuse treatment generally, noted the tendency of most dissemination packages to be fairly limited in scope and to bear relatively limited resemblance to what the research suggests is effective. A review of the MI literature suggests that similar conclusions are warranted.

Miller et al. (2004) note that learning via reading the MI book and watching videotapes is insufficient to improve practitioner skills. However, it may be an important precursor step in knowledge acquisition. Miller and colleagues (2006) refer to this as the *ground school for flying* where important foundation skills are learned, but the person is not ready to fly without flight instruction.

The prototypic introduction to MI concepts involves a 2-day workshop with a blend of didactic, observational, experiential, and practice activities. Although studies support this combination of modalities, there has been little research that describes the specific elements needed. However, skill practice appears important.

Shafer, Rhode, and Chong (2004) note that knowledge can be increased via distance learning methods, but that clinician behavior change was more difficult to achieve. Although provision for skill practice was included in this innovative approach, technical, logistical, and local skill levels appeared to limit the amount and quality of skill practice. Many researchers (e.g., Baer et al., 2004, 2009; Forrester, McCambridge, Waissbein, Emlyn-Jones, & Rollnick, 2008; Miller & Mount, 2005; Miller et al., 2004; Moyers et al., 2008) report skill gains after a 2-day workshop that includes skill practice.

A few studies have pointed out additional elements that may improve training outcomes. Miller et al. (2004) report that either feedback or coaching and feedback produced acquisition, improvement, and maintenance. Interestingly, the study did not find that coaching alone was sufficient; only coaching and feedback together led to increased levels of client change talk. In contrast, Smith et al. (2007) note that providing "real-time" coaching did improve performance after workshop attendance. The real-time coaching, accomplished via a "bug in the ear" telephone connection, allowed the trainer to provide intervention suggestions as the session unfolded. There were also opportunities for coaching during a session break and postsession. Although some gains were modest for this very intensive training, these results did show skill gain and maintenance at 3 months posttraining. The gains were most evident in basic MI skills (e.g., ratio of reflections to questions).

However, the addition of these MI training services does not necessarily guarantee sustained changes nor does it lead to significant differences in skill gain. For example, Moyers et al. (2008) did not find that an enriched follow-up program that included coaching and feedback produced better skill maintenance than workshop alone. Similarly, Bennett et al. (2007) did not find that a combination of postworkshop training activities (i.e., weekly self-review of taped client sessions, worksheets, additional coaching, and the availability of coding feedback on tapes) produced greater skill gains than a simple booster session (i.e., a 6-hour review of concepts, feedback on assessment interviews, and viewing a video demonstration of MI) for previously trained MI clinicians.

In all of these studies a challenge was noted. Practitioners often do not take up the offer of additional feedback or coaching. Forrester and colleagues (2007) noted that although coaching improved clinician skills, very few social workers took up their offer for free coaching, and the maximum number of sessions completed was three of the five offered. Moyers et al. (2007) also reported low levels of compliance in participants completing the enriched condition. Bennett et al. (2007) noted that the modal number of tape self-review, coaching calls, and submission of tapes for review was one. This finding matches the anecdotal observations of MINT trainers, which indicate that the offer of follow-up coaching is rarely accessed, unless the organization actively encourages or mandates it.

The benefit of specific methods of skills training remains less well established. For example, Rollnick, Kinnersley, and Butler (2002) have advocated for using contextualized training that includes the use of standardized patients or actors to portray clients. These researchers note promising anecdotal findings. However, the empirical support for this approach remains lacking. Mounsey, Bovbjerg, White, and Gazewood (2006) failed to note any additional benefit from using actors versus role-playing participants. Lane, Hood, and Rollnick (2008) also did not find that use of standardized patients improved skill acquisition any better than role-playing between medical care providers. Nor was perceived applicability or general acceptability different across either method.

Our investigative group recently completed a test of Rollick's model, which we referred to as context-tailored training (CTT), using a small randomized controlled trial (RCT) to compare a standard 2-day workshop to CTT (Baer et al., 2009). We employed a spaced practice model for the CTT, which occurred over 9–10 weeks and used a standardized patient during intervening sessions to practice skills. Trainers scored and provided feedback on the percentage of open-to-closed questions, reflection-to-question ratio, and MI spirit. Both groups had significant skill gain, but they also evidenced a shift back toward baseline skill levels 3 months after the conclusion of training. There was slightly greater satisfaction noted by participants in the CTT method. Thus, there did not appear to be any additional gains or maintenance of gains from a training designed to more carefully address goodness of fit to clinician practice.

There are some reports of other innovative techniques. For example, Villaume, Berger, and Barker (2006) describe a script-writing exercise for a virtual patient prototype. The script-writing process required pharmacy students to write responses to patient statements and then anticipate likely client responses. This iterative process resulted in greater understanding of MI and why it might work, and facility in developing MI-consistent responses, than did a lecture-and-observation-alone method used in the prior year. Carpenter, Watson, Raffety, and Chabal (2003) describe the use of a computer-based tutorial that assesses clinician competence and delivers targeted training in MI concepts. Initial results suggest that after a 45-minute tutorial, volunteers can produce more MI-consistent responses to smoking cessation scenarios than at baseline.

There are additional considerations in thinking about learning and practicing MI skills. Miller et al. (2006) note that levels of organizational readiness (Simpson, 2002) and support of new practices influence skill acquisition. Our research hints that MI "champion activity" may influence skill maintenance (Hartzler, Baer, Dunn, Rosengren, & Wells, 2007). That is, the presence of someone who actively promotes the use of MI through activities within an agency leads to greater skill maintenance at short-term follow-up. These activities can vary widely. Examples of champion activities include posting signs reminding people of MI skills, apportioning times of staff meetings for MI discussion, sending out e-mail reminders, writing MI columns in agency newsletters, and arranging for additional training review or skill practice. This research is preliminary and therefore insufficient to indicate what types of activities may be essential, though it does suggest that the greater the number of activities, the more skills are retained.

Research indicates that MI may fit well across cultures. For example, Miller et al. (2008) recently report that African American, Native American, and Spanish-speaking addiction treatment providers show as large or larger skill gains in learning MI than had been found with non-Hispanic white providers. Although there were methodological issues that limit generalization from this study, the findings do suggest that cross-cultural dissemination of MI is possible.

There is little additional research to guide this area, but in a query to the MINT listserve, most trainers suggest that some trainees are more receptive and better equipped to learn MI than others. However, these trainers also caution against making the same reasoning error we as practitioners can sometimes make when clients don't improve because of our clinical efforts. That is, we may "blame" the client rather than assessing our clinical method. Similarly, trainers can "blame" their trainees for failure to learn when a more thorough evaluation of our methods might be warranted. That is, the problem does not lie with the trainee, but rather in how we teach the methods.

With that caution in mind, Miller and Moyers (2006), in their recent discussion of learning stages in MI, suggest that clinicians who work from a deficit model of treatment (e.g., "My clients are in denial, lack knowledge, insight, or skills") may have a harder time learning MI. Our research group (Hartzler et al., 2007) found data that clinicians who endorse a disease model of addictions, which incorporates many of those deficits views, do not differ in their acquisition of MI skills, but do tend to revert to prior behaviors more at 3-month follow-up. One interpretation of these findings is that the lack of fit between the MI model and participants' preexisting belief system may make it hard for them to adopt this new skill set. Still, there is much more research needed before we may draw firm conclusions about this area.

Does the Degree of MI Proficiency Matter in Terms of Client Outcomes?

A recent study by Thrasher et al. (2005) indicates that the researchers could differentiate the quality of MI sessions and that greater MI quality did predict greater adherence in antiretroviral therapy under some conditions, but not all. Moyers et al. (2008) have also noted that the better the quality of MI, the more client change talk was observed and that this change talk did predict client behaviors. These findings suggest that the quality of MI is important to outcome.

Moyers and Martin (2006) describe the development of a sequential processing system that allows them to look at how practitioner behavior influences the subsequent likelihood of a particular client behavior. They note that if practitioners act in an MI-consistent manner, the likelihood of change talk being the next statement from a client increases, while also noting that MI-inconsistent behavior increases the likelihood of resistance or sustain talk. The MI model predicts these relationships.

Moyers et al. (2008) extend these findings by demonstrating that the presence of change talk then predicts subsequent outcomes for amount and frequency of drinking. They also note that client change talk is not related to one therapy method alone and can be observed in other methods (i.e., cognitive-behavioral therapy and 12-step facilitation) with the same type of predictive power evident. They are also quick to caution that this remains a correlation and thus can*not* be used to explain a cause-and-effect relationship.

What Do We Recommend for the Learning of MI, Based on These Findings?

There is a blueprint available as we consider this question. Miller and Moyers (2006) describe an eight-stage model for learning MI:

- Stage 1: Conveying the spirit of MI
- Stage 2: Teaching OARS: Client-centered counseling skills
- Stage 3: Recognizing and reinforcing change talk
- Stage 4: Eliciting and strengthening change talk
- Stage 5: Rolling with resistance
- Stage 6: Developing a change plan
- Stage 7: Consolidating client commitment
- Stage 8: Switching between MI and other counseling methods

This model is intuitively devised, though there is some empirical support for Miller and Moyers's decision making. For example, there is some research to suggest that MI spirit is an important predictor of other MI skills (Moyers, Martin, Manuel, Hendrickson, & Miller, 2005) and therefore should be a logical initial focus for training. The model allows both a learner of MI and a teacher/trainer to develop methods geared toward each stage and to assess where they are in the learning process. Madson, Loigon, and Lane (2008) recently completed a systematic review of studies about learning MI and noted that the studies can be assessed for the eight learning tasks, based on the study descriptions.

Although the general categories presented by Miller and Moyers seem very appropriate, there are problems with making this a stage-based approach. For example, stages require establishment of a correct order and assume that completion of one stage presupposes the start of the next. From my perspective as both a researcher and trainer, it's unclear if learning the OARS skills helps one better acquire MI spirit, or if the reverse is true. It seems that a more useful way of thinking about these stages would be to reconceptualize them as tasks of learning MI. This semantic change would eliminate the concerns noted and allow people to work simultaneously or bidirectionally on tasks, while still noting that all seem to be important elements in learning MI. Perhaps in recognition of some of these challenges, Miller, in his most recent description (Arkowitz & Miller, 2008), describes these as "Eight Skills." Regardless, as Miller and Moyers readily acknowledge, this model requires empirical validation, including development of instruments to test these different areas. Madson and colleagues (2008) make suggestions as to how this research might be accomplished.

In terms of guiding learning efforts, my recommendations are consistent with those that our research team has suggested previously (Hartzler, Rosengren, & Baer, 2009).

First, reading written materials and watching videos of MI practice may be an important preliminary step. It can be self- or other guided and for some—particularly early adopters of MI—this was how they became interested in the method. However, this preliminary is not sufficient to acquire MI skillfulness and may not be a necessary first step. Still, it might help prepare learners for the next recommendation, especially for those learners who are analytic and verbally oriented.

Second, in order to gain basic skills in MI, a minimum of 2 days of training appears to be needed. Fewer then 2 days appears inadequate. The research suggests that this training should include skill practice, but it's less clear how much knowledge acquisition is necessary. That is, do all of the accompanying cognitive materials associated with the basic MI "tasks" need to be taught, or is a subsample sufficient? Whether in its entirety or a subsample, having a coherent cognitive framework to understand and direct these skills seems consistent with other research that suggests adherence to a theoretical framework improves client outcomes (e.g., Messer & Wampold, 2002).

Third, after a 2-day training, participants are likely to have beginning MI proficiency (Miller et al., 2008; Rosengren et al., 2008). Acquiring greater skill proficiency will require additional skill practice, coaching, and feedback. There appear to be multiple ways to acquire these components (e.g., distance learning, telephonic supervision, taped observation, real-time observation), with some perhaps being more effective individually than others. However, preliminary research suggests that coaching and feedback in combination are best, though offering coaching and feedback seems to be insufficient to cause most busy practitioners to avail themselves of these services. The research is also unclear about how long this needs to continue before expert levels of proficiency are attained, though experience training in research settings suggests at least 3 months to build up skill habit and comfort.

Finally, skill maintenance and skill proficiency are not the same, though they seem to rely on similar processes. That is, skill maintenance also seems to require coaching and feedback. Institutional support may be necessary condition for maintaining skills. Also, learners coming from a skill deficit model may require additional attention, though the method for delivering this attention is not clear.

Final Thoughts

Many questions about learning MI remain (Arkowitz & Miller, 2008; Madson et al., 2008). Perhaps the biggest is, *What is needed beyond a 2-day training to build practitioner proficiency?* However, this is not the only question. *What elements are essential in learning MI, and which are superfluous? What are the best ways to learn specific skills? Do certain practitioner groups respond best to certain types of training? How much skill is acquired from a particular training length? Does the trainer make a difference?* The answers to all of these questions would provide useful data to inform methods for teaching and learning MI.

Bill Miller has used the analogy more than once that learning MI is like learning to play the piano (e.g., Arkowitz & Miller, 2008). Typically, he uses this analogy in the context of a brief (e.g., 2-hour) presentation and then assuming readiness to "do MI." It seems the analogy may extend to completing a workbook as well. Although some people may complete a workbook and have learned the essential basics of piano playing, it is typically through the tutelage of an experienced piano teacher that the skills come to life.

Still, there is an interesting twist to this analogy. What of the self-taught musician? Some people seem to have natural aptitudes in making music. They sit down at the piano and seem to understand intuitively how to make it work, experiment with it, and through independent practice develop these skills. Similarly, I have observed people in my trainings who aren't trained as counselors but who nonetheless seem to have excellent native skills, and this training provides labels and a cognitive structure to what has come to them intuitively. They seem particularly in tune to the MI spirit and/or using the microskills of MI. It is like a duck to water watching them adopt these skills. The use of this workbook may aid them in what is an already unfolding internal process. For the vast majority of learners, this workbook can serve as an adjunct that extends and deepens understanding or skills, and works in harmony with an initial training experience, coaching, feedback, and ongoing institutional support. In either event, I hope that this workbook has been helpful in further developing your interest and skill in MI.

And what's the next step if you try all of these things and your client still explodes with anger? Begin by recognizing that MI is generally effective, but not always. Some clients are very angry and looking for reasons to be angry with practitioners; this may be the case for you. Try other MI-consistent approaches with the client and if this is still ineffective, change what you're doing. A former professor used to say, "If what you're doing isn't working, for God's sake don't do more of it. Do something else. Stand on your head if you have to, but don't do more of the same!"

On the other hand, if many of your clients are reacting that way, then there are probably some things that you are doing that need some alteration. Although you could practice the microskills in the workbook again, you might find it a better use of your time to seek out expert review and coaching. You can find someone near you by going to the MINT website (*www.motivationalinterview.org*). You may also be able to do this type of coaching via distance learning methods (e.g., online or telephone coaching, tape review). You can also visit my website (*www.2sft.com*) for additional learning opportunities.

Some of you may be interested in evaluating your MI skillfulness more formally. There is one method available, with more on the horizon. The VASE-R (Rosengren et al., 2008) is a system that does not require a real client encounter, but instead asks clinicians to respond to a series of videotaped vignettes and standardized prompts with written responses. The VASE-R can be done independently. A rating manual and copies of the VASE-R are available free, though learning the scoring materials does require some time investment. The Appendix B lists resources where you can access these materials.

A web-based system is also currently being developed by Jeff Allison and Rik Bes, called MI Campus, that will allow evaluation of MI skillfulness over the Internet. It is a fee-based service and will require electronic submission of tapes. Once completed, the practitioner will receive certification of MI proficiency that will be renewable.

Establishing an MI Learning Group

In addition to using a partner, you might consider setting up an MI learning group. You do not need to be an expert in MI to lead this group, but rather someone who is willing to make the group happen. In our research, we refer to this as being an MI champion. Because there is a broad array of settings in which this type of learning group might occur, the recommendations are also broad. You will need to adapt these to your setting.

Being an MI Champion

You will need to accomplish a few basic tasks to start a learning group. First, decide that you are enthusiastic about learning more and improving your MI skills. Your purchase of this book indicates that you may already be well on the path. Second, communicate your enthusiasm to others. Although e-mailing is a great way to send information en masse, we have found that it does not generate the type of response and commitment that a personal connection does. So, call or talk to your coworkers or colleagues about your idea of starting a learning group. Once they indicate interest, then you can follow-up with e-mail. Third, set up an initial meeting time with interested parties; discuss your aspirations for the group and solicit potential group members' interests. Encourage attendance at this meeting as a chance for participants to decide if they want to join, not as a commitment to be a part of the group. Fourth, establish the parameters of the meetings (e.g., when, where, how often, agenda or agenda making) and have someone take notes. Finally, send out a follow-up communication indicating the parameters and the first meeting time. Invite those who aren't able to attend this initial meeting to join if still interested.

There are a few things you will need to do as a champion to maintain the group. To begin, you need to schedule the meeting place, then send out reminders or post information as the time for the meeting approaches. Ensure that the materials you need will be present. For example, if you choose to listen to a tape, make sure that a tape recorder is present and that there are coding forms to use (these can be found on the MI website, *www.motivationalinterview.org*). Then start the meeting on time, end on time, and keep your group on track. This does not mean that you have to control the meeting, only that your colleagues or coworkers feel that time spent has been productive and useful. Meetings that digress lose steam quickly. Again, as champion, you are not expected to be an MI expert, just someone who is enthusiastic and willing to take the lead in helping to form a group learning experience. Making your facilitator role explicit to the group can help all avoid misunderstandings.

Structuring an MI Learning Group

Here some ideas that MINT trainers have shared about structuring an MI learning group.

Schedule Regular Meetings

The sole purpose of this group should be to strengthen MI skills. Don't let administrative details or other agenda fill the time. An hour meeting twice a month would be one possibility. Less than monthly is probably not often enough to maintain group momentum or cohesion. Weekly is often more time than most work units will accommodate, and members may find it burdensome.

Have an Agenda, But Be Flexible

It will feel more productive if participants know what will happen during the meeting. This book would be one way to structure an agenda, with each meeting devoted to a specific chapter. Members would be asked to read the chapter in advance of a meeting. This method would allow the learning process to follow a complete sequence of MI skills.

An alternative approach would be to use the sequence suggested by Miller and Moyers (2006) in their article on eight stages in learning motivational interviewing. Your training sequence could follow these stages and progress as participants feel competent to move forward.

A third approach would be to use other reading material in initial meetings. The group could discuss topics of particular interest and then choose a different topic for the next meeting. There is a rapidly growing list of books and articles on the MI website from which to select. For those particularly interested in research on MI, a "journal club" of 20 minutes could be used at the beginning or end, or even added on to the meeting. Journal articles can be found through the website or the *MINT Bulletin*, also found on the website. The bulletin is a useful resource on which to find new thoughts about MI, which have not yet reached the traditional media outlets.

Practice Is Important

Consider using some of the exercises from this book or those you experienced in your initial training. Talk about the exercises. Have some prompts to use for debriefing. Think about these ahead of time. What went well? What was a challenge? Where would you like to do some refining?

Review Tapes of Expert MI Practice

Resources are available for free, such as *Body & Soul*, which is produced by the National Cancer Institute. Ordering information can be found in Appendix B. The VASE-R is a free assessment instrument that the group could use, score, and discuss. You could also use the VASE-R to provide standard prompts for skill practices. A variety of MI videos for purchase can also be found in Appendix B. Different tapes will offer different learning opportunities. If no specific skills are targeted in the tape, select a focus for the group ahead of time and attend to that element. This can be fun—for example, using Steve Berg-Smith's Drumming for Change Talk activity described in Chapter 5 when listening to tapes.

Code Tapes

Rather than simply listening to a tape, make use of some structured coding tools. These tools help tune your ears to specific types of activities and keep you focused on the process of the interaction. Coding systems can range from the very basic to the more elaborate. Here are some examples:

- Counting questions and reflections
- Coding OARS
- Coding depth of reflections (simple vs. complex)
- Counting client change talk, and noting what preceded it
- Tracking client readiness for change during the session, and key moments of shift

Coding forms can be found on the MI website. Participants can use the same coding form and compare findings or use different coding forms to attend to different aspects of the session.

Listen to Your Own Tapes

A key learning tool is to listen to, and discuss together, your own and other participants' tapes of MI sessions. For people unused to this type of public view of their work as part of professional training, this can be a challenging idea. Yet, it is immensely helpful in learning and improving technique. Here are a few ideas to help move past this discomfort. First, don't begin with this activity, unless the group is used to this type of practice. Allow the group to develop some cohesiveness and trust doing some of the other activities already discussed. Second, as MI champion, be willing to show your tape first. Third, provide clear tasks in the review. Fourth, always begin the discussion of a recording by focusing on the practitioner who showed the work. Ask him or her what went well, what he or she would like to have done differently or more of, and then invite other members to contribute. Then add your feedback. Finally, keep in mind that this endeavor is about learning and not about achieving perfection. Practitioners receiving feedback generally feel vulnerable, so although the comments should be honest, they should also be supportive.

There are a few logistical pointers to consider in terms of managing the taping process. You will need a recording device. Experience suggests that external microphones work best, though some of the smaller digital recording equipment has become quite impressive. Higher-quality sound aids the learning process. Set up a rotation schedule so that practitioners know when their turn is coming and can make recordings. Try listening to and discussing one tape per session. A 20-minute segment of tape is probably sufficient. Finally, you will need to obtain written permission from clients to use this type of recording. This permission should explain how the tape will be used, who will hear it, how and when the tape will be destroyed, and confidentiality agreements with the listeners.

Miller suggests a couple of other ideas as important with this type of tape review. When introducing the background of the recording, the practitioner should indicate what target(s) for behavior change were being pursued. Without this information, it is not possible to identify change talk, which is goal-specific. Discussion of each tape should also include the ways in which the session is and is not consistent with the spirit and method of MI. Again, it is useful for the person who did the interview to lead off this discussion with his or her comments. Participants can ask each other, "What might have been done to make this session more MI consistent?"

Consult about Challenging Clients

Bring up clients whom you are finding difficult and receive input from your colleagues about how you might use MI ideas to work with them. Sometimes it is helpful to role-play a difficult client, with the practitioner portraying the client.

Consider Additional Targeted Training

Increasingly, MI trainers are offering distance learning activities. Perhaps it would be possible to do a conference call with an MI trainer that targets a particular area. Prepare ahead of time by carefully articulating what you would like to see addressed and how during this activity.

Structure the End of Your Meeting

Make sure you leave time to confirm when the next meeting will occur, what the agenda will be, and who is responsible for what; then send reminders. Even for highly valued activities, other tasks come into play. Remind people, especially those who have a role (e.g., their turn to show a tape). If your meetings are monthly, the MI champion might send out a reminder midmonth.

There are a few other odds and ends to consider. If your workplace is too small to support its own MI learning group, consider joining forces with another group in the area. If you are a private-practice individual, contact other practitioners in your area to see if there would be interest in this type of activity. You should decide whether the group will be time limited or open-ended, whether the membership is open to new members, and there are any expectations for attendance. These types of discussions at the front end will reduce problems later. Finally, as any 4-year-old can remind us (adults), we learn more when we're having fun. So, make sure this group is enjoyable!

Additional Resources

General MI

Arkowitz, H., Westra, H. A., Miller, W. R., & Rollnick, S. (Eds.). (2008). *Motivational interviewing in the treatment of psychological problems.* New York: Guilford Press. [Book]

> This book is a must-have for all mental health clinicians integrating MI into their treatment setting. It provides information on frequently encountered clinical problems, including anxiety, posttraumatic stress disorder, obsessive–compulsive disorder, depression, suicidal behavior, eating disorders, and schizophrenia. It also contains information on gambling addictions and dual diagnoses. The chapters review the research base, clinical applications, and provide rich clinical examples.

Dartmouth Evidence-Based Practices Center. *IDDT introductory and practice demonstration video.* [DVD]

> This is a training DVD that accompanies the *Integrated Dual Disorders Training* (IDDT) manual. Produced and distributed by The Dartmouth Evidence-Based Practices Center in New Hampshire (from the National Implementing Evidence-Based Practices Project), the DVD provides an introduction (somewhat basic) to IDDT- and MI-consistent skills. To order or download, use the website (*www.mentalhealth. samhsa.gov/cmhs/CommunitySupport/toolkits/cooccurring*) or contact Karen Dunn via e-mail (*Karen. Dunn@Dartmouth.EDU*).

Kistenmacher, B. *MI road map.* [Document]

> The director of addictions treatments at Bronx-Lebanon Hospital Center developed a road map to guide trainees in their thinking about what decisions to make during a client interaction. It is particularly useful when coding a video tape. In particular, Dr. Kistenmacher uses Tape B from the Learning MI video series and a handout to illustrate the decision-making process that guides MI work. These materials can be obtained via e-mail at *bkistenmacher@yahoo.com*.

Mash, R. *MISA training.* [DVD]

> This double DVD is produced by MI trainers from the Motivational Interviewing in Southern Africa (MISA) network and is designed to meet the need for a local training resource that looks and feels like it belongs to Southern Africa. A variety of typical counseling scenarios are used, such as a pregnant mother in the HIV clinic, a drug addict in an outpatient treatment center, an alcoholic mother with a child who has fetal alcohol syndrome, and an asthmatic patient in primary care. There are 22 different segments, which are mainly filmed in English, but Afrikaans and a mixture of Xhosa and Zulu are also used. Both

guiding and directing styles are illustrated, and the actors share feedback on their experience of the sessions. To order a copy or for further information, please contact Ms. Loren Human by phone at 083-258-5989, e-mail at *loren@kwplace.com*, or by fax at 021-790-8055.

Mason, P., & Gilligan, T. *Engaging motivation* (2006) [DVD]; *Engaging motivation 2* (2008) [DVD]; and *Motivational interviewing: An introduction to the theory* [CD-ROM].

Two DVDs are available as an adjunct to training services. Each DVD contains six demonstrations using MI in several different settings. The second DVD also provides skills demonstrations. The third set of materials is an interactive CD-ROM that provides a description of the basic tenets of MI.

These recordings are primarily for use as adjuncts to MI courses. They provide demonstration material relevant to the work lives of course participants in Britain, and that would provoke discussion and understanding of MI principles. The material is not intended to be self-explanatory or to be used as a stand-alone teaching aid. The authors anticipate that it might be useful for trainers and training participants.

The *Engaging Motivation* (2006) DVD offers six scenarios each 15–20 minutes long: two take place in the Criminal Justice System, two in health care settings, one in a drug agency, and one in a youth counseling context. The scenes are unscripted role plays using professional actors as clients.

The second DVD, *Engaging Motivation 2* (2008), is divided into four sections that illustrate concepts in key areas. The first section contains scenarios in health promotion, criminal justice, vocational training, and mental health. Subsequent sections contain portions of these scenarios to illustrate key aspects of MI, including core MI skills, strategies and principles, and client change and sustain talk.

The CD-ROM of *Motivational Interviewing: An Introduction to the Theory* is an interactive course intended to complement attendance at a training workshop and supervised practice. The CD-ROM describes key elements of the theory of MI using text and static images. The course can normally be completed within an hour. Ten questions are embedded within the course to test comprehension. Students who answer them correctly can apply for a certificate.

To order, contact: Pip Mason Consultancy Limited, 116 Watford Road, Kings Norton, Birmingham B30 1PB; phone: 0121-604-7399; e-mail: *info@pipmason.com*; and web: *www.pipmason.com*.

Miller, W. R., & Rollnick, S. (2002). *Motivational interviewing: Preparing people for change* (2nd ed.). New York: Guilford Press. [Book]

This is the second edition of the MI book. It was entirely rewritten from the first edition. Anyone who owns the first edition of this book should add this to their wish list. This book provides the most comprehensive and detailed description of MI and its clinical application. It truly is a seminal work and belongs on the bookshelf of anyone doing, or training others to do, MI.

Miller, W. R. (2000). *Motivational interviewing with Dr. William R. Miller.* [DVD]

This tape is part of the Brief Therapy for Addictions Series. It contains an interview with Bill Miller describing MI, then an extended interaction with a real client, followed by a discussion with a studio audience. This video shows a master working his craft and is filled with examples of OARS, eliciting change talk, and rolling with resistance. You can find it at Psychotherapy Net: *www.psychotherapy.net/video/miller_motivational_interviewing*.

Rhode, R., *Sample counseling sessions.* [CD]

Dr. Rhode created a CD that contains seven short examples of counselors talking to clients. Two examples are adapted from a role play. The others are rerecordings of real counselors with real clients (voices disguised). Some are consistent with MI principles, and some are less consistent. You can play the examples straight through or you can play them, interchange by interchange, to look at what the counselor is doing and whether it facilitates change. You can hear the example only, see the text only, or hear and see it. Most people use the CD to begin recognizing MI-consistent skills or to practice coding interchanges. Contact at *rrhode@u.arizona.edu* or 520-615-7623.

University of New Mexico. (1998). *Motivational interviewing professional training.* [DVD]

The MI series by Miller, Rollnick, and Moyers is well done and inexpensive. Originally published as a six-tape volume, the series has been remastered onto a single DVD. It provides a wealth of information about MI and demonstrations of MI techniques by master trainers, including Bill Miller, Steve Rollnick, and Terri Moyers. It is available through the University of New Mexico. Ordering information is available through the MI website at *www.motivationalinterview.org/training/videos.html.*

MI Spirit

Roberts, M. (2004). *Join-up.* [DVD]

An example of the MI spirit is found in the world of horse training. Renowned horse trainer Monty Roberts produces great results in training horses using a sophisticated and humane approach that incorporates a special knowledge of the "language" of horses (Equus). By studying the behaviors that horses naturally express (flight, cooperation, and obeisance), Roberts designed a training system in harmony with these behaviors. His style, evident in video and live demonstrations, is respectful, optimistic, and strikingly in harmony with the needs of the horse.

These tapes describe his training method and contain demonstrations of horse "starting" (as opposed to "breaking")—that is, training horses who have never before had a saddle, bridle, or rider. *Join-Up* is an excellent video demonstration of this approach. Audiences find this video a powerful metaphor for the work of MI, as well as a hypnotic look at the process of engaging another in change. His video can be ordered through the website *www.montyroberts.com.*

OARS

National Cancer Institute. (2005). *Body and soul.* [DVD]

Body & Soul is a health program developed for African American churches by the National Cancer Institute. The program encourages church members to eat a healthy diet rich in fruits and vegetables every day for better health. One pillar of the program, peer counseling, has church members talk with their peer counselors about how eating more healthily relates to their life goals and personal values. The peer counseling of *Body & Soul* is based on principles of MI. It offers one-on-one attention and support to those who need it. This interactive DVD provides examples in the context of developing a peer counseling training program for improving eating habits. To order a copy of this training DVD, phone 800-422-6237.

Rosengren, D., Hartzler, B., Baer, J. S., Wells, E. A., & Dunn, C. (2008). *Video Assessment of Simulated Encounters—Revised (VASE-R).* [DVD]

Our research team developed a DVD assessment system, *Video Assessment of Simulated Encounters— Revised (VASE-R)*, which allows users to view video vignettes and then write and score their responses. The tape focuses on MI skills, including OARS, and can be readily adapted for training purposes. This video is available free by e-mailing John Baer, PhD, at *jsbaer@u.washington.edu.*

Stout, D. *OARS crib notes.* [Document]

Ms. Stout, along with a former student, created documents that list a series of open-ended questions, suggested affirmations, etc., for use in group OARS-building exercises. Ms. Stout uses these in her trainings so that participants aren't "put on the spot" when practicing or demonstrating skills. These can be obtained by contacting Dee-Dee Stout, MA, CADC II, at *ddstoutrps@aol.com*, or through the web at *www.responsiblerecovery.org.*

Change Talk

Allison, J. (2006). *MI in practice: The Edinburgh interview.* [CD]

> Mr. Allison created an MI CD that contains an audio-recorded session of a real MI encounter between a man who has decided to drink himself to death and an alcohol service worker. The CD provides a rolling transcript that reflects the dialogue being heard. This interactive CD also contains commentaries from the worker, the client, and Mr. Allison. It provides rich opportunities for recognizing, reinforcing, and eliciting change talk. The CD can be obtained through either Mr. Allison's e-mail (*info@jeffallison.co.uk*) or website (*www.jeffallison.co.uk*).

HBO series. (2007). *Addiction.* [DVD]

> This 14-part HBO series provides excellent examples of people articulating their struggle with change. You can purchase these materials through the HBO website (*www.hbo.com*).

Resolving Ambivalence

Engle, D. E., & Arkowitz, H. (2006). *Ambivalence in psychotherapy: Facilitating readiness to change.* New York: Guilford Press. [Book]

> This well-written book describes the concepts of resistance and ambivalence from four theoretical perspectives and then provides practical tips for their resolution. It will certainly deepen your understanding of the concepts.

Motivational Interviewing Resources. *The values card sort.* [Document]

> The values card sort is a technique used to help resolve ambivalence. It can be obtained through the MINT website. (Instructions and description of its use can be found in Chapter 8.) The specific location is *www.motivationalinterview.org/library/valuescardsort.pdf.*

Steinberg, J. (2008). *Sizwe's test: A young man's journey through Africa's AIDS epidemic.* New York: Simon & Schuster. [Book]

> This book documents the struggles of a South African man as he stands at the crossroads of his traditional culture and the benefits of retroviral medications, deciding if he should be tested for HIV. It is a powerful example of the factors within and outside individuals that create and maintain ambivalence.

Supervision and Coding

Lane, C., & Rollnick, S. (2001). *Behavior change counseling index.* [Document]

> The Behavior Change Counseling Index (BECCI) was developed to assess how practitioners are engaging in discussions about health. It can be obtained through the MI website: *www.motivationalinterview.org/library/BECCIManual.pdf.*

Madson, M. *Motivational Interviewing Supervision and Training Scale* (MISTS); *Client Evaluation of Motivational Interviewing* (CEMI); and *Motivational Interviewing Self-Efficacy Scale—Dietetics Version* (MISES-DV). [Documents]

> MISTS is a coding scale designed to assist in the training and supervision of therapists implementing treatments utilizing MI as a core element of their interventions. Raters observe a session (live or audio/videotaped) and use the scale to rate adherence to, and competence in, MI-related skills. It provides a reliable and valid assessment of MI skills. Raters require minimal training if versed in MI.
>
> CEMI is a client feedback measure aimed for use in training and supervision to provide the client

perception of therapist adherence to the spirit and principles of MI. The 35-item measure is session specific and can be administered after each session in which a therapist intended to use MI. Initial psychometric data suggest good reliability and face validity.

MISES-DV is a brief self-report measure that provides dietetics trainees and trainers with an understanding of their perceived level of self-confidence in using MI with their patients. The first subscale provides a global assessment of self-confidence, and a second scale helps to identify potential roadblocks for using MI. The measure can be administered individually or in a group setting.

Dr. Madson and students created these three instruments for evaluating MI practice. Contact Dr. Madson directly to receive a copy of these instruments (*michael.madson@usm.edu*).

Martino, S., Ball, S., & Carrol, K. (2007). *Independent Tape Rating Scale* (ITRS). [Document]

Martino and colleagues have developed an MI adherence and competence measure. More information about this instrument can be obtained from the lead author at *steve.martino@yale.edu*.

Miller, W. R., Moyers, T., Ernest, D., & Amrhein, P. (2003). *Motivational Interviewing Skill Code—Version 2* (MISC 2.0) *Scale*. [Document]

The MISC was originally developed in 1997 as a method for evaluating the quality of MI from audio and videotapes of individual counseling sessions. The MISC contains three reviews of each tape, which include global spirit ratings, behavioral counts, and talk time. Because it codes both practitioner and client behavior, it allows for sequential coding of the interaction between clients and practitioners. It also facilitates documentation of counselor MI adherence, evaluation of MI training, and prediction of treatment outcome. The MISC 2.0 coding manual—a third generation is about to be released—can be found at *www.motivationalinterview.org/training/MISC2.pdf*.

Moyers, T., Martin, T., Manuel, J. K., & Miller, W. R. (2006). *Motivational Interviewing Treatment Integrity* (MITI) *scale*. [Document]

A companion instrument to the MISC is the MITI scale, which permits a more efficient method of rating therapist adherence to MI methods. Derived from factor analysis of the MISC, this is a briefer instrument that uses only a one-pass review and provides fewer behavior counts. Version 3.0 will expand the number of global scales from two to four.

NIDA/SAMHSA-ATTC Motivational Interviewing Blending Team. (2006, revised 2007). *Motivational Interviewing Assessment: Supervisory Tools for Enhancing Proficiency* (MIA-STEP). [Mixed media]

A product of the NIDA's Clinical Trial Network, MIA-STEP is a package of resources to help supervisors, peer mentors, and counselors improve and maintain their skills in the use of MI methods and strategy. It includes exercises, brief didactics, tips for supervisors, a rating scale for reviewing counselor sessions, and, in the hardback form, DVDs for skill demonstration. The manual can be downloaded for free from a variety of websites. The Mid Atlantic Addiction Technology Transfer Center also has Clinical Trials Network blending products for MI, as well as the MIA-STEP, at *www.mid-attc.org/mia.htm*. The Alcohol and Drug Abuse Institute at the University of Washington also has a link for these materials (*adai@u.washington.edu*). Lastly, there is a printed manual with DVDs. Here is a link for ordering those materials: *ctndisseminationlibrary.org/display/146.htm*.

Applications of MI to Health Issues

Dunn, C. *Motivation: Behavior change counseling in chronic care*. [DVD]

Chris Dunn, PhD, using a Robert Wood Johnson grant, developed a brief DVD that demonstrates microskills and strategies in the context of working with diabetes care. It is available for a nominal fee from Dr. Dunn (*cdunn@u.washington.edu*).

Dunn, C., & Rollnick, S. (2003). *Rapid reference to lifestyle and behavior change: Rapid reference series.* London: Elsevier Health Sciences. [Book]

This is a brief text written for health care providers interested in learning the basics of behavior change counseling (BHC). It provides an overview of concepts, a review of three primary components in BHC, and practical dos and don'ts for the practitioner.

Rollnick, S., Mason, P., & Butler, C. (1999). *Health behavior change: A guide for practitioners.* London: Churchill-Livingstone. [Book]

Although Rollnick and Miller have rethought the use of the term *health behavior change*, this book remains a very useful little text on the practical application of communication skills in the context of health behavior consultations. It is filled with practical tools, tips, and dos and don'ts. I continue to refer to my copy.

Rollnick, S., Miller, W. R., & Butler, C. (2008). *Motivational interviewing in health care: Helping patients change behavior.* New York: Guilford Press. [Book]

This highly readable text continues in the tradition of the health behavior change book. It explains the core concepts of MI and then applies them in a variety of health situations. If people buy only one MI book, this is the one I send them to—regardless of whether or not they work in a medical setting. It also contains an excellent reference section divided by topic areas.

Transtheoretical Model (Stages of Change) and Addiction

APA Video Series, *Psychotherapy Videotape Series—III. Behavioral Health and Health Counseling: Drug and Alcohol Abuse with William R. Miller.* [DVD]

Hosted by Jon Carlson, PsyD, EdD, this video again features a discussion with William R. Miller, PhD, and a demonstration of MI. In this video, Dr. Miller works with Debbie, a polysubstance abuser of many years with multiple issues. Already in therapy, she has begun making changes in her life that include some changes in substance use. She has now considered stopping alcohol, but remains committed to using marijuana. Available through *www.apa.org/videos/4310585.html*.

Cannabis Youth Project Research Project. (2007). *Motivational enhancement therapy and cognitive behavioral therapy for adolescent cannabis users (MET-CBT-5).* [DVD]

This DVD is designed for training treatment professionals. It contains nearly 4 hours of video vignettes illustrating concepts from the MET-CBT-5 manual developed as part of the Cannabis Youth Treatment Research project. Therapists are shown demonstrating techniques from the MET-CBT-5 sessions with adolescent "clients." The first two individual sessions show the use of MI principles with adolescent clients; the three group sessions demonstrate the integration of MI with CBT.

The DVD is intended to be used as a supplement to classroom MET-CBT-5 training. This is a curriculum written for anyone providing training in this protocol and is published by the Mid-Atlantic Addictions Technology Transfer Center (ATTC). The curriculum uses the DVDs and materials from the Motivational Interviewing Network of Trainers TNT. This DVD can be ordered through a link on the MI website (*www.motivationalinterview.org*).

Connors, G. J., Donovan, D. M., & DiClemente, C. C. (2001). *Substance abuse treatment and the stages of change: Selecting and planning interventions.* New York: Guilford Press. [Book]

Connors, Donovan, and DiClemente provide a scholarly look at the integration of stages of change into treatment planning and interventions for substance abuse treatment.

DiClemente, C. C. (2003). *Addiction and change: How addictions develop and addicted people recover.* New York: Guilford Press. [Book]

I highly recommend this book for the reader interested in the research basis for the transtheoretical model. Although a few years old now, it is a complete review of the transtheoretical model and the research that supports it. It also describes the application of the stages of change model to the acquisition of addictive behaviors.

Illinois Higher Education Center. *Maximizing brief interventions for college drinkers.* [DVD]

This DVD provides background and instructional video on using MI with college students and young adult drinkers and is designed to be used as an adjunct to training. The Illinois Higher Education Center sells the DVD at cost. Contact IHEC, Eastern Illinois University, 600 Lincoln Avenue, Charleston, IL 62901, 217-581-2019.

Lewis, J., Carlson, J., & Norcross, J. (2000). *Stages of change for addictions with Dr. John C. Norcross: Brief therapy for addictions.* Columbus, OH: Allyn & Bacon Professional. [DVD]

This video, which includes a demonstration by John Norcross, PhD of the transtheoretical model, is part of the Brief Therapy for Addictions series hosted by Judy Lewis, PhD, and Jon Carlson, PsyD. The series is published by Allyn & Bacon/Prentice Hall and can be ordered through the Pearson website at *www.pearsonhighered.com/educator*. This DVD has an ISBN of 0-205-31544-5.

Miller, W. R. (1999). TIP 35: *Enhancing motivation for change in substance abuse treatment.* Rockville: Substance Abuse and Mental Health Services Administration. [Book or document]

The Center for Substance Abuse Treatment (CSAT) invites experts in an area to create a state-of-the-art manual for use by treatment professionals. These *Treatment Improvement Protocol* (TIP) manuals provide conceptual information as well as treatment service information. An expert panel, led by Bill Miller, created TIP 35, which integrates stages of change concepts with MI. This resource can be ordered by calling the National Clearinghouse for Alcohol and Drug Information (NCADI) Hotline at 800-729-6686 or through the Substance Abuse and Mental Health Services Administration (SAMHSA) website at: *www.samhsa.gov*. Once at this webpage, click on the "Clearinghouses" button and then on the "NCADI" button.

Prochaska, J. O., Norcross, J. C., & DiClemente, C. C. (1994). *Changing for good.* New York: Harper-Collins. [Book]

Although originally published more than a decade ago, this remains an excellent self-help book that provides a highly readable introduction to the concepts of the transtheoretical model. It includes information about how to help a loved one, as well as yourself, work through the stages of change. This book also provides a nice discussion for professionals who are less interested in the research basis for the model.

Velasquez, M. M., Maurer, G. G., Crouch, C., & DiClemente, C. C. (2001). *Group treatment for substance abuse.* New York: Guilford Press. [Book]

This manual provides session-by-session outlines of how to apply the transtheoretical model in a group intervention setting. The discussion includes information about required materials, forms, and step-by-step instructions for conducting sessions.

Walters, S. T., & Baer, J. S. (2006). *Talking with college students about alcohol: Motivational strategies for reducing abuse.* New York: Guilford Press. [Book]

MI training slides and suggested training formats, adapted from this book, are available at *www.guilford.com/walters2*. The slides and instructions are designed to assist readers in presenting material discussed in the book.

Foreign-Language Resources

Daeppen, J., *French-speaking motivational interviewing.* [DVD]

This DVD provides an introduction to MI (including spirit of MI, definition of MI, stages of change, and four principles) and Phase I and Phase II skills. For information and ordering, contact Jean-Bernard Daeppen at *jean-bernard.daeppen@chuv.ch.*

Harai, H., MD, *Japanese version motivational interviewing professional training videotape series (DVD); Korean version motivational interviewing professional training videotape series.* [DVD]

Directed by Dr. Harai, this DVD follows the organization of the *Motivational Interviewing Professional Training Videotape Series* (1998), Tapes A and B, by Miller, Rollnick, and Moyers. Ordering should be sent to *ocd2004@gmail.com,* Japanese Obsessive Compulsive Disorder Foundation.

The Korean version, which is subtitled in Korean, also follows the organization of the *Motivational Interviewing Professional Training Videotape Series* (1998), Tapes A and B by Miller, Rollnick, and Moyers. Ordering information can be obtained from the publisher, Sigma Press, at *www.spress.co.kr/.*

Yahne, C., PhD, *La entrevista motivacional: Preparación para el Cambio.* [DVD]

This 90-minute Spanish-language DVD is directed by Carolina Yahne, PhD, and done in collaboration with William R. Miller, Ph.D.. It provides three clinical examples (tobacco, cocaine, and diabetes management), as well as introductory materials By Drs. Yahne and Miller. The video/DVD may be ordered from UNM CASAA 2650 Yale SE, Albuquerque, NM 87106 USA.

Websites

The best site for all things MI is the official webpage of the MI Network of Trainers at *www.motivationalinterview.org,* which is hosted by the Atlantic Addictions Technology Transfer Center (ATTC). This website contains a treasure trove of information, including an extensive MI bibliography, a listing of MI trainers and MI training events, and links to individual web pages of MI trainers. It also contains recommendations about training lengths and goals, as well as important points to consider when hiring an MI trainer. Here are a few other resources to consider:

- You can get your MI questions answered by Dr. Rollnick himself at *www.stephenrollnick.com.*
- The Institute for Motivation and Change specializes in utilizing MI in health care settings. It has a free newsletter and tip sheet that you can sign up for at *www.miinstitute.com.*
- The Centre for Motivation and Change provides excellent information about international training and events. It can be found at *www.motivationalinterview.nl.*
- Hiroaki Harai, MD, offers a Japanese-language website for the general public at *homepage1.nifty.com/hharai/mi/index.htm.*

Other Resources

Field, A., *Group MI curriculum.* [Document]

Ms. Field has developed a group curriculum for MI. She describes it as follows: "This motivational group model has broad application for all treatment providers, counselors, therapists, educators, and other human service practitioners. It allows for the facilitation and implementation of motivational interviewing strategies within five group sessions." It can be obtained through her website at *www.hollifieldassociates.com*. Ms. Fields also notes that this curriculum is being translated into Spanish and Korean and that she is currently completing a DVD that complements these materials.

Walters, S. T., Clark, M. D., Gingerich, R., & Meltzer, M. L. (2007). *A guide for motivating offenders to change.* [Document]

These authors have put together a comprehensive guide for learning and implementing MI in the criminal justice setting. An excellent resource, it is available free of charge via download at *nicic.org/Downloads/PDF/Library/022253.pdf.*

References

Allison, J. (2006). Resistant ramblings: Feedback on a consensus statement on change talk. *MINT Bulletin, 13*(1), 4–5. Available at *motivationalinterview.org/mint/MINT13.2.full.pdf.*

Amrhein, P., Miller, W. R., Moyers, T. B., & Rollnick, S. (2005). A consensus statement on change talk. *MINT Bulletin, 12*(2), 3–4. Available at *motivationalinterview.org/mint/MINT12.2.full.pdf.*

Amrhein, P., Miller, W. R., Yahne, C. E., Knupsky, A., & Hochstein, D. (2004). Strength of client commitment language improves with training in motivational interviewing. *Alcoholism: Clinical and Experimental Research, 28*(5), 74A.

Amrhein, P., Miller, W. R., Yahne, C. E., Palmer, M., & Fulcher, L. (2003). Client commitment language during motivational interviewing predicts drug use outcomes. *Journal of Consulting and Clinical Psychology, 71*, 862–878.

Arkowitz, H., & Miller, W. R. (2008). Learning, applying and extending MI. In H. Arkowitz, H. A. Westra, W. R. Miller, & S. Rollnick (Eds.), *Motivational interviewing in the treatment of psychological problems* (pp. 1–25). New York: Guilford Press.

Arkowitz, H., Westra, H. A., Miller, W. R., & Rollnick, S. (Eds.) (2008). *Motivational interviewing in the treatment of psychological problems.* New York: Guilford Press.

Baer, J. B., Wells, E., Rosengren, D. B., Hartzler, B., Beadnell, B., & Dunn, C. (2009). Context and tailored training in technology transfer: Evaluating motivational interviewing training for community counselors. *Journal of Substance Abuse Treatment, 37*(2), 191–202.

Baer, J. S., Rosengren, D. B., Dunn, C. W., Wells, E. A., Ogle, R. L., & Hartzler, B. (2004). An evaluation of workshop training in motivational interviewing for addiction and mental health clinicians. *Drug and Alcohol Dependence, 73*, 99–106.

Bandura, A. (1997). *Self-efficacy: The exercise of control.* New York: Freeman.

Barth, T. (2006). Consensus and change talk: Feedback on a consensus statement on change talk. *MINT Bulletin, 13*(1), 5.

Bem, D. J. (1967). Self-perception theory: An alternative interpretation of cognitive dissonance. *Psychological Review, 74*, 183–200.

Bennett, G. A., Moore, J., Vaughan, T., Rouse, L., Gibbins, J. A., Thomas, P., et al. (2007). Strengthening motivational interviewing following initial training: A randomised trial of workplace-based reflective practice. *Addictive Behaviors, 32*(12), 2963–2975.

Brug, J., Spikmans, F., Aartsen, C., Breedveld, B., Bes, R., & Ferieria, I. (2007). Training dietitians in basic motivational interviewing skills results in changes in their counseling style and lower saturated fat intakes in their patients. *Journal of Nutrition Education and Behavior, 39*, 8–12.

Burke, B. L., Arkowitz, H., & Dunn, C. (2002). The efficacy of motivational interviewing: What we know so far. In W. R. Miller & S. Rollnick, *Motivational interviewing: Preparing people for change* (2nd ed., pp. 217–250). New York: Guilford Press.

Carbonari, J. P., & DiClemente, C. C. (2000). Using transtheoretical model profiles to differentiate levels of alcohol abstinence success. *Journal of Consulting and Clinical Psychology, 68*(5), 810–817.

Carpenter, K. M., Watson, J. M., Raffety, B., & Chabal, C. (2003). Teaching brief interventions for smoking cessation via an interactive computer-based tutorial. *Journal of Health Psychology, 8,* 149–160.

Carroll, K. M., Kadden, R. M., Donovan, D. M., Zweben, A., & Rounsaville, B. J. (1994). Implementing treatment and protecting the validity of the independent variable in treatment matching studies. *Journal of Studies on Alcohol, 12,* 149–155.

Center for Substance Abuse Treatment. (1999). *Enhancing motivation for change in substance abuse treatment* (Treatment Improvement Protocol [TIP] Series, No. 35; DHHS Pub. No. [SMA] 99-3354). Washington, DC: U.S. Government Printing Office.

Chossis, I. C., Lane, C., Gache, P., Michaud, P. A., Pecoud, A., Rollnick, S., et al. (2007). Effect of training on primary care residents' performance in brief intervention: A randomized controlled trial. *Society of General Internal Medicine, 22,* 1144–1149.

Connors, G. J., Donovan, D. M., & DiClemente, C. C. (2001). *Substance abuse treatment and the stages of change: Selecting and planning interventions.* New York: Guilford Press.

Curry, S., Wagner, E. H., & Grothaus, L. C. (1990). Intrinsic and extrinsic motivation for smoking cessation. *Journal of Consulting and Clinical Psychology, 58,* 310–316.

Daniels, J. W. (1998). *Coping with the health threat of smoking: An analysis of the precontemplation stage of smoking cessation.* Unpublished doctoral dissertation, Psychology Department, University of Maryland, MD, Baltimore.

Davison, R. (1998). The transtheoretical model: A critical overview. In W. R. Miller & N. Heather (Eds.), *Treating addictive behaviors* (2nd ed., pp. 25–38). New York: Plenum Press.

De Shazer, S., Berg, I., Lipchick, E., Nunelly, E., Molnar, A., Gingerich, W., et al. (1986). Brief therapy: A focused solution development. *Family Process, 25,* 207–222.

Diabetes Control and Complications Trial Research Group. (1993). The effect of intensive treatment of diabetes on the development and progression of long-term complications in insulin-dependent diabetes mellitus. *New England Journal of Medicine, 329*(14), 977–986.

DiClemente, C. C. (1991). Motivational interviewing and stages of change. In W. R. Miller & S. Rollnick, *Motivational interviewing: Preparing people to change addictive behavior* (pp. 191–202). New York: Guilford Press.

DiClemente, C. C. (1999). Motivation for change: Implications for substance abuse. *Psychological Science, 10*(3), 209–213.

DiClemente, C. C. (2003). *Addiction and change: How addictions develop and addicted people recover.* New York: Guilford Press.

DiClemente, C. C., & Prochaska, J. O. (1998). Toward a comprehensive, transtheoretical model of change: Stages of change and addictive behaviors. In W. R. Miller & N. Heather (Eds.), *Treating addictive behaviors* (2nd ed., pp. 3–24). New York: Plenum Press.

Donovan, D. M., Rosengren, D. B., Downey, L., Cox, G. B., & Sloan, K. L. (2001). Attrition prevention with individuals awaiting publicly funded drug treatment. *Addiction, 96,* 1149–1160.

Downey, L., Rosengren, D. B., & Donovan, D. M. (2000). To thine own self be true: Self-concept and motivation for abstinence among substance users. *Addictive Behaviors, 25,* 743–757.

Engle, D., & Arkowitz, H. (2006). *Ambivalence in psychotherapy: Facilitating readiness to change.* New York: Guilford Press.

Festinger, L. (1957). *A theory of cognitive dissonance.* Palo Alto, CA: Stanford University Press.

Forrester, D., McCambridge, J., Waissbein, C., Emlyn-Jones, R., & Rollnick, S. (2008). Child risk and parental resistance: Can motivational interviewing improve the practice of child and family social workers in working with parental alcohol misuse? *British Journal of Social Work*, *38*, 1302–1319.

Gordon, T. (1970). *Parent effectiveness training*. New York: Wyden.

Handmaker, N. S., Hester, R. K., & Delaney, H. D. (1999). Videotape training in alcohol counseling for obstetric care practitioners: A randomized control trial. *Obstetrics and Gynecology*, *93*, 213–218.

Hartzler, B., Baer, J. S., Dunn, C., Rosengren, D. B., & Wells, E. A. (2007). What is seen through the looking glass: The impact of training on practitioner self-rating of motivational interviewing skills. *Behavioural and Cognitive Psychotherapy*, *35*(4), 431–445.

Hartzler, B., Rosengren, D. B., & Baer, J. S. (2009). Motivational interviewing. In L. M. Cohen, F. L. Collins, A. Young, D. E. McChargue, & T. Leffingwell (Eds.), *The pharmacology and treatment of substance abuse: Evidence- and outcome-based perspectives*. Mahwah, NJ: Erlbaum.

Hecht, J., Borrelli, B., Breger, R. K. R., DeFrancesco, C., Ernest, D. A., & Resnicow, K. (2005). Motivational interviewing in community-based research: Experiences from the field. *Annals of Behavioral Medicine*, *29*, 24–29.

Hettema, J., Steele, J., & Miller, W. R. (2005). Motivational interviewing. *Annual Review of Clinical Psychology*, *1*, 91–111.

Janis, I. L., & Mann, L. (1977). *Decision making*. New York: Free Press.

Jones, E. E., & Harris, V. A. (1967). The attribution of attitudes. *Journal of Experimental Social Psychology*, *3*, 1–24.

Lane, C., Hood, K., & Rollnick, S. (2008). Teaching motivational interviewing: Using role-play is as effective as using simulated patients. *Medical Education*, *42*, 637–644.

Lane, C., Johnson, S., Rollnick, S., Edwards, K., & Lyons, M. (2003). Consulting about lifestyle change: Evaluation of a training course for diabetes nurses. *Practicing Diabetes International*, *20*, 204–208.

Leake, G. J., & King, A. S. (1977). Effect of counselor expectations on alcoholic recovery. *Alcohol Health and Research World*, *11*(3), 16–22.

Leffingwell, T. R., Neumann, C. A., Babitske, A. C., Leedy, M. J., & Walters, S. T. (2006). Social psychology and motivational interviewing: A review of relevant principles and recommendations for research and practice. *Behavioural and Cognitive Psychotherapy*, *35*(1), 1–15.

Madson, M. B., Campbell, T. C., Barrett, D. E., Brondino, M. J., & Melchert, T. P. (2005). Development of the motivational interviewing supervision and training scale. *Psychology of Addictive Behaviors*, *19*, 303–310.

Madson, M. B., Loigon, A. C., & Lane, C. (2009). Training in motivational interviewing: A systematic review. *Journal of Substance Abuse Treatment*, *36*(1), 101–109.

Martino, S., Ball, S. A., Ceperich, S., del Mar Garcia, M., Gallon, S., Hall, D., et al. (2006). *Motivational interviewing assessment: Supervisor tools for enhancing proficiency (MIA-STEP)*. Available at *ctndisseminationlibrary.org/display/146.htm*.

Martino, S., Ball, S. A., Nich, C., Frankforter, T. L., & Carroll, K. M. (2008). Community program therapist adherence and competence in motivational interviewing. *Drug and Alcohol Dependence*, *96*, 37–48.

Martino, S., Haeseler, F., Belitsky, R., Pantalon, M., & Fortin, A. H. (2007). Teaching brief motivational interviewing to year three medical students. *Medical Education*, *41*, 160–167.

Messer, S. B., & Wampald, B. E. (2002). Let's face facts: Common factors are more potent than specific therapy ingredients. *Clinical Psychology: Science and Practice*, *9*(1), 21–25.

Miller, W. R. (1983). Motivational interviewing with problem drinkers. *Behavioural Psychotherapy*, *11*, 147–172.

Miller, W. R. (2005). Toward a theory of motivational interviewing. *MINT Bulletin*, *12*, 14. Available at *motivationalinterview.org/mint/MINT12.1.supplement.pdf*.

Miller, W. R., Benefield, R. G., & Tonigan, J. S. (1993). Enhancing motivation for change in problem drinking: A controlled comparison of two different styles. *Journal of Consulting and Clinical Psychology, 61*(3), 455–461.

Miller, W. R., & C' de Baca, J. (2001). *Quantum change: When epiphanies and sudden insights transform lives.* New York: Guilford Press.

Miller, W. R., & Heather, N. (Eds.). (1998). *Treating addictive behaviors* (2nd ed.). New York: Plenum Press.

Miller, W. R., Hendrickson, S. M. L., Venner, K., Bisono, M. S., Daugherty, M., & Yahne, C. E. (2008). Cross-cultural training in motivational interviewing. *Journal of Teaching in the Addictions, 7*(1), 4–15.

Miller, W. R., & Mount, K. A. (2005). A small study of training in motivational interviewing: Does one workshop change clinician and client behavior? *Behavioural and Cognitive Psychotherapy, 29*, 457–471.

Miller, W. R., & Moyers, T. (2006). Eight stages in learning motivational interviewing. *Journal of Teaching the Addictions, 5*, 3–17.

Miller, W. R., Moyers, T. B., Amrhein, P., & Rollnick, S. (2006). A consensus statement on defining change talk. *MINT Bulletin, 13*(2), 6–7. Available at *motivationalinterview.org/mint/MINT13.2.full.pdf.*

Miller, W. R., & Rollnick, S. (1991). *Motivational interviewing: Preparing people to change addictive behavior.* New York: Guilford Press.

Miller, W. R., & Rollnick, S. (2002). *Motivational interviewing: Preparing people for change* (2nd ed.). New York: Guilford Press.

Miller, W. R., & Rollnick, S. (2009). Ten things that motivational interviewing is not. *Behavioral and Cognitive Psychotherapy, 37*, 129–140.

Miller, W. R., Sorensen, J. L., Selzer, J. A., & Brigham, G. S. (2006). Disseminating evidence-based practices in substance abuse treatment: A review with suggestions. *Journal of Substance Abuse Treatment, 31*, 25–39.

Miller, W. R., & Sovereign, R. G. (1989). The check-up: A model for early intervention in addictive behaviors. In T. Løberg, W. R. Miller, P. E. Nathan, & G. A. Marlatt (Eds.), *Addictive behaviors: Prevention and early intervention* (pp. 219–231). Amsterdam: Swets & Zeitlinger.

Miller, W. R., Yahne, C. E., Moyers, T. B., Martinez, J., & Pirritano, M. (2004). A randomized trial of methods to help clinicians learn motivational interviewing. *Journal of Counseling and Clinical Psychology, 72*(6), 1050–1062.

Miller, W. R., Yahne, C. E., & Tonigan, J. S. (2003). Motivational interviewing in drug abuse services: A randomized trial. *Journal of Consulting and Clinical Psychology, 72*, 1052–1062.

Miller, W. R., Zweben, A., DiClemente, C. C., & Rychtarik, R. (1992). *Motivational enhancement therapy manual: A clinical research guide for therapists treating individuals with alcohol abuse and dependence (Project MATCH Monograph Series, Vol. 2).* Rockville, MD: National Institute on Alcohol Abuse and Alcoholism.

Mounsey, A. L., Bovbjerg, V., White, L., & Gazewood, J. (2006). Do students develop better motivational interviewing skills through role-play with standardized patients or with student colleagues? *Medical Education, 40*(8), 775–780.

Moyers, T. B., Manuel, J. K., Wilson, P. G., Hendrickson, S. M. L., Talcot, W., & Durand, P. (2008). A randomized trial investigating training in motivational interviewing for behavioral health providers. *Behavioural and Cognitive Psychotherapy, 36*, 149–162.

Moyers, T. B., & Martin, T (2006). A conceptual framework for transferring research into practice. *Journal of Substance Abuse Treatment, 30*, 245–251.

Moyers, T. B., Martin, T., Christopher, P. J., Houck, J. M., Tonigan, J. S., & Amrhein, P. C. (2007). Client language as a mediator of motivational interviewing efficacy: Where is the evidence? *Alcoholism: Clinical and Experimental Research, 31*(S3), 40S–47S.

Moyers, T. B., Martin, T., Manuel, J. K., Hendrickson, S. M. L., & Miller, W. R. (2005). Assessing competence in the use of motivational interviewing. *Journal of Substance Abuse Treatment, 28*, 19–26.

Moyers, T. B., Martin, T., Manuel, J. K., & Miller, W. R. (2003). *The motivational interviewing treatment integrity code* (Version 2). Retrieved June 20, 2008, from *www/casa.unm.edu/download. miti.pdf.*

Moyers, T. B., Miller, W. R., & Hendrickson, S. M. L. (2005). How does motivational interviewing work?: Therapist interpersonal skill predicts client involvement within motivational interviewing sessions. *Journal of Consulting and Clinical Psychology, 73*, 590–598.

Patterson, G. R., & Forgatch, M. S. (1985). Therapist behaviors as a determinant of client noncompliance: A paradox for the behavior modifier. *Journal of Consulting and Clinical Psychology, 53*, 846–851.

Poirier, M. K., Clark, M. M., Cerhan, J. H., Pruthi, S., Geda, Y. E., & Dale, L. C. (2004). Teaching motivational interviewing to first-year medical students to improve counseling skills in health behavior change. *Mayo Clinic Proceedings, 79*, 327–331.

Prochaska, J. O., & DiClemente, C. C. (1984). *The transtheoretical approach: Crossing the traditional boundaries of therapy.* Malabar, FL: Kreiger.

Prochaska, J. O., & DiClemente, C. C. (1998). Comments, criteria, and creating better models. In W. R. Miller & N. Heather (Eds.), *Treating addictive behaviors* (2nd ed., pp. 39–46). New York: Plenum Press.

Prochaska, J. O., DiClemente, C. C., & Norcross, J. C. (1992). In search of how people change: Applications to addictive behaviors. *American Psychologist, 47*, 1102–1114.

Prochaska, J. O., Norcross, J. C., & DiClemente, C. C. (1994). *Changing for good: The revolutionary program that explains the six stages of change and teaches you how to free yourself from bad habits.* New York: William Morrow.

Prochaska, J. O., Velicer, W. F., Rossi, J. S., Goldstein, M. G., Marcus, B. H., Rakowski, W., et al. (1994). Stages of change and decisional balance for twelve problem behaviors. *Health Psychology, 12*(1), 39–46.

Project MATCH Research Group. (1997a). Matching alcoholism treatment to client heterogeneity: Project MATCH posttreatment drinking outcomes. *Journal of Studies on Alcohol, 58*, 7–29.

Project MATCH Research Group. (1997b). Project MATCH secondary a priori hypotheses. *Addiction, 92*, 1671–1698.

Project MATCH Research Group. (1998a). Matching alcoholism treatment to client heterogeneity: Project MATCH three-year drinking outcomes. *Alcoholism: Clinical and Experimental Research, 23*(60), 1300–1311.

Project MATCH Research Group. (1998b). Matching alcoholism treatment to client heterogeneity: Treatment main effects and matching effects during treatment. *Journal of Studies on Alcohol, 59*, 631–639.

Rogers, C. (1980). *A way of being.* New York: Houghton Mifflin.

Rokeach, M. (1973). *The nature of human values.* New York: Free Press.

Rokeach, M. (Ed.). (1979). *Understanding human values.* New York: Macmillan.

Rollnick, S., Heather, N., & Bell, A. (1992). Negotiating behaviour change in medical settings: The development of brief motivational interviewing. *Journal of Mental Health, 1*, 25–39.

Rollnick, S., Kinnersley, P., & Butler, C. (2002). Context-bound communication skills training: Development of a new method. *Medical Education, 36*, 377–383.

Rollnick, S., Mason, P., & Butler, C. (1999). *Health behavior change: A guide for practitioners.* London: Churchill-Livingstone.

Rollnick, S., Miller, W. R., & Butler, C. (2008). *Motivational interviewing in health care: Helping patients change behavior.* New York: Guilford Press.

Rosengren, D. B., Baer, J. S., Hartzler, B., Dunn, C. W., & Wells, E. A. (2005). The Video Assessment of Simulated Encounters (VASE): Development and validation of a group-administered method for evaluating clinician skills in motivational interviewing. *Drug and Alcohol Dependence, 79,* 321–330.

Rosengren, D. B., Hartzler, B., Baer, J. S., Wells, E. A., & Dunn, C. W. (2008). The Video Assessment of Simulated Encounters—Revised (VASE-R): Reliability and validity of a revised measure of motivational interviewing skills. *Drug and Alcohol Dependence, 97*(1–2), 130–138.

Ross, L. (1977). The intuitive psychologist and his shortcomings: Distortions in the attribution process. In L. Berkowitz (Ed.), *Advances in experimental social psychology* (Vol. 10, pp. 173–220). New York: Academic Press.

Saitz, R., Sullivan, L. M., & Samet, J. H. (2000). Training community-based clinicians in screening and brief intervention for substance abuse problems: Translating evidence into practice. *Substance Abuse, 21,* 21–31.

Schoener, E. P., Madeja, C. L., Henderson, M. J., Ondersma, S. J., & Janisse, J. J. (2006). Effects of motivational interviewing training on mental health therapist behavior. *Drug and Alcohol Dependence, 82,* 269–275.

Shafer, M. S., Rhode, R., & Chong, J. (2004). Using distance education to promote transfer of motivational interviewing skills among health professionals. *Journal of Substance Abuse Treatment, 26,* 141–148.

Silver, H. F., Strong, R. W., & Perini, M. J. (2000). *So each may learn: Integrating learning styles and multiple intelligences.* Trenton, NJ: Silver Strong.

Simpson, D. D. (2002). A conceptual framework for transferring research into practice. *Journal of Substance Abuse Treatment, 22,* 171–182.

Simpson, D. D., & Joe, G. W. (1993). Motivation as a predictor of early dropout from drug abuse treatment. *Psychotherapy, 30,* 357–368.

Smith, J. L., Amrhein, P. C., Brooks, A. C., Carpenter, K. M., Levin, D., Schreiber, E. A., et al. (2007). Providing live supervision via teleconferencing improves skill acquisition of motivational interviewing skills after workshop attendance. *American Journal of Drug and Alcohol Abuse, 33,* 163–168.

Steele, C. M. (1988). The psychology of self-affirmation: Sustaining the integrity of the self. In L. Berkowitz (Ed.), *Advances in experimental social psychology* (Vol. 21, pp. 261–302). San Diego, CA: Academic Press.

Thijs, G. A. (2007). GP's consult and behavior change project: Developing a programme to train GPs in communication skills to achieve lifestyle improvements. *Patient Education and Counseling, 67,* 267–271

Thomas, C. P., Wallack, S. S., Lee, S., McCarthy, D., & Swift, R. (2003). Research to practice: Adoption of naltrexone in alcoholism treatment. *Journal of Substance Abuse Treatment, 24,* 1–11.

Thrasher, A. D., Golin, C. E., Earp, J. A., Tien, H., Porter, C., & Howie, L. (2005). Training general practitioners in behavior change counseling to improve asthma medication adherence. *Patient Education and Counseling, 58,* 279–287.

Tober, G., Godfrey, C., Parrott, S., Copello, A., Farrin, A., Hodgson, R., et al. (2005). Setting standards for training and competence: The UK alcohol treatment trial. *Alcohol and Alcoholism, 40,* 413–418.

Villaume, W. A., Berger, B. A., & Barker, B. N. (2006). Learning motivational interviewing: Scripting a virtual patient. *American Journal of Pharmacy Education, 70*(2), 1–9.

Voss, J. D., & Wolf, A. M. (2004). Teaching motivational interviewing in chronic care: A workshop approach. *Journal of General Internal Medicine, 19,* 213.

Walters, S. T., Matson, S. A., Baer, J. S., & Ziedonis, D. M. (2005). Effectiveness of workshop training of psychosocial addictions treatment: A systemic review. *Journal of Substance Abuse Treatment, 29*(4), 283–293.

Werch, C. E., & DiClemente, C. C. (1994). A multi-component stage model for matching drug prevention strategies and methods to youth stage of use. *Health Education Research: Theory and Practice, 9*(1), 37–46.

Index